POWER JUICES SUPER DRINKS

Quick, Delicious Recipes to Prevent & Reverse Disease

STEVE MEYEROWITZ

KENSINGTON PUBLISHING CORP
http://kensingtonbooks.com

Edited by Jens Jensen and Renée Betar
Illustrations rendered by Mary Giddens

Acknowledgments: Thanks to editor Jens Jensen, research editor Renée Betar, copy editor Ellyne Raueber, research assistant Deborah Kinney, artist and page formatter Mary Giddens, and administrative assistant Martha Lorentzen.

Special thanks to Warren Brassel and the health and natural healing research experts at Nutrition Works and Hyperhealth (www.hyperhealth.com). Thank you to the Alumni Library at Simon's Rock College for their resources and hospitality.

Disclaimer: The information in this book is not intended to be a prescription for the user. This book does not claim to cure anything; it does not offer medical advice. Instead it presents research and nutritional information regarding the use of plants and vegetables in harmony with natural laws for good health and healing. Please do not use this book is you are unwilling to assume the sole responsibility of evaluating and choosing your own diet/lifestyle or treatment program. Because each person's health condition is unique, the author urges the reader to consult a qualified health professional before undertaking any suggestions described in this book. Good luck and good health.

KENSINGTON BOOKS are published by

Kensington Publishing Corp.
119 West 40th Street
New York, NY 10018
http://kensingtonbooks.com

ISBN-13: 978-0-7582-6712-2
ISBN-10: 0-7582-6712-6
First Printing: April, 2000.

30 29 28 27 26 25 24 23 22

Printed in the United States of America

POWER JUICES SUPER DRINKS

Contents

Ailments and Conditions

Foods and Herbs

Foreword

The Value of Fresh Juices and Drinks

by Dr. Gabriel Cousens, M.D.

Power Juices and Super Drinks by the Sproutman fills a most interesting niche in health literature. In a very delightful and informative way, Steve Meyerowitz opens up a bountiful kitchen cupboard of nutritious and medicinal power juices and live food super drinks. This book shows how to tap the secret healing powers of natural foods: vegetables, fruits, herbs, nuts, seeds, and live-food concentrates to feed the cells and to heal and detoxify the body by using juices and power drinks.

The advantage of juices is that they focus and concentrate the energy of enzymes, minerals, vitamins, and phytonutrients. Juices carry the amplified healing energy of fruits and vegetables plus added food concentrates such as chlorella. Fruit juices act primarily as cleansers. Citrus fruits, for example, have solvent actions; apples contain malic acid and galacturonic acid, which are detoxifiers; pineapples have a high bromelain content, which has many healing and anti-inflammatory effects. Fruits—and fruit juices even more so—help to cleanse and purify the organs. Vegetable juices have more of a tonic effect that heals, stabilizes, and builds the body. Like fruit juices, each vegetable has a specific power to heal a particular organ. For example, beets and dandelions help heal the liver. Green juices contain chlorophyll, which is a tonifier that leads to incredible healing experiences for many.

The nice thing about juices is that they make it very simple and easy to take in the nutrition and the healing powers of nature. They make a wonderful and fun shortcut that amplifies the healing forces in our foods.

What is the secret healing power of juices and power drinks? How are they different from the vitamins, minerals, and other supplements taken in capsules or tablets? The major difference is that juices are living foods in one of their most potent and easily accessible forms. To fully understand the depth of this book, we need to understand more about the principles of live-foods.

The essence of understanding living food is this: If it ain't broken, don't fix it. Living, or raw, foods are those that have not been cooked, processed, or treated with pesticides or herbicides. They represent the unbroken wholeness of the original creation and nutritional gift of the Divine. The food we eat is an energetic whole that is greater than the sum of the parts. This understanding reflects a quantum mechanical view of nutrition versus the classical Newtonian approach.

Research by Dr. Brekhman of the former Soviet Union showed that when he gave whole, live-foods to animals, their endurance was 2-3 times greater than when he gave the same foods that had been cooked. From a traditional nutritional perspective, this should not make a difference, since cooked and raw foods have the same amount of calories and, therefore, the same amount of energy. Once we recognize how cooking affects the whole food, however, Brekhman's results can be easily understood. Thorough cooking destroys the ecological balance of food. It makes 50% of the protein unavailable and destroys 60-70% of the vitamins. It also destroys up to 96% of the B12 and eliminates many lesser factors such as gibberellins, anthrocyans, as well as many other phytonutrients, which boost the immune system and other bodily functions. Cooking foods also disrupts the bioelectrical structure and destroys the bioluminescence of the original food. All of these factors are important for building and maintaining our life forces, energy, and health.

The European physician Dr. Bircher-Brenner started the first live-food clinic in 1897. He understood that eating raw foods could help restore a diseased body and the mind's ability to heal. Many healers who use living foods with their clients have gotten fantastic results. One of the most famous examples was Dr. Gerson, who healed Dr. Albert Schweitzer of diabetes and Schweitzer's wife of tuberculosis. Dr. Gerson used live-foods to heal hundreds of documented cancer cases.

There has been some interesting research to validate Dr. Bircher-Brenner's insights. Dr. Hans Eppinger of the First Medical Clinic at the University of Vienna found that the micro-electrical potential of the cells in a disease process would decrease and that their ability to absorb nutrients and excrete toxins would be diminished. He found that live-foods are the only type of food that can restore the cells' micro-electrical potential. Eppinger's work correlates with that of Dr. Kollath from Sweden. Dr. Kollath found that when he fed animals the typical cooked food of an affluent Western diet, they developed what he called meso-health. This is a condition in which the animals appear to be as healthy as those living on raw food, but they had less resistance to illness and developed chronic, degenerative diseases at an earlier age than those eating live-food. He found that raw food was able to restore their health and slow the aging process, whereas giving them specific vitamin and mineral doses did not.

In their book *The Dark Side of the Brain,* Harry Oldfield and Roger Coghill describe, through research involving Kirlian photography, how live-foods were surrounded by a considerably stronger bioluminescent field than were cooked foods. This field was associated with cell bioelectricity and life force. The implication of this research is that cooking food destroys its bioluminescent field.

The enzymes in live-foods are also destroyed by cooking. Enzymes seem to be connected to life force, health, and longevity. Ann Wigmore, the mother of the raw-foods movement, felt that enzyme preservation is the secret to health. Enzymes are living biochemical factors that activate and carry out all the biological processes in the body, such as digestion, nerve impulses, detoxification processes, RNA/DNA functions, the repair and healing of the body, and even brain functions. There are natural enzymes in raw food, which minimize the enzymes that the body needs to secrete for digestion. The preserved body enzymes are then converted and can be used for the processes of detoxification, repair, and overall healing. We preserve our body's enzymes by eating live foods, and this seems to play an important role in slowing the aging process. With age there seems to be a significant drop in our enzyme reserves. Live-foods, and particularly fresh juices, give back to the body a high concentration of bio-active enzymes, which builds the body's enzyme reserve, thus healing and rejuvenating the whole human organism.

By cooking our food, we may also change the molecular structure of its components and consequently impair our health. For example, researchers found that Eskimos who eat about two pounds of raw blubber a day had no heart disease or atherosclerosis. But when this same community of Eskimos began to eat the same amount of blubber that had been cooked, they developed high rates of heart disease and atherosclerosis. Since then, other researchers have found that cooking fats changes their molecular structure in a way that disrupts cell structure and impairs cellular function.

Satya Sai Baba, one of the few Indian spiritual teachers who has transcended his cultural food tradition, explains why people may be slow in switching to diets high in live-foods. He says, "Out of all the species … man alone tries to cook and change his food. A seed when planted will sprout to life.., but when cooked, the life is destroyed.… Man does not like to partake of food as God created it. He is the victim of his tongue, which he wants to be satisfied in terms of taste, and so his own likes and dislikes come in the way of what he should eat.… Because he is exterminating the life-giving forces in the food available to him, he is increasingly subjecting himself to disease." This quote brings us back to the statement: *If it ain't broken, don't fix it.*

I am very excited about this book, *Power Juices Super Drinks*, because it puts the power and life-giving energy of live-foods into the hands of many who would otherwise find such a transition too difficult. Meyerowitz has done an excellent job of organizing this material in such a way that people can easily find what they need to enhance their health and well-being. His medicine chest of power drinks for the body, mind, and longevity and his phytonutrient review of foods and herbs is outstanding. This book is a boon to health seekers. I am recommending it to all my clients and students.

Salute to your health,

Gabriel Cousens

Gabriel Cousens, M.D., Patagonia, AZ

Dr. Cousens is the director of the "Tree of Life Rejuvenation Center" in Patagonia AZ and author of "Conscious Eating" and "Spiritual Nutrition and The Rainbow Diet." (See "Resources")

Power Drinks Basics

The How-To for Making Your Power Juices and Super Drinks

How to Wash Your Fruits and Vegetables

It is a sad comment on our times. Washing fruits and vegetables is no longer just a simple act of rinsing off soil. Today, it is a compulsory obligation if we wish to avoid downing the residues of pesticides, insecticides, and herbicides. As if these synthetic adversaries were not enough, we must also scrub away the bugs. Potential contamination from bacteria such as E-coli and salmonella are additional hazards for those who choose not to cook every vegetable they eat. If you are growing vegetables in your own back yard, you may not need to fret so much about such concerns. But, if you purchase produce from the market, here are a few methods for ridding the pests from your produce.

Grapefruit Seed Extract (GSE). This is the volatile citrus oil of grapefruit seeds. It is a potent antimicrobial and is used instead of iodine by some outdoor enthusiasts to purify water. Ten drops per 8 ounce glass of water is enough to kill detrimental bacteria. Since it is itself an oil, it can also break down oil-based pesticides. You should allow about ten minutes for GSE to work its wonders, then rinse it off before consuming your vegetables.

Lemon Juice Bath. Fill your sink with cold water, add four tablespoons of salt and the juice from 2-3 lemons. Soak the fruits and vegetables for ten minutes then rinse under cold water.

White Vinegar Bath. Follow the same instructions as for lemon juice, but add ½ cup or more of white vinegar.

Boil Bath. This is suitable for all but the most fragile vegetables. It kills microbes but does not remove pesticides. First bring a pot of water to a boil. Dip your vegetable into it one at a time for approximately 5-30 seconds. You can dip as long as 30 seconds for hearty vegetables like zucchini, but only 5-10 seconds for delicate greens such as lettuce. This "flash pasteurization" is enough to kill most germs. Immerse your vegetables or fruits with tongs, or throw them in the pot whole and then drain. This is also a great way to remove waxes on fruits and vegetables.

Chlorine Bath. This is what the government uses to kill giardia, salmonella, and other microbial threats to municipal water supplies. Use one tablespoon of household bleach per quart of water. Let your produce sit in the solution for 10 minutes, then drain and soak again in fresh water for another five minutes. If there is still a bleach odor after rinsing, rinse once more and let the produce air out before consuming.

Bleach is very effective, but because of the environmental hazards of chlorine it is also controversial. Nevertheless, many nutritionists recommend it. In addition to killing parasites and their eggs, this aggressive oxidizer can improve color, flavor, and freshness. It extracts pesticides like a chelating agent. Even pesticide workers use it to clean their equipment. If you do use bleach, rinse your vegetables thoroughly and let them air out. One good thing about bleach is that it dissipates quickly, so if there is no odor, it has already escaped into the air, leaving you with pure food.

Organic Produce — The Better Alternative

Pesticides are actually a relatively recent addition to commercial agriculture, coming as a result of efforts to expand agricultural production during WWII. Although they never used the term, our grandparents and their ancestors farmed with organic methods. Today, the organic farming movement is expanding rapidly and making inroads into mainstream agriculture. But there are still far too many chemicals in our food. America's favorite vegetable, the one we eat more of than any other, is the potato. According to the USDA data, 78% of our potatoes have pesticide residues. Why does an underground vegetable require so many chemicals? The potato's greatest enemy is the tiny Colorado potato beetle. For organic farmers, this pest is no problem. They merely send out their ladybugs to nest nearby. These colorful ladies love to eat the eggs of the Colorado beetle. Organic farming uses creativity instead of chemicals.

We should support organic farming just because it protects our environment; but organic food also tastes better. Experiment for yourself. Juice a pound of organic and a pound of commercial carrots and compare the results. You will be amazed at the dramatic difference.

If You Can't Find it Organic, Sprout It

Sprouting is indoor organic farming. This does not mean just sprouting beans in a jar, but real "kitchen gardening" in professional sprouters that allow you to harvest pounds of sprouts of many different varieties every week. Your sprouts will be 100% organic, because you are the farmer. Sprouts grow in voluminous quantities making them perfect for juicing, and they are among the most nutritious vegetables in the world. Where else can you find such an abundance of organic produce for only pennies per pound? With a good setup, sprouts are easy to grow and fun for the whole family. Liven up your cuisine with the wonderful flavors of fresh buckwheat lettuce, baby sunflowers, alfalfa, garlic, chives, onion, cabbage, pea shoots, broccoli, and radish, just to name a few. Use them as substitutes for many common vegetables. If a recipe calls for broccoli, for example, use broccoli sprouts. Also you can juice them together with carrots or other veggies. Sprouting is especially economical and nutritious when making juices, but it is a valuable adjunct to any diet.

Basic Sprouting Instructions

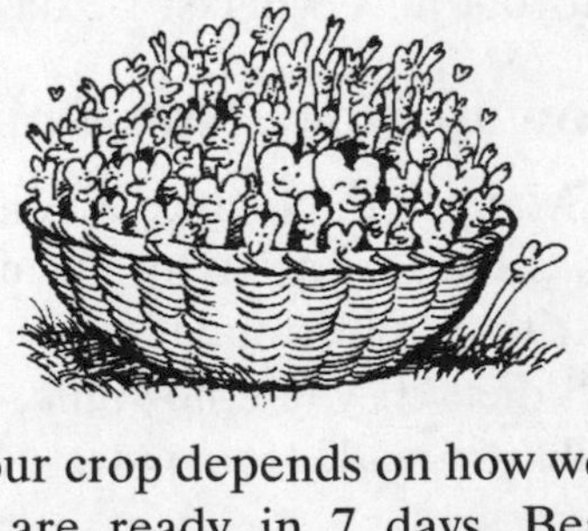

First, obtain a good home sprouter *(see "Resources")*. Soak your seeds for approximately 8 hours or overnight. Pour the seeds into the sprouter, rinse, and then rinse well twice daily. Rinsing is your main job, since the success of your crop depends on how well you rinse. Most green leafy sprouts are ready in 7 days. Bean sprouts are ready in 3–5 days. Green sprouts like a bright spot but not direct sun. Bean sprouts will grow in either a light or dark area. Sprouts will also grow under artificial light when necessary *(For more about sprouting, read "Sprouts The Miracle Food" by this author.)*

How to Store Fresh Juices & Blended Drinks

The best storage place for a freshly squeezed fruit and vegetable juice is in your stomach! Drink these juices right away to get their maximum nutritional benefit. But because you will not want to bother with your juice machine more than once a day, it is both convenient and desirable to make a few drinks at a time. Save the extra drinks for later or take one to the office. Here are some ideas for extending the life of your juices and blended drinks.

Cold Storage. Cold is the best preservation environment. Pour your fresh juice or smoothie into a quart jar and place it in your freezer for 15 to 30 minutes. Be careful; the goal is to chill the juice, not freeze it. If you have a food thermometer, you can test your juice and aim at reducing its temperature to 35-40°F. Keep the juice refrigerated at this point. A dark glass jar is preferable.

Portable Thermos Method. Purchase a glass or stainless steel thermos that holds enough to satisfy your needs. Stainless steel is especially resistant to breakage in situations that require daily portability, such as to and from work. Pre-chill your thermos by filling it temporarily with plain water and placing it in the freezer or fridge and leaving it uncapped so the cold air can enter. Next, chill your juice or blended drink following the instructions for the cold storage method. Empty the chilled thermos and fill it with the chilled juice. At 40°F, juice should stay cold all day. Surrounding temperatures influence the thermos, so don't leave it in the hot sun. When stored in a refrigerator, your juice will last 1-3 days.

How to Make Non-Dairy Milks

Many of the recipes in this book use alternative milks. These faux milks have a variety of advantages, including fewer allergens, more nutrition, and suitability to the restrictions of various health needs and diets. If you enjoy milk, there is no need to go without it. Faux milks are made from nuts, seeds, beans, or grains.

Basic Nut Milk

If you love nuts and seeds, this is the milk for you. Nut milk is easy to prepare, requires no cooking, and is alive with enzymes. The basic process is simple. Blend the nuts with water or juice and, using a fine sieve, strain out the nut meal. The ratio of water to nuts is approximately 3 to 1. Refrigerate the drink and use within a few days.

Here is the recipe for basic nut milk that uses almonds. Other nuts and seeds may be substituted, although the ratio of nuts to water will vary. It yields 4 cups.

1 cup of almonds
3 cups pure water
2 tablespoons maple syrup, honey, or your favorite sweetener

Because almonds are the hardest of the nuts used for making milk, it is best to soften almonds by soaking them in the pure water for 3-6 hours. Once soft, thoroughly blend the almonds in water and pass the mixture through a fine sieve or strainer. Now add your favorite sweetener, stir and drink. You will be surprised at how creamy and sweet it is. The sweetener is optional.

Sunflower Seed Milk

Follow the basic almond milk recipe above. Sunflower seeds are so small, however, that it is not necessary to pre-soak them. Just put the cup of raw, shelled (silver-colored) sunflower seeds in a blender and start whipping. First, blend them dry to the consistency of nut meal. Now blend in the water, and if you like your milk thick, do not strain out the seed pulp. This gives your drink a milkshake consistency. However, straining gives you a lighter, smoother milk. You may also adjust the consistency by increasing or decreasing the amount of water.

Cashew Milk

One of the most seductive members of the nut kingdom is the ever-sensuous cashew. Grown in exotic faraway lands like Mozambique and Brazil, this succulent ambrosia is in fact not a nut at all, but the seed of the cashew apple. It makes a wonderful faux milk because of its smooth texture, milky color, and unique taste. Blend it with 3 to 4 parts water and add a tablespoon of maple syrup, honey, or other sweetener, and you are on your way to nondairy heaven.

Like sunflowers, cashews do not require a pre-soaking stage. Prepare them just as you would sunflower or almond milk, with one exception: this milk does not need to be strained. In fact, because the cashew has such soft fiber, it refuses to be strained. When you drink cashew milk, you are drinking a purée of cashews and water. This contrasts with almond milk, from which the pulp is removed and only the water extract is consumed.

These are the most popular nuts and seeds for milk, but once you have perfected your milk-making skills, you may want to experiment with sesame and pumpkin seeds, both of which are prepared just like sunflower milk and are very satisfying.

Grain & Bean Milks

Milk can also be made from oats, rice, and soybeans. Health food stores carry several brands of each, but you can also make them at home. Below is the basic recipe for oat milk, since it is the easiest. Soy milk can be made at home but is more complicated. However, appliances for making soy milk are now available, and they make the process easier. *(See "Resources: Juicers and Other Equipment")* Rice milk is best made with "sweet" rice. It involves cooking the rice with extra water, then pressing and straining out the milk.

Oat Milk

1-2 Tbsp	Oats, quick cooking
1 cup	Pure Water
½-1 tsp	Vanilla Extract
1 Tbsp	Maple Syrup

Here is the basic one-cup recipe for making oat milk at home. Place one or two tablespoons of quick cooking oatmeal oats in one cup of boiling water. Cook for just a few minutes, then cool and blend until smooth in your blender. Now you have a choice. You can pour the resulting milk through a strainer to make it lighter and smoother, or use it unstrained for a richer consistency. When strained and served hot, it could be called oat "tea." Oat milk flavor is enhanced with a half/whole teaspoon of vanilla extract and your favorite sweetener. If you choose a viscous sweetener such as honey, or rice syrup, add a teaspoon of it while the oat milk is still hot so it will melt in. Maple syrup or stevia can be added straight into the blender. Oats are a rich source of carbohydrates that convert easily into energy and increase stamina. Serve hot or cold.

How to Make Herbal Teas

Brewing tea is simple, but here are a few basic rules to ensure the optimum therapeutic benefits.

Green Tea and Black Tea. Heat your water up to but do not boil (170-185°F). Gather 1-2 teaspoons of loose tea or 1 tea bag and place them in an empty teapot. Pour in the hot water over the tea bag or leaves. Brew for 3-5 minutes. This process of tea making is called an infusion. These teas should not be reheated, and over-brewing ruins them. However, green tea leaves can be used twice, but black tea only once. These teas, along with Indian and Chinese tea, contain caffeine.

Twig Teas. Simmer these teas for about 5 minutes, straining them into a cup. Add a dash of tamari for an invigorating warm-up drink after vigorous outdoor activities.

Herbal Teas. Unlike green, black, and twig teas, most herbal teas do not contain caffeine. They encompass a wide variety of plant leaves, flowers, twigs, and barks.

Leaves. Leaves are delicate things. You should not boil spearmint, peppermint, sage, chamomile, hops, mullein, and the many other leafy herbs mentioned in this book. Steep them just as you would green and black teas—the infusion method.

Roots, Seeds and Barks. Ginseng, ginger, licorice, cloves, all-spice, and wild cherry are some examples of roots, seeds and barks. They need to boil and steep longer to extract their therapeutic compounds. Steeping time ranges from 10-20 minutes, depending on the variety. This process of tea-making is called a decoction.

About the Recipes in This Book

Units of Measure

Following recipes is an art. If a recipe calls for 1 apple, the apple could yield 1 to 3 ounces of juice, depending on its size and juiciness. The same is true of carrots. Eight medium-size carrots should yield 12 ounces of juice; but what is a medium-size carrot? By their nature, recipes are unscientific. For this reason, the juice and blended drink recipes in this book are designated in ounces of juice. Thus, if a recipe calls for 12 ounces of carrot juice, juice enough carrots to yield 12 ounces of juice. This is the best way to ensure your recipe will result in a balanced and delicious taste.

Taste is another very unscientific area. What the author deigns tasty may not suit you. Wheatgrass juice, for example, is an acquired taste and often unpalatable to the uninitiated. Some folks will down anything that is a potential remedy for their health; others simply cannot. Some of the recipes in this book may not be sweet enough for your taste. Here is a confession: your faithful author is prejudiced against sweets. It stems from a philosophy that blames excess sweets for sending too many people down the path of ill health. But you, the recipe user, should always feel free to add another carrot, another ounce of apple juice, another teaspoon of honey, and so on. The recipes in this book are elastic. The therapeutic ingredients are there in a good general balance, and you can stretch them to suit your taste.

Teas. "Bag" means a tea bag. Many herbal tea recipes in this book use herbs that are readily available in tea bags, which are convenient and protect the herb's therapeutic properties. In many cases, you do not have to use loose herbs unless you want to. Generally, a teaspoon of loose herbs is close to the amount found in a tea bag. Thus, the recipe ingredients offer you a choice of *"1 tsp or bag."*

Recipe Symbols

Every recipe in this book has a title accompanied by symbols. The symbols represent the type of recipe.

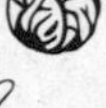 *These Symbols represent fresh vegetable juices* 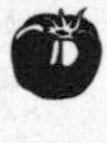

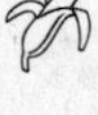 *These Symbols represent blended drinks or smoothies* 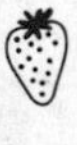

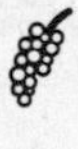 *These Symbols represent fruit juices* 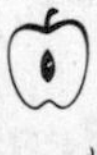

 *These Symbols represent herbal teas* 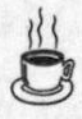

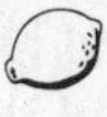 *These Symbols represent fresh citrus juices* 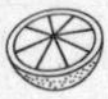

 *These Symbols represent other types of special drinks* 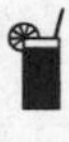

Juices & Drinks vs. Foods

Why You Should Make Power Juices and Drinks a Cornerstone of Your Diet

This book by no means suggests that you stop eating. Juices and blended drinks, however, are the fastest way to supercharge your bloodstream with powerful plant medicines and concentrated nutrients. When you drink these potent elixirs, you will feel their synergistic power and live enzymes push you through your day. No time to sit for a decent meal? Are you reaching for the french fries or chips? Have a blended drink instead. A delicious super smoothie will satisfy your hunger and help you lose weight besides. Your fruit and vegetable juicer will become your medicine chest. With the power juices and super drinks in this book, you will tap into a natural energy source that helps you sleep, clears thoughts, strengthens digestion, and builds immunity. They provide you with a lifetime of health benefits.

Liquid Acupuncture

Healing takes energy. Nutrients are great, but to work they must get into the cells. Theoretically, given enough quality nourishment, your cells can perform everything they are genetically capable of doing. But they must also process that nourishment, and they invariably function at different levels of performance. It is a matter of subtle energies. A dying person may be fed the world's healthiest food, but it still won't help. At that point, one doesn't have the energy to assimilate that good nutrition. Too many systems have been damaged. The "wires" to the cells are frayed and broken and no longer able to deliver nutrients. Such a person lacks the energy needed to push the nutrients through to their destination.

But it is not too late for you. Many of us, however, are running on low batteries. We could use more bioelectricity to deliver those good nutrients. Greater energy improves the capacity of our cells to process nutrition. In other words, our cells will perform at higher levels. Optimum cell performance means optimum overall health.

The energy we are discussing is the same subtle vibrations that exist throughout nature. It is the prana of the yogis and the chi of the ancient Chinese. It is the modus operandi behind the effectiveness of homeopathy, acupuncture, laying on of hands, and Bach flower remedies.

Plants contain this subtle energy just as people do. When we eat raw fruits and vegetables or drink their juices, we are imbibing a dose of their electrochemical energy. In other words, it enlivens us. We are more alive and less fatigued. It is like liquid acupuncture, flowing up and down the body's meridians. Raw-foodists even claim they need less sleep.

Glug–Zoom! Quick Energy

Perhaps you have already experienced the feeling of raw juices instantly supercharging your body. Why do you get this quick jolt of energy? In addition to their bioelectric energy field, raw nutrients are more viable than cooked nutrients. Nutrients such as vitamin C, most B-complex vitamins, and enzymes simply cannot survive the heat. Proteins may be altered in a way that makes them indigestible, and fats can degrade into carcinogenic aldehydes and peroxides. But when you consume these foods in a more natural state, you get nearly 100% of their nutrients and cofactors, including the phytochemicals and enzymes that assist in their digestion. This increased digestibility means you get to use more of what you eat. Since it takes less energy to digest the meal, you have more left over and you feel it. You become more efficient! You need less sleep, have more energy, more stamina, less fatigue, and do a better job of fighting disease.

Fresh juices digest even more easily than blended drinks, because the juicer eliminates the cellulose. The resulting fruit and vegetable extract passes right through the stomach and is absorbed within minutes. For this reason, juices are predigested food. The juicer machine is like an external digestive system. And who couldn't use a spare stomach! Our digestion breaks down food into a liquid nutrient mass that is small enough to travel into the bloodstream. Usually, a lot of work and energy is expended to get to that point, but juicing provides the same result. While conserving your body's energy, juices deliver an instant nutritional charge into your bloodstream.

Better Digestion and Assimilation

How many people do you know who fall asleep after a big meal? A big meal can be very taxing, especially when you consider that a turkey dinner with all the trimmings can take up to 3-4 hours to digest. Even vegetables, when cooked in complex sauces and oils, can take 2-3 hours. But a typical meal of raw fruits and vegetables takes one hour, and you can feel the burst of energy from juices within minutes.

Let's face it, you just can't stomach all the fruits and vegetables you would need to treat arthritis, lower cholesterol, reduce allergies, or prevent cancer. You would have to eat 8 medium sized carrots to match the equivalent beta-carotene in a 12 oz glass of carrot juice. Try digesting that! And this is assuming that you have good digestion. Most of us are a sad set of pipes, trucking food in and out and absorbing as little as 10% of the food we eat. But with fresh squeezed juices, we get all the benefits of pounds of produce concentrated into a single glass. Juices enhance our digestion by getting more nourishment into our cells and rebuilding our health and strength.

The Magic of Phytochemicals

The National Cancer Institute (NCI) and the U.S. Dept of Health and Human Services recommends eating 5 or more servings of fruits and vegetables every day. They define one serving as a piece of fruit, a cup of raw leafy vegetables, or a 12-ounce glass of juice. (They also include canned fruits and vegetables.) But we are falling short. In a recent study of adults, more than 50% had less than a single serving of fruit per day. They did eat vegetables, but potatoes exceeded all other vegetables by far with french fries and chips being the most popular form.[1] That is not what the NCI had in mind!

Fresh fruits and vegetables contain marvelous plant compounds that stimulate your immune system, and they are proven fighters of diseases such as arthritis, heart disease, and cancer. Even plain and common foods have these phytochemicals. **Broccoli** has glucosinolates that are converted by enzymes into isothiocyanates and indoles. All of them obstruct the formation of cancer cells. **Carrots** contain alpha- and beta-carotene, the quintessential antioxidants whose ability to quench the appetite of free radicals provides numerous anti-aging and health benefits. **Spinach** contains the carotenoid lutein (along with beta-carotene), which fights colon and lung cancers, cataracts, and age-related macular degeneration. **Tomatoes** are our best source of lycopene, the oxygenated red carotenoid that has a special thirst for single-oxygen free radicals and, according to Dr. Edward Gioavannuci of Harvard University, can reduce the risk of prostate cancer by 34 percent. And, after years of studies, the USDA officially agreed in 1999 that **Soy Protein** lowers the risk of heart disease by 20%.

Whole Foods — Nature Makes the Best Vitamins

The natural nutrient complexes in fruits and vegetables outperform synthetic or extracted supplements, and at much lower concentrations. Albert Szent-Györgyi, the Nobel prize winning bio-chemist who discovered Vitamin C, found that the complex structure of C in peppers was more effective than chemically isolated C. When we start adding various isolated vitamins to our diet, it is an attempt to replicate nature through nutrition by the numbers. But a whole food is a complex bundle of thousands of chemicals. Squeezing isolated nutrients from whole food dissipates its magic. The many cofactors, micro-nutrients, and phytochemicals found in foods synergistically enhance the delivery and function of nutrition. The USDA's minimum daily requirements (MDR) for vitamins and minerals were established on the basis of using supplements. But real foods are effective at lower concentrations. Although supplements have their place, they are not a substitute for whole foods and fresh juices. The perfect supplements are inside these foods, stored in nature's ideal package.

Lose Weight

If you incorporate the blended drinks and juices in this book as part of a weight-loss program along with regular exercise, you will have the only diet you'll ever need to slim down and charge up. You'll be cutting thousands of calories and never feel deprived. How is this possible? Juices contain so much concentrated nourishment, they automatically quench hunger. Many of the green juice recipes, like wheatgrass for example, actually suppress appetite. The blended drink recipes in this book are rich in fiber that will fill you up and function as a meal substitute. They are thick and nourishing and make you feel full. They are low in calories, and because they are full of indigestible fiber, most of that bulk passes right through you. Fiber is food that is not absorbed by the body. What a concept! Fiber absorbs lots of water, makes you feel full, keeps the intestinal tract moving, and lowers your risk of colon cancer. It has other benefits, too, such as lowering cholesterol and reducing the risk of heart disease.

A whole food is a complex bundle of thousands of chemicals. Squeezing isolated nutrients from food dissipates its magic.

What About the Lack of Fiber in Juice?

Many people complain about the extraction of this valuable fiber in fresh juices. Sure it is extracted, but juices have a different purpose. Juicers function like our digestive tracts, eliminating fiber and sending the juice into our bloodstream. They concentrate pounds of produce into the best kind of natural whole foods supplements. Just as vitamins do not substitute for foods, there is a role for eating and a role for juicing. This book acclaims the wholesome benefits of fiber and has many blended drinks that are rich sources of it.

Folks who juice can also benefit from the many inedible portions of foods that are simply discarded when we eat. This includes water melon rinds (one of our finest natural diuretics), orange skins (rich in volatile oils that dissolve gallstones), and grape seeds (one of our best natural antibiotics). Since we get all this good stuff when we juice and throw them away when we eat, juicing gives us a "whole foods" advantage.

What's Wrong with Store-Bought Bottled Juice?

Bottled juices must be pasteurized for longer shelf life. This boiling process sanitizes the juice to protect against salmonella, E. coli, and other harmful organisms. Unfortunately, enzymes and many vitamins are also destroyed in the process, and other nutrients are altered in ways that reduce their bioavailability. Generally speaking, the vitality of the fresh product is gone and, along with it, all the magnetism and bioelectricity that engender fresh foods with their healing power. Many commercial juices, are, in nutritional terms, processed down to sugar, flavor, and water. Read the labels. Some of them are labeled "juice drinks." They are not real juices but recipes using water, flavoring, and frozen juice concentrates. None of these are a match for the freshly squeezed version. Preserve human life, not shelf life. Juice: it's the real thing.

Preserve human life, not shelf life.

What's Wrong with Soft Drinks

Think before you drink. Soft drinks are responsible for the term "empty calories." These calories lack vitamins, minerals, fiber, and phtyo-nutrients. Most soft drinks contain high fructose corn syrup, a concentrated form of fructose. True, fructose is fruit sugar, but despite the fact that "fruit" sounds healthy, it is still sugar and soft drinks contain more fructose than a glass of orange juice. They also contain large amounts of caffeine, a central nervous system stimulant that, after an initial pickup, zaps your energy and depletes your B vitamins. Studies indicate that long-term, soft-drink drinkers may be accelerating their rate of aging, especially through the loss of the collagen in their skin.[2]

Raw fruit and vegetable juices and blended drinks are the most powerful and effective nutrient vehicles you can put in your body. Follow the recipes in this book to experience quick energy, improve digestion and stamina, prevent disease, beat cancer, and slow your body's aging process. You will enjoy a lifetime of health benefits. Not only that, they taste great, are fun to make, and are great for the whole family.

Juicers, Blenders & Water Purifiers

See "Resources" for manufacturers from whom you can get more information.

About Juicing Machines

A fruit and vegetable juicer can be the most important nutritional appliance in your home. As a dispenser of vitamins and minerals alone, this machine will provide hundreds of dollars worth of vitamins and minerals. And that does not count all the fun you and your family will have using it. A juicer is a magic thirst-quenching, fountain-of-youth machine that conjures all kinds of flavors and colors to interest even the most soda-pop minded family member. If you are committed to the pursuit of health, get a good juicing machine and watch it become your personal drug store and medicine chest for all that ails you.

All juicers are not equal. Good juicing machines generally cost about $200. True, there are machines for under $100, but they are likely to be inefficient and too weak to suit the serious juice fan. These juicers are usually products of large, general appliance manufacturers, some of which are more famous for home electronics and portable stereos. Contrast this to a dedicated juice manufacturer who specializes in juicers.

The Different Types of Juicers

There are four different methods for extracting nutrients from fruits and vegetables. The first and most common of these is the centrifugal-force juicer. These juicers cut vegetables into tiny pieces and spin them in a basket at high speed—3,000-7,000 rpms. The juice is extracted by the sheer power of centrifugal force, just as wet clothes are relieved of excess water in a washing machine's spin cycle. As you may have guessed, these machines are circular in shape.

The second method is known as "trituration." It operates by chewing, or ripping, the vegetables and then forcing the minced pulp against a screen with the pressure of the rotating cutter. This ripping action distinguishes triturators from centrifugal machines. Theoretically, they tear open the plant's cell membranes exposing their deep seated nutrients and enzymes. On the other hand, the blades of a centrifugal juicer, as the theory goes, slice the vegetables into tiny pieces that do not penetrate as deeply. A triturator also operates at a slower speed (about 1,700 rpms). Unlike centrifugal machines, triturators do not whip anything around. Therefore, there is less oxidation of nutrients. These manufacturers argue that their juice is nutritionally superior. While claims from manufacturers are by nature controversial, all agree that slower speeds and less oxidation yield more nutrition.

Another method of extraction is the old reliable worm gear juicer. Many are cast iron affairs, similar to the old table top, hand-crank meat grinders that were popular during the mid-twentieth century. These machines are good for fruits and leafy vegetables, but are most popular for juicing wheat grass. They come as manual or motorized machines. Manual machines range in price from $50–$150, and the motorized ones cost $300–600. Even the motorized machines turn a gentle 100 rpms, which is ideal for protecting fragile nutrients.

The newest juicing system is the twin gear masticator. This technology is both innovative and unique. Two gears fold inward on each other, squeezing the vegetables pushed through between them. The crushed veggie is then forced against a fine sieve, squeezing out its juice. The gears' 90-rpm speed is as slow as hand cranking, which eliminates the heat caused by the friction of faster machines as well as the oxidation caused by the high-velocity blades. Crushing, or mastication, is the best way to break open the plant's cell walls to extract deeply entrenched nutrients. Twin-gear machines are also versatile; they will juice wheat grass in addition to common vegetables. Thus, if you want to explore the wonders of wheat grass, you don't have to find space for two machines. Twin-gear machines sell for approximately $500.

Some of these machines are pulp-ejectors. They save a lot of time by expelling the pulp continuously during the juicing. This means you can juice more than half a gallon without stopping to clean the machine. A non-ejecting juicer, on the other hand, collects the pulp in a spinning basket, which must be emptied after juicing approximately two quarts. On the plus side, many non-ejecting juicers come with paper filters that make clean-up easier, faster, and neater.

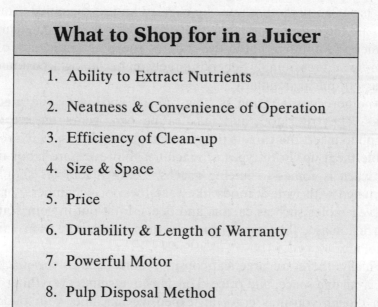

What to Shop for in a Juicer

1. Ability to Extract Nutrients
2. Neatness & Convenience of Operation
3. Efficiency of Clean-up
4. Size & Space
5. Price
6. Durability & Length of Warranty
7. Powerful Motor
8. Pulp Disposal Method

All of these machines can juice citrus fruits, although some come with specially designed citrus juicing attachments. These attachments operate like a stand-alone citrus juicer, in which the fruit cut in half rides atop a ridged dome that rips into the fruit, sending its juice down through a sieve. If you do not have this attachment, simply cut and peel the fruit into 4-8 parts and stuff them down the juicing chute as you would a carrot. Be sure to include the pulpy part of the fruit, since it contains a wealth of flavonoids. This method makes for a smoother and creamier juice than the stand-alone citrus juicers. Stand-alone citrus juicers, however, range in price from only $15–$40, an inexpensive and worthwhile investment.

When it comes to using a juicer, convenience of operation and ease of clean-up are probably the most important factors. If you are discouraged by the set-up and clean-up of your juicer, you will probably use it less. An unused juicer does nothing for your health. Regular use is the secret to unleashing the power of juice therapy.

All machines must be assembled and disassembled for each use. They all have a cutter blade or a gear, a cover, a screen, and a housing or juicer body, all of which must be removed and cleaned. They typically have 3–5 parts that must be cleaned and reassembled. You can compare the differences in handling these parts from one machine to another ad infinitum, but in the end, the speed and efficiency of this clean-up and reassembly depends largely on becoming accustomed to doing it by juicing regularly.

Another consideration is how quickly and easily the machine works. The triturators and masticating twin gears require more oomph to insert the carrots than centrifugal machines, which readily gobble them up. Both types of machines, however, are labor-intensive when it comes to juicing greens. Leafy vegetables should be alternated with watery foods like tomatoes, or cucumbers, or with stiff vegetables such as carrots and beets. First put in your spinach, then a tomato, then more spinach, then cucumber, then spinach again, etc.

Finally, there are practical considerations such as the machine's size, available space, and price. This may determine everything, since even though you may crave an expensive machine, your budget is what it is. Whatever juicer you choose, it all drizzles down to this question: Will I use it? Choose a machine that you can use conveniently and maintain on a daily basis.

Can't Buy A Juicer?

If you do not have a juicer and cannot buy one now, here are some alternatives. Invest in a good citrus juicer. Even the electric models are affordable, and they will serve you well. Visit your local juice bar. Juice bars and many health food stores offer freshly squeezed fruit and vegetable and wheatgrass juice. Purchase a good blender. With a blender and a citrus juicer you can still enjoy many of the recipes in this book—for example, blended drinks, teas, broths, powdered juices, fresh apple cider, and homemade citrus juice.

About Blenders

A blender is arguably the workhorse of the American kitchen. Pour in your ingredients, hit the switch, and watch the blender whip and emulsify your drink into a creamy, liquid meal sent from heaven. After one of these velvety feasts, you may not want any other kitchen appliance.

So, what are the main differences between juicing and blending? Juicing extracts the liquid from a fruit or vegetable, and separates it from its fiber or pulp. Blending uses the whole fruit and liquefies it into a buoyant, fiber-rich purée. Blenders can incorporate a broader selection of foods than juicers. Juicers are limited primarily to fresh fruits and vegetables. Blenders can mix powders, granules, hot liquids, nuts, seeds, ice cubes, oils, spices, vegetables, fruits, herbs, and extracts. They do everything but the wash!

Getting a good blender is a top priority. Prices span the Atlantic, from $20 to $400, but inexpensive blenders have a weak heart. They struggle and strain over every grain and can choke to death on an oversized banana. Some blenders come with a legion of buttons, looking very official but signifying nothing. Purée, whip, mix, frappé ... what does it all mean? The professionals don't understand it, either. They use the $200 $400 blenders with only one switch for high, low, and pulse. When they turn their tiger on, it grabs onto the counter and roars into action. In contrast, the fancy multi-button affairs whir like pencil sharpeners and dance the rhumba right off your counter.

Avoid bad landings for your blender. Buy the best one you can afford. Choose a powerful motor with a solid heavy base. Blenders throw food upward, so start every recipe by pulsing the ingredients or using low power until the food is cut into smaller bits. Then add a little liquid and rev up the engine to high for a smooth, creamy finale. Blenders aerate their ingredients making them fluffy, light, and silky. Food processors cannot blend your drinks. They beat, chop, shred, slice, and grind, but they cannot liquefy. They fail to create that ethereal emulsification of ingredients. Suffice it to say that a blender is a valuable part of your nutrition program. It is an efficient, timesaving asset that will deliver a wide variety of liquid meals and feathery fantasies that your palate will find hard to resist.

Drink Pure Water

Next to air, water is our most vital ingredient. Our blood is 96% water, and our heart and brain are 75% water. We are walking sacks of fluid! Some health professionals consider dehydration the underlying cause of many human disorders and claim that it is a silent epidemic. While juices and raw fruits and vegetables are rich sources of water, they do not replace the need to drink plain water, just as vitamins do not replace our need for food. Water is the primary ingredient of the recipes in this book. So, in addition to a juice machine and blender, a method of obtaining pure water is of vital importance.

Our kidneys make great water filters. They work decade after decade cleaning our blood and our water. Why should they have to remove nitrates, fluoride, lead, arsenic, mercury, aluminum, chlorine, E. coli bacteria, giardia, and industrial wastes? The replacement cost of a good charcoal filter cartridge is about $50. Compare that to the price of a kidney replacement. Look around the planet and you will see that water is the essential ingredient of life. Flush your kidneys, colon, and blood daily with the purest water possible, and hydrate your cells so they will function at optimum efficiency.

Sadly, this precious commodity has become polluted everywhere we look. From Chernobyl to Love Canal to the quaint back hills of New England, no stream, no river, no well, no reservoir has escaped contamination. It is a sad comment on our civilization that citizens of an evolved society must worry about their water.

Dioxin, PCBs, radioactive waste, pesticides, cyanide, giardia, acid rain, petrochemicals, and other industrial waste have polluted our waterways worldwide. Some of these chemicals never break down and are so dangerous that they must be "contained" forever in the hope that they will not infect our ground (drinking) water. In the 1970s, many of us assumed that only the big cities had a water pollution problem. But today, PCBs are found even in the Antarctic ice, and the problem has arrived at everyone's tap.

While governments struggle with pollution cleanup, the best solution is to take action yourself—at your tap. Sure, buying spring water is good, but juggling all those jugs in and out of your house week after week is inconvenient. Besides, not all spring water is equal. Often, "spring water" does not even come from a spring, and some are no cleaner than what comes out of our tap. Further, water not distributed across state lines is not regulated by the FDA.

Mechanical Purifiers

Mechanical filters are one way to purify water right at your tap. Almost all of these units use activated charcoal as the primary cleaning agent. Charcoal is famous for absorbing bad odors and tastes. But the simplest units, costing in the $50 range, do little more. In fact, worse, they can breed bacteria.

Space-age technology has created highly compressed carbon blocks. These filters are so dense that their microscopic pores are smaller than a red blood cell. Bacteria cannot penetrate these devices, which allows them to be labeled "purifiers." Unlike germ-killing bactericides such as silver and iodine, these filters physically block microorganisms. Such filters range in price from $200–$400.

In addition to germs such as E. Coli and giardia, high-end, carbon-block purifiers remove bad odor, color, taste, dirt, algae, toxic metals like lead, chlorine and pesticides, and hundreds of cancer causing chemicals like chlorine and its by-products like THMs. They do an excellent job of restoring good water to its original pristine condition. Their weakness, however, is in removing inorganic chemicals such as nitrates, fluorides, and sodium. If the latter are of major concern to you, then you ought to consider a water distiller.

Distillers

Distillation is the oldest and most thorough method of water purification. Rain is natural distillation, and distillers mimic this process. They boil water into steam, capture the steam, and condense it back to water. During this transformation from liquid to gas to liquid again, anything with a molecular weight heavier than steam is removed. Only some gaseous pollutants remain in distilled water, but this weakness can be compensated for.

Distillers are not as popular as mechanical filters and purifiers because they cost more, take hours to make a gallon, and remove minerals. Distilled water is laboratory-pure and may be too clean for some. The public worries: Is sterile water "healthy?"

The controversy over distillation is about the loss of minerals. On the other hand, if purity is your top priority, there is no purer water than distilled. Fortunately, the minerals in natural water are abundantly available from fresh fruits and vegetables and their juices. In fact, it would take approximately 100 glasses of spring water, for example, to equal the calcium in one glass of fresh carrot juice. Our diet is a far more substantial source of minerals and trace minerals than water. That being said, we must still drink plain water for cleansing and hydration. If you want both pure water and minerals, try remineralizing distilled water. You can add mineral tablets or just a few mineral rich whole grains to this ultra-pure water. For example, six grains of rice will turn one gallon of distilled water into a living mineral water.

Distillers can be expensive. They can range in price from $225 to $1500 for household use. The more expensive units do not necessarily produce purer water. Mostly, they produce water at a faster rate, and are automated. Select a distiller that meets the needs of your household now and in the future. If your household averages 1-1½ gallons of cooking and drinking water per day, a low output distiller would be adequate. However, since a distiller can last for decades, you may want to plan ahead.

Other Purification Methods

Other methods of water purification include reverse osmosis, ozonation, and ultraviolet light. Many swimming pools are ozonated. Los Angeles used this method to purify the Olympic swimming pool during the international Olympic games held there in 1984.

While it is not within the scope of this book to evaluate all water purification methods, you can research them to be a more informed shopper. Make the choice that best suits you, but make sure you choose to drink pure water.

Power Drinks for the

Physical Body

Better Athletic Performance, Sexual Health, Physical Energy & Stamina

This chapter is about the foods, herbs, and nutrients that promote optimum physical performance for athletes and heighten sexual performance and general good health. These are the foods, nutrients, and herbs that provide optimum energy, improve fertility, counteract impotence, boost sexual vigor, keep joints flexible, stimulate muscle growth and repair, and, in general, enhance energy and physical strength.

Please keep in mind that foods, herbs and nutrients are not drugs. They nourish our cells in a way that enables higher, long term functioning. Chemicals can pump us up, but ultimately they may burn us out. Real improvement takes time and persistence, and regular consumption of the good nutrients and foods described in this chapter will help accomplish your goals. *(For more information about specific foods and nutrients mentioned here, see "Nutrient Sources and the Glossary.")*

Foods for Optimum Physical Performance

Whey Protein contains the branched-chain amino acids (BCAAs) needed to recover from muscle fatigue and increase stamina after a body has been taxed by endurance (cardiovascular) exercise or weight training. Once the muscles have been tapped for BCAAs, fatigue sets in. Whey, the liquid that separates from the curds during cheese production, is full of amino acids. Whey protein is the concentrated extract of whey and has the highest concentration of

BCAAs (approximately 24%) of any food. Not only can whey protein prevent muscle loss, it can actually promote muscle growth and repair damaged muscles.[1]

Wheat Grass Juice. Because wheat grass is a combination of the concentrated nutrients that give life to grain, it produces tremendous energy. Wheat grass is rich in minerals, vitamins, and chlorophyll and acts as a potent antioxidant. There is an abundance of anecdotal evidence about the capacity of wheat grass to increase performance. As an overall, energizing tonic, wheat grass juice benefits many systems within the body, and its universal appeal stems from the ability to enhance oxygen absorption. See what juicing with wheat grass does for improving your performance and shortening your time to the finish line.[2]

Wheat Germ. This is the kernel of life, from which a new wheat plant is grown. Wheat germ is rich in carbohydrates, B and E vitamins, and fatty acids, and it is high in performance minerals such as iron, zinc, and magnesium. Wheat germ oil has been known to increase stamina because of its octacosanol content, a lipid that stimulates the production of androgens and muscle growth.

Algae. Composed primarily of protein and carbohydrates, algae are active, vital contributors to peak performance. Muscle maintenance and algae go hand-in-hand. Muscles are made up of 22% protein and need high-quality, rich sources of protein such as algae. Choose any of the three types of algae (described below) according to personal taste and experience. Nutritionally, they are all "super." *(For more, see "Algae.")*

Spirulina is a powerhouse of amino acids, carotenoids, enzymes, lipids, protein, glycogen, minerals, and vitamins. What more could you ask for! In fact, structurally, spirulina resembles DNA, which is where it got its "spiral" name. More specifically, spirulina is a superb source of beta carotene and 10 other carotenoids, as well as antioxidants and the phytochemicals phycocyanin, chlorophyll, glycolipids, and sulfolipids. For this reason, spirulina has been praised as an immune system booster. It is also rich in the essential fatty acid GLA (gamma linolenic acid) with lots of easy-to-absorb iron. As a source of vitamin B12 (200 mcg/100g), this food is superior to liver (80mcg) and all other animal foods (cheese is 2mcg). And, at 60%

protein, it is arguably the most concentrated protein food on the planet. For athletic performance, higher glycogen levels in muscles translate into higher performance. Spirulina is claimed to be the only known dietary source of glycogen.

Chlorella is highest of all foods in chlorophyll, which is why they call it chlorella. This single-cell plant has the unique ability to self-reproduce. The Chlorella Growth Factor (CGF) holds the promise of assisting in the repair and regeneration of human tissue. Its nucleus contains lots of nucleopeptides as well as cell growth factors such as RNA and DNA. This is the fundamental stuff needed for the creation of life at the cellular level, and chlorella is our best food source. With its high-grade plant protein, chlorella is a superb food for optimizing mineral absorption and bone density, two critical factors in achieving peak performance.

Blue-Green Algae differs from spirulina and chlorella in that it is not cultivated in artificial ponds by "farming" but harvested from natural lakes by "fishing." But not in just any lake. The largest available natural algae lake in the world is Klamath Lake in Oregon. Famous as a brain food, blue-green algae is rich in neuropeptides that have low molecular weights and can pass freely through the blood-brain barrier. There they help strengthen neurotransmitters and improve mental functioning by increasing alertness and concentration, two factors that keep the athletic performer out in the front of the pack.

Other Foods. *Oats,* as a source of carbohydrates that is easily converted into energy, increase stamina. *Sunflower seeds* convert glycogen into glucose, a readily available source of energy. And *green peas* have been known to impede the process of conception because of their high m-xylohydroquinone content.[3]

Water. Muscles are made up of 70% water, so adequate amounts of pure water are essential for keeping the body free of injuries and in good condition. Super-oxygenated water has also been known to improve athletic performance. Eighty-three percent of runners who used water that had seven times more oxygen added to it prior to a 5-kilometer race clocked running times 31 seconds shorter than their normal times.[4]

Nutrients for Physical Performance

Vitamins

When your body is under the stress of intense exercise or other performance demands, vitamins may be your answer. They act as antistress factors for muscles, nerves, and circulatory functions. In addition to neutralizing free radicals, antioxidant vitamins such as C and E help speed recovery from exercise stress. Vitamin C is helpful for strengthening connective tissue and vitamin E aids circulation, which also helps with male sexual impotence. B-complex vitamins, a balanced blend of several B vitamins, are necessary for releasing the energy contained in carbohydrates, preventing muscle cramping, and promoting nerve health. Other vitamins that help with the metabolism of carbohydrates include lipoic acid and vitamin K, while B6 helps release glycogen from the liver and muscles, and helps restore mobility to swollen joints. Foods rich in vitamin C include acerola juice, wheat grass, black currant, parsley, broccoli, orange and lemon with peel, strawberry, and spinach. Brown rice, barley, rye, wheat germ, green leaves, nuts, and legumes are all high in vitamin E. Brewer's yeast is an excellent source of B vitamins as are soy beans and nuts.

Vitamin B12 concentrates in the testes, increasing sperm counts and aiding male fertility.[5] Vegetarians and especially those adhering to vegan diets can get B12 only from algae, brewer's yeast, and acidophilus rich, fermented foods. Consequently, strict diet management or supplementation is essential. Brewer's yeast, algae, peanuts, pecans, wheat germ, wheat bran, soybeans, sunflower seeds, and royal jelly add vitamin B5, which can increase stamina. Nicotinic acid, a form of Vitamin B3, facilitates orgasm by triggering histamine release. It can be found in brewer's yeast and spirulina.

Amino Acids

Athletes get amino acids–protein building blocks–from protein, but eating too much protein can actually promote osteoporosis and kidney disease. Amino acid supplements may be a better way to get the extra boost required by athletes. Improved muscle mass, stamina, and sexual function can result from amino acids that include **BCAAs (branched-chain amino acids)** such as valine, isoleucine, and leucine, as well as carnitine, l-dopa, and arginine. It should be noted that excessive use of specific amino acids can produce side effects and too much protein can overwork the kidney. Before taking high doses, consult with your nutritionist and take the time to investigate possible side effects.

When a body is taxed by exercise, muscle fatigue is delayed and stamina is increased by providing BCAAs. Once the BCAAs are tapped out in a muscle, fatigue sets in. BCAAs from whey, eggs, or supplements help delay muscle fatigue and build muscle mass.[6]

Leucine is a branched-chain, essential amino acid with many very desirable performance properties, offering both metabolic and musculoskeletal benefits. Leucine stabilizes blood sugar levels and produces energy. It can also prevent exercise-induced loss of muscle (overtraining), promote muscle growth, repair damaged muscle tissue, and expedite the healing of bones.[7]

Carnitine increases aerobic stamina by strengthening the heart and circulatory system and is especially helpful for endurance events. It boosts energy within the body, specifically in the muscles. *Acetyl-L-Carnitine,* a form of carnitine, may increase a runner's capacity for speed.[8]

L-Dopa possesses antioxidant properties and stimulates the central nervous system, thereby increasing stamina, sexual desire, and performance.

Arginine, due to its nitric oxide content, can help increase muscle mass and improve both male and female sexual performance. Possible benefits include more frequent erections and endurance for males and increased ability to reach orgasm for females.

Creatine is an amino acid manufactured in the liver, kidneys, and pancreas. It relies on beef, chicken, and certain fish to stimulate its production. Creatine monohydrate is the supplemental form of creatine. Because this supplement improves muscle fibers, delays fatigue, and speeds recovery time, creatine monohydrate can contribute to better athletic performance. Weightlifters benefit from its capacity to reduce lactic acid levels in muscles by up to 41%.[9] Lactic acid is the end result of anaerobic respiration and can cause muscle weakness, cramping, and fatigue.

Coenzymes

Coenzyme Q10 is the most important coenzyme for humans. It acts as a catalyst for energy production and release. Found throughout the body, this antioxidant increases stamina and improves athletic performance by enhancing the flow of oxygen to the cells, and its effects are noticeable after only four weeks of use! This near-miracle supplement benefits athletes by prolonging the time until exhaustion and reducing muscle damage. It is also a potential aid for male infertility. Coenzyme Q10 can be added to the diet via spinach, broccoli, cabbage, carrot, sweet potato, peanuts, sesame, and fish, or may be taken as a supplement.[10]

NADH. Another coenzyme that is especially helpful to athletic performance is NADH, also known as coenzyme Q1. Intricately involved in the energy-producing processes within each cell, NADH has added advantage for athletes because of its role in the final step of the process that oxidizes glucose from dietary carbohydrates, fats, and proteins. Supplements of NADH increase energy production and reduce fatigue.[11]

Minerals

Minerals increase bone density, speed and endurance and are essential for optimal performance. Potassium is important for the conversion of glucose to glycogen, and magnesium is important for the storage and release of glycogen. More glycogen in the muscles often translates into better athletic performance. Potassium and magnesium relieve muscle fatigue and prevent the buildup of lactic acid. Phosphorus also reduces lactic acid levels. Magnesium is also important for good muscle contraction and relaxation, for nerve functions, and for regulating blood pressure. Adequate levels of chromium and zinc help regulate blood sugar, energy production, and tissue repair, while calcium, magnesium, and zinc prevent muscle cramping and protect bones. Iron transports oxygen, which is critical for optimal aerobic performance. Sulfur helps improve the condition of joints. MSM, a type of sulfur produced by the body, reduces the lactic acid built up by exercise. *(See "Nutrient Sources" for dietary sources of these minerals.)*

Fats

Triglycerides are dietary fats and oils used to fuel the body and energize the metabolism. Triglycerides with medium carbon chains (MCTs) aid the athletic performer by increasing stamina and providing a rapid burst of energy, especially when consumed with glucose. Additionally, MCTs increase the body's absorption of calcium and magnesium, two minerals that are particularly important for endurance and performance.

Gamma Oryzanol. Gamma oryzanol is a phytosterol, a type of fat derived from plant sources that is helpful for the serious athlete. Endurance exercise releases a hormone called cortisol, which helps relieve inflammation in tissues, nerves, or muscles. However, too much cortisol negatively affects optimal performance by breaking down muscle tissue, which, in turn, leads to muscle weakness and fatigue. Gamma oryzanol controls the release of excessive cortisol, thereby extending the time of optimal muscle function.

As a natural alternative to steroids to increase testosterone, gamma oryzanol may also have properties that increase muscle strength for weight lifters. Additionally, gamma oryzanol has antioxidant properties and can be applied to the skin as a sun screen, providing both internal and external aid for the outdoor endurance athlete.[12]

Rice Bran and rice bran oil are the best sources of gamma oryzanol. Cereal grains such as rice, oats, barley, and wheat also deliver this valuable phytosterol, which is also available as a supplement.

Linoleic Acid. The healthy fat that surrounds muscles needs linoleic acid (LA), which substantially shortens the recovery time for muscles after intensive exercise. Linoleic acid also helps transport oxygen into cell tissue and may also increase male fertility. Oils with high percentages of linoleic acid include safflower, grape seed, sunflower, soybean, and corn. Fennel is also a source of linoleic acid.

Alpha-Linolenic Acid shortens the recovery time of muscles following intense exercise. When your muscles are fatigued by exertion, try taking some flaxseed oil to rejuvenate them more quickly.

Other Nutrients

Antioxidants. Athletes need extra protection against free radicals, because there is a direct relationship between the production of free radicals and strenuous exercise. Antioxidants stop the damaging effects of free radicals and may help during the exercise recovery phase. Antioxidants increase oxygen use in the blood, tissues and brain.[13]

Pyruvate, also known as pyruvic acid, is essential in the metabolic process. It increases energy and stamina and decreases fatigue. Although some fruits, vegetables, wines, and cheeses contain limited amounts of pyruvic acid, taking it as a supplement is the most practical way to gain these effects.[14]

Glucosamine Sulfate. Glucosamine is the amino sugar of glucose and is found naturally in human joints. It helps cartilage and connective tissue health and also maintains flexible joints. Glucosamine sulfate is glucosamine bound to sulfur. The combination makes the supplement extremely easy to absorb. It has been consistently proven to reduce joint pain and inflammation, and it helps repair damaged joints (especially knee cartilage), while promoting tendon and ligament health. This supplement is a must-have for anyone who exercises and even for non-exercisers who are plagued by joint injury or osteoarthritis.[15]

Dopamine. The central nervous system uses dopamine as a neurotransmitter to relay messages of sexual desire in the male. Found in the penis, dopamine has been linked to erection and ejaculation, and it stimulates the production of testosterone indirectly.

Herbs for Physical Performance

Ginseng boosts energy and endurance. Siberian and Asiatic ginseng (also known as Korean ginseng) increase stamina. Both Siberian and Asiatic ginseng enhance the body's use of oxygen, providing support for aerobic activities, casual exercise, performance training, and sexual vigor. Benefits related to athletic performance, however, seem to favor Asiatic ginseng.[16] Asiatic ginseng has characteristics that raise dopamine utilization, fostering the growth and repair of tissues, and increasing male sexual desire and stamina.

For quick, temporary energy, try ginseng instead of coffee for a stimulating effect that won't make you jumpy. Most people find that tea made with Siberian ginseng is more pleasant tasting than the Asiatic tea. Like many herbs, potency and quality can vary depending on the source and storage method.

Ginkgo Biloba, Gotu Kola, and Yohimbe. These herbs enhance sexual performance. Ginkgo biloba can help some men who experience impotence or reduced sexual desire. Due to its ability to help blood circulation, ginkgo biloba has produced significant improvement for blood flow in erectile tissue. Similar to Asiatic ginseng, ginkgo biloba increases the body's use of dopamine, thereby increasing male sexual desire. The triterpenoid saponin content in gotu kola increases sexual desire and yohimbine, the active compound in yohimbe, can improve sexual performance in males.[17]

Other Herbs. Herbs that increase energy due to their caffeine content or caffeine-like effects include *yerbamaté* and *guaraná*. The antioxidant properties of *astragalus* improve athletic performance and decrease fatigue by increasing energy production. *Garlic* has also been known to increase stamina.

Burdock reputedly reduces inflammation and calcification in the joints. **Cocoa** acts as a tonic for the muscles due to its calcium and potassium content, both of which help muscle contraction.

Helpful Foods, Nutrients & Herbs

For more information, see "Nutrient Sources" & "Glossary"

Foods

Alfalfa Sprouts
Barley
Blue-Green Algae
Brewer's Yeast
Broccoli
Cabbage
Carrots
Chlorella
Citrus Fruit & Peel
Corn Oil
Fennel
Grape Seed Oil
Green Leaves
Kelp
Legumes
Nuts
Oats
Rice Bran
Rice Bran Oil
Safflower Oil
Soybean Oil
Spinach
Spirulina
Strawberries
Sunflower Seeds
Sunflower Oil
Super-Oxygenated Water
Sweet Potatoes
Wheat Grass
Wheat Germ & Oil
Whey Protein

Nutrients

Arginine
B-Complex
BCAAs
Bee Pollen
Carnitine
Chromium
Coenzyme Q10
Creatine Monohydrate
Dopamine
Gamma Oryzanol
Glucosamine Sulfate
Iron
L-Dopa
Leucine
Lipoic acid
Magnesium
MCTs
NADH
Phosphorus
Potassium
Pyruvate
Royal Jelly
Sulfur
Vitamin K
Vitamin B3
Vitamin E
Vitamin B6
Vitamin C
Vitamin B12
Vitamin B5
Zinc

Herbs

Asiatic Ginseng
Astragalus
Burdock
Cocoa
Garlic
Ginkgo Biloba
Gotu Kola
Guaraná
Siberian Ginseng
Yerbamaté
Yohimbe

Recipes

Rise and Shine

1 bag or tsp	Yerbamaté
1 bag or tsp	Guaraná

Are you looking for a coffee alternative? Guaraná is a low-caffeine, South American herb also known as Brazilian cocoa. It makes a perfect combination with yerbamaté, another Spanish and South American caffeine tea. These teas increase metabolic rate, which will keep your motor going, eliminate fatigue, and improve stamina.

Muscle Tissue Tune-Up

3 oz	Cranberry Juice
3–5	Strawberries or Raspberries
3 oz	Orange Juice
½–1	Lime or Lemon, juiced

The bioflavonoids, vitamin C, and sulfates in this juice are just what you need to stimulate muscle growth, repair damaged muscle and connective tissue, and reduce inflammation in tissues, nerves, or muscles. Cranberries, strawberries, and raspberries are good sources of the sulfur necessary for producing glucosamine sulfate, which is found naturally in joints and promotes tendon and ligament health. Vitamin C, found in citrus fruits, fortifies connective tissue and supports muscle growth and strength.

Blend the berries into the juices for a delicious antioxidant cocktail. Don't forget to scrape out some of the white orange or lemon pulp to reap their bioflavonoids. Use organic ingredients whenever possible.

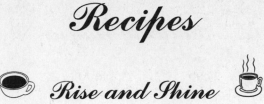

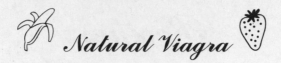

Natural Viagra

½–1 cup	Apple Juice
2–3 Tbsp	Tahini, raw
2 Tbsp	Wheat Germ
1 Tbsp	Spirulina Powder
1 Tbsp	Brewer's Yeast
To taste	Pure Water

If you wish you had a prescription for Viagra, this is your dream drink. The vitamin E in wheat germ increases fertility rates in males. Vitamin B12, more concentrated in spirulina than in any other food, increases sperm count. Spirulina and brewer's yeast contain nicotinic acid, a form of niacin that facilitates orgasm. Tahini (ground sesame seeds) is rich in coenzyme Q10, which prolongs endurance.

Blend the first 2 ingredients for about 15 seconds or until smooth. Add the powders and water and blend again. Add more water if needed to achieve your desired consistency. This drink will work even if you have to leave out one of the powders. Use organic ingredients whenever possible.

Battery Recharge

8 oz	Carrot Juice
1 clove	Garlic, juiced
1 tsp	Ginseng Powder

Here is a quick pick-me-up that provides long-term energy and is easy to make. Carrot juice is a great source of beta-carotene, the famous antioxidant that athletes need to protect against the damaging effects of exercise and to increase oxygen in the blood, tissues, and brain. Ginseng is renown for providing strength and energy, and garlic, among its many other benefits, increases stamina.

Juice the carrots and garlic and stir in the ginseng powder or granules. Ginseng is available at health and oriental food stores. Use organic carrots for the best tasting juice.

Legal Steroids

½ cup	Pure Water
1 cup	Soy, Rice or Oat Milk
1 Tbsp	Barley Malt or Rice Syrup
2 Tbsp	Rice Bran
1 Tbsp	Ginseng Granules
1 Tbsp	Brewer's Yeast
1 Tbsp	Blue-Green or other Algae
1 Tbsp	Wheat Grass Powder

If power is your pursuit, you'll devour this. Rice bran is a superb source of gamma oryzanol, a natural steroid alternative that increases testosterone and muscle mass for weight lifters. Algae and soy are two of our finest sources of the protein needed for muscle development. Asiatic ginseng increases dopamine, which is utilized in the growth and repair of muscle tissue. Wheat grass is our best source of the potassium we need for muscle growth. Brewer's yeast is the number one source of chromium, necessary for the uptake of creatine into our muscles. Creatine improves muscle fibers and reduces lactic acid buildup.

First, blend your choice of sweetener in water until it dissolves. These grain-derived sweeteners provide long lasting energy. If neither sweetener is on hand, use honey. Add the remaining ingredients slowly, blending after each one. Choose a flavored soy milk such as vanilla or chocolate. This drink will work even if you have to leave out one of the powders.

Remember, herbs and nutrients are not drugs. They nourish your cells in a way that enables higher, long term functioning. Chemicals may pump you up, but ultimately they leave you burned out. Real enhancement takes time. Regular consumption of the good nutrients in this drink and others will accomplish your goals.

Heavy Lifter

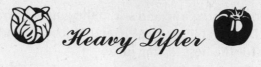

5 oz	Celery Juice
2 oz	Spinach Juice
2 oz	Kale Juice
1 oz	Alfalfa Sprouts Juice
1 oz	Cabbage Juice
1 tsp	Ginseng Powder
1 tsp	Brewer's Yeast
1-2 Tbsp	Tamari or Soy Sauce

Spinach, kale, and cabbage juices make this juice a tonic for muscles because of their calcium and potassium content, which enables muscular contraction. All three are also high in glucosamine sulfate, the amino sugar of glucose, which boosts energy. The magnesium from alfalfa sprouts is important for the storage and release of glycogen and for preventing the buildup of lactic acid. Yeast is our best source of chromium, which facilitates the uptake of creatine into the muscles. Creatine improves muscle fibers. Asiatic ginseng promotes stamina and endurance. This drink will work even if you have to leave out one of the powders. Use organic ingredients whenever possible.

Virilit Tea

1 bag or tsp	Ginkgo Biloba
1 bag or tsp	Asiatic Ginseng
1 ml	Yohimbine Fluid Extract (1 dropperful)

Turn on the music. These herbs build sexual vigor! Ginkgo biloba improves blood circulation in the male genitals, remedying impotence. Ginseng is a 3,000-year-old aphrodisiac, and yohimbine is an extract of the yohimbe mushroom, which increases sexual performance in males. This tea is herbal therapy. Results show after 2-3 weeks of regular administration. If yohimbe is not readily available as an extract, take it in tablet form.

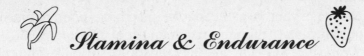

Stamina & Endurance

1 cup	Apple Juice
1	Banana
2 Tbsp	Oat, Rice, or Wheat Bran
1 Tbsp	Spirulina, Chlorella, or Blue-Green Algae
8–12	Almonds
To taste	Pure Water

Banana and spirulina are good sources of potassium, important for the conversion of glucose to glycogen for energy. Magnesium (from bran, almonds, and spirulina) is important for the storage and release of glycogen. Almonds are also a high energy food, producing 6 calories per gram. Adequate levels of chromium (from bran and banana) and zinc (from spirulina) help balance blood sugar regulation and therefore energy production.

Blend the banana and the bran in the juice until smooth. Add the spirulina or other algae powder. For best digestion, almonds should be softened by pre-soaking them for several hours. If you like a crunchy, chewy drink, add the almonds at the end and just chop or blend them briefly. Otherwise, blend until smooth. If you don't pre-soften the almonds, be prepared for a machinc gun sound effect when you blend them! Use organic ingredients whenever possible.

Muscle Milk

1 cup	Oat or Soy Milk
1 tsp	Whey Protein Powder
1 Tbsp	Cocoa Powder
1 tsp	Honey

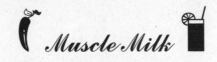

Oats provide a rich source of carbohydrates that are easily converted into energy. Oats increase stamina and are particularly fortifying for the heart muscle. Oat milk is available in health food stores, or you can make your own. Steep a heaping tablespoon of oats in 8 oz of hot water for 10 minutes; strain and cool. *(For more, see "Power Drinks Basics.")* Or, you may substitute soy milk. The calcium contained in cocoa acts as a muscle tonic and helps with muscular contraction. Whey protein is the richest dietary source of BCAAs, a form of amino acids that builds muscle mass. Whey protein prevents muscle loss and promotes muscle growth and repair. Honey provides glucose, a source of quick energy.

Serve hot or cold. If drinking hot, stir the cocoa powder and whey into the hot milk. Heat up to, but do not boil. If drinking cold, shake or blend the powders and honey thoroughly into the milk.

Power Drinks for the
Mind

Information and Recipes to Aid in Mental Performance, Memory Recall, Alzheimer Prevention, Focus and Concentration, Stress Relief.

Some people compare the human brain to a computer. But at only three pounds, this walnut shaped organ weighs a lot less than even a small laptop computer. Nevertheless, the brain stores decades of memories and can create monumental works like Hamlet or the theory of relativity, all while simultaneously directing our biological functions. There is much we do not understand about the brain, but we have determined that its complex functions and those of its switchboard—the central nervous system—require certain nutrients. These nutrients serve two roles: architectural and functional. The architectural nutrients are like the wood used to build a house and the functional nutrients are like the fuel that heats it. Think of these two types of nutrients in terms of construction and maintenance.

This chapter will help you identify various foods, nutrients and herbs that constitute the brain's architecture and enable it to function optimally. *(See the glossary for definitions of technical words used here, such as neurotransmitter, acetylcholine, steroid, etc. For more information related to the mind see "Fatigue," "Depression," "Headache," and "Menopause.")*

Food for the Brain

Flaxseed Oil, Hemp Seed Oil, Evening Primrose Oil. Fats are arguably the brain's most important nutrient category. Up to half of the walls in our brain cells are made from fats, which keep these cell walls permeable. Eight international food and health organizations recommend that children and adults consume between 500 mg to 2,000 mg daily of the essentially fatty acid omega-3. But since America is on a fat-free binge these days, we take in an average of only 150mg. Flax, hemp, and evening primrose oils are superb sources of omega-3 essential fatty acids. These acids are essential, because our bodies cannot manufacture them. In other words, we must obtain them through our diet.

Flaxseed Oil has been used effectively for the treatment of depression and has improved mental function for the elderly. Evening primrose oil alleviates the symptoms of multiple sclerosis because of its high gamma-linolenic acid. Hemp oil has the best balance of different essential fatty acids of any vegetable food. Other vegetarian sources of these essential fats are soybean, canola, and wheat germ oils. Sources of omega-6 fatty acids are grapeseed, safflower, corn, sunflower, and sesame oils. *(See "Lipids" later in this chapter for information on the role of these fats in the functioning of the brain.)*

Fish Oils, Eggs, Organ Meats. Fish oils and the fats from red meat, eggs, and organ meats are excellent sources of the popular DHA, the most abundant fat in the brain *(see DHA this chapter)*. Some of the best sources of fish oils are salmon, mackerel, sardines, rainbow trout, herring, canned white albacore tuna, oysters, halibut, and anchovies. Be careful to avoid fish that may contain environmental or chemical pollutants. Animal organs may also contain residues of tranquilizers, antibiotics, and the hormones used to fatten them up. The purest food is always the lowest source on the food chain. Fish get these oils from eating microalgae. Vegetarians should eat microalgae to get their DHA *(see below)*, and all of us should buy organic foods whenever possible.

Lecithin. This is a phosphorus-rich fat common in plants and animals. It is essential for breaking down fats in the body. Lecithin is found in the liver, nerve tissue, bile, and blood. The best dietary sources are lecithin, soybeans, egg yolks, and corn. Soy lecithin granules are widely available. Its high phospholipid content enhances intelligence. It has demonstrated the ability to retard the progression of Alzheimer's disease by stimulating the production of the neurotransmitter acetylcholine. Even 80-year-olds remember better on a diet including lecithin.[1] Lecithin is also the primary source of phosphatidylserine (PS) and phosphatidylcholine (PC). *(See PS and PC this chapter.)*

Algae—Spirulina, Blue-Green, & Chlorella. Algae are water-borne plants. Macro-algae, such as kelp, hijiki, dulse, nori, wakame, and the like, are seaweeds with roots and leaves and are similar to plants. But *micro*-algae such as spirulina, chlorella, and blue-green algae are single cell, microscopic organisms that actually have more in common with bacteria than plants.

These mysterious and amazing aquatic, plant-like organisms have the unique distinction of being the planet's first food, dating back 3.5 billion years. They are also our richest source of chlorophyll—the blood of plants—being 1-3% chlorophyll, higher than that contained in alfalfa or grass. And at 50-60% protein, they are also our finest source of protein, surpassing meat and poultry (16-18%) and soybeans (26%).

As protein-rich foods, they are superb sources of the nucleic acids RNA and DNA. The quantity of nucleic acids stored in the brain decreases with age, and this depletion is associated with impaired learning. RNA improves memory retention and has been helpful in treating Alzheimer's disease.[2] These algae are a rich source of neuropeptides, which repair, rebuild, and strengthen neurotransmitters. The neuropeptides in algae have a low molecular weight, which means they are small enough to pass through the blood-brain barrier. This is one reason why many users claim an increase in alertness and concentration and clearer communication shortly after consuming algae.

Malic Acid Foods. Malic acid is a proven chelation agent for aluminum. It binds and removes it from the brain and other vital organs.[3] Prunes have the highest amount of naturally-occurring malic acid of any fruit. Stone fruits in general are excellent sources. Wine also contains large amounts of malic acid added as a flavoring agent.

Foods Rich in Malic Acid

Rhubarb	Apples	Cherries	Limes
Lychees	Peaches	Prunes	Apricots
Nectarines	Plums	Grapes	Tomatoes
Strawberries	Pears	Cornsilk	Fennel

Carbohydrates. Sugar has a direct effect on the brain and nervous system. Glucose, which is the name for the kind of sugar that ends up in our blood, is a source of energy for the brain. Galactose is another simple sugar (carbohydrate) that can be converted to sugar in the liver. It is a major component of the myelin sheaths that cover the axons of the brain's neurons. Carbohydrates are fuel for the brain.

Nutrients for Brain Power

Oxygen. Although the brain comprises only 2% of the body's weight, it consumes 20% of the body's oxygen intake. Fresh air and exercise increase the circulation and oxygenation of the blood. Subjects who inhaled pure oxygen immediately before a memory test had a higher rate of recall. Inverted platforms or yoga postures such as headstands, handstands, and shoulder stands all ensure that oxygen, as well as the other valuable nutrients discussed here, will travel to the brain. No matter what you add to your diet, you cannot achieve a healthy brain without sufficient oxygen.[4]

DHA (Docosahexaenoic Acid) is a polyunsaturated fatty acid and is the most abundant fatty acid in the brain. It is the primary architectural nutrient of the brain and the retina. It is crucial for brain and vision development in infants.[5] DHA concentrates in the cell membranes of the brain where it attracts the oxygen needed for the chemical activities of neurons. DHA is related to the architecture and size of the brain and our ability to learn, judge, and concentrate. Children with ADD (Attention Deficit Disorder) commonly exhibit low levels of DHA. Cold water fishes such as mackerel, trout, salmon, herring and sardines are the best sources of this nutrient. Algae is the best vegetarian source.

PS (Phosphatidylserine) is the major phospholipid in the brain. It is present in all the cell membranes. Whereas the brain can manufacture PS, its production can be inhibited by deficiencies of essential fatty acids, and vitamins such as B12 and folic acid can also inhibit its production. PS has demonstrated the ability to positively influence a wide range of memory, mood, and mental conditions. It has been helpful in treating Alzheimer's, dementia and Attention Deficit Disorder (ADD). It also reduces apathy, lengthens attention span, and improves concentration. In a short term memory study with 55–80 year-olds suffering from early dementia, it improved their ability to learn and recall names and telephone numbers, locate misplaced objects and concentrate while reading.[6] Soy lecithin is the best food source.

Phosphatidylcholine (PC), another component of lecithin, prevents age associated memory impairment (AAMI) by nourishing the myelin sheaths surrounding neurons and increasing the levels of acetylcholine.[7] Fifteen to 30 grams per day alleviates manic depression[8] and 10-20 grams per day in a six month double blind study stabilized the memory of patients with Alzheimer's disease.[9] In general, neurons require large amounts of PC for repair and maintenance.

Coenzyme Q10. This is a fat soluble enzyme similar in structure to vitamin E. It has demonstrated effectiveness in treating schizophrenia and Huntington's disease and protects neurons from the damage that leads to Alzheimer's disease.[10] Best dietary sources are oily fish *(see Fish Oils)*. Best vegetarian sources are peanuts, sesame seeds, and walnuts.

Amino Acids

L-Tryptophan is integral to the production of the neurotransmitter serotonin. Serotonin has demonstrated sedative and sleep-promoting qualities. Bananas, milk and sunflower seeds are sources of L-tryptophan. But the US Food and Drug Administration (FDA) recalled it in 1989 because of reported neuromuscular side effects. Although these effects were later traced to a bacterial contaminant from a single manufacturer, the FDA has not withdrawn the ban.

5-HTP (5-Hydroxytryptophan) is manufactured within the body from Tryptophan. If L-tryptophan is unavailable, you can use 5-HTP, which is a close relative and has many of the same benefits. It is the precursor necessary for the production of serotonin. It has numerous mental and nervous system effects, including the control of aggression and anxiety and the alleviation of depression and insomnia, and it has been used successfully in the treatment of Parkinson's disease, Down's Syndrome, and epilepsy.

L-Tyrosine is a precursor to the neurotransmitters norepinephrine and dopamine. These chemical messengers promote mental acuity and alertness. L-tyrosine improves mood, behavior, reaction times, and thinking.[11] Dietary sources for L-tyrosine are all protein foods, such as meat, poultry, seafood, nuts, seeds, algae, and tofu.

Carnitine is also present in the brain, and confusion is one result of a deficiency. Carnitine also protects neurons from the degeneration caused by ammonia. Its derivative **Acetyl-L-Carnitine (ALC),** has been widely studied and demonstrates numerous benefits, such as relief from sleep disorders and stress, improved mood control and attention span, and healthier nerves and neurons. ALC is also beneficial for Down's Syndrome, Parkinson's, short- and long-term memory loss, and Alzheimer's disease. ALC increased alertness, attention span, and short-term memory in Alzheimer's patients, as verified with nuclear magnetic resonance imagery (MRI).[12]

Another important amino acid is **Spermine,** which has a major presence in neurons. It measurably increases brain activity and improves memory by stimulating the production of RNA. **Cysteine** protects the brain from the toxic effects of alcohol and tobacco smoking. **Glutamine** increases some aspects of human intelligence, and it functions as a stimulant when it converts to its amide, glutamic acid, thus exciting neurons and accelerating their communication. **Histidine** is necessary for the maintenance of the myelin sheaths and promotes tranquility by producing alpha-wave activity within the brain via the neurotransmitter histamine. Dietary sources are all protein foods.

Hormones

Although these hormones are widely available as nutritional supplements, they should not be consumed as zealously as vitamins. Treat them with the same precaution as prescription drugs and consult your health professional about their dosage.

DHEA (Dehydro-epiandrosterone) is six and a half times more concentrated in the brain than in other body tissues and is also present in spinal fluid. Persons with dementia routinely display abnormally low levels of DHEA. It has numerous functions, including deepening sleep, reducing anxiety and stress, and alleviating major depression. It also alleviates amnesia and can increase the quantity of neurons.[13]

Melatonin is the famous sleep hormone produced mostly by the pineal gland. Dosages as low as 0.3mg alleviate most sleep disorders without incurring next-morning drowsiness. It improves jet-lag and generally enhances learning ability. Melatonin relieves headaches and migraines. In one study, 100% of the subjects had improvement and 50% had a total cessation of cluster headaches.[14]

Human Growth Hormone (HGH) is our primary hormone for growth produced in our pituitary gland. It declines naturally with age. HGH is currently generating a lot of excitement in the arena of anti-aging. Users claim it improves concentration, mood, eyesight, muscle tone, sleep, and counteracts stress. It has demonstrated improvement for both short term memory and long term memory and numerous studies are underway.[15] It is available in micro-dosage sublingual and homeopathic formulas.

Estrogens improve various brain functions. Soy and alfalfa derived *phytoestrogens* are chemically similar to animal estrogens and may provide a dietary source for this hormone.

Adrenaline dilates the blood vessels that supply the brain, and cortisone helps to regulate the brain's utilization of glucose.

Lipids — Fats

The bully who called you "fathead" in grade school was biochemically correct. At least half of the brain cell walls are made from fat. Fats keep the cell walls of our brain flexible and permeable. DHA (docosahexaenoic acid) is the most abundant fatty acid in the brain. The brain and the retina of the eye use DHA as building blocks.

Essential Fatty Acids are unsaturated fats that cannot be manufactured by the human body and must be provided by the diet. They are popularly known as omega-3 and 6. In general, they provide cell membranes their fluidity. Alpha-linolenic acid (LNA) is essential for the normal development of the brain in children. It enhances brain function because it is a precursor for DHA. A lack of omega-3 can result in poor coordination. Chia, flax, and hemp seeds and evening primrose are the finest dietary sources of this oil. Linoleic acid (LA or omega-6) is a component of phospholipids, like PS and PC *(see above)*, and helps to prevent degeneration of the brain. It is abundant in many common vegetable oils, such as corn, soybean, and safflower.

Cholesterol is essential for correct brain function. It increases the number of receptors in the brain for serotonin and makes up the myelin sheaths that protect our neurons. Too much cholesterol, however, makes cell membranes rigid. Just as with heart disease, we have to learn to differentiate between good cholesterol and bad cholesterol in the diet. Avoid the bad fats in fried foods and rancid oils. Keep oils refrigerated or in dark bottles and increase your intake of some of the oil rich foods mentioned in this chapter.

Phospholipids are waxy compounds manufactured by the liver and are especially prevalent in the cells of the brain. They are essential to the formation of all other fats discussed here. Oily fish, cod liver oil, and soy lecithin are the best sources.

Vitamins

B Vitamins. The B vitamin family plays several roles in the brain. Children with vitamin B1 thiamine deficiency exhibit lower IQ levels. Vitamin B3, nicotinic acid, increases blood circulation to the brain and improves memory in normal, healthy middle-aged adults by 10-40%.[16] Vitamin B12 improves IQ and memory. It plays an important role in the formation of the myelin sheaths around nerve fibers. Deficiencies result in nerve dysfunction such as poor reflexes and depression. Algaes such as spirulina, brewer's yeast, and acidophilus rich foods such as yoghurt are the best sources of B12 and B-vitamins in general.

Vitamin C & E. The brain contains the second highest concentration of vitamin C in the body, and 6-8 grams of supplemental vitamin C per day noticeably increases brain wave activity. Students who consumed high amounts of vitamin C scored better on IQ tests than those with lower vitamin C consumption. Large doses of vitamin C over an extended period increased the IQ of mentally retarded people by 15-20 points.[17] Vitamin E protects polyunsaturated fatty acids in the brain from oxidative damage. Hot red peppers, acerola juice berries, and wheat grass are the top food sources of vitamin C. Wheat germ and sunflower seeds are some of the best sources of vitamin E.

Herbs for the Brain

Ginkgo Biloba is the world's oldest species of tree. Western and Chinese herbalists have traditionally used ginkgo for age-related memory loss and diminished mental functioning. Ginkgo does three things for the brain: It increases blood circulation; expands its supply of oxygen; and helps to prevent damage to the brain's neurons by free radicals.[18] Even the conservative and prestigious *Journal of the American Medical Association* (JAMA) agrees. In their October 1997 double-blind study, ginkgo demonstrated results that make it at least as effective as any Alzheimer drug on the market. It is "capable of stabilizing and…improving the cognitive performance and the social functioning of demented patients."

Ginseng has a direct influence on the hypothalamus and pituitary glands, creating numerous benefits. It affects various mental functions, helping to alleviate insomnia and depression and improve concentration and attention span in the elderly. In one study it increased overall blood circulation to the brain in 90% of the people tested.[19]

Saint John's Wort significantly reduces anxiety and aggressiveness and is famous for its successful mitigation of depression.[20] It prevents certain oxidative enzymes from destroying neurotransmitters and has other functions similar to Prozac-type drugs. It has also been an effective treatment for insomnia and Seasonal Affective Disorder (SAD).

Huperzine is a natural ingredient of **Chinese Club Moss** (Huperzia serrata). Several clinical trials show that huperzine improves memory, concentration, learning, and the symptoms of Alzheimer's disease. It functions by inhibiting the enzyme that blocks the neurotransmitter acetylcholine and is effective in crossing the blood-brain barrier.[21]

Golden Root *(Rhodiola rosea from the Orpine or Crassulaceae family)* improves general mental function by improving blood circulation to the brain. This includes improving attention span and concentration and counteracting the toxic effects of stress.

Garlic. Extracts of aged garlic improve memory retention in mice.[22]

Astragalus improves memory by inhibiting an enzyme that degrades the most abundant neurotransmitter in the brain—acetylcholine.

Sage Tea also improves memory by inhibiting the enzyme that degrades the major neurotransmitter acetylcholine.

Corn Silk and **Raspberry Leaf** bind and remove aluminum from the brain because they are excellent sources of malic acid.

Substances that are Toxic to the Brain

Recreational Drugs
Overindulgence of Alcohol
Free Radicals (from stress & diet)
CO2 Carbon Dioxide (from cars)
Aluminum (from cooking utensils)
Cigarettes
Copper, Nickel, Lead
Lack of exercise
Mercury (from dental fillings)

Helpful Foods, Nutrients & Herbs

For more information, see "Nutrient Sources" & "Glossary"

Foods

Apples
Apricots
Blue-Green Algae
Brewer's Yeast
Celery
Cherries
Chlorella & Spirulina
Eggs
Fish Oils
Flaxseed
Grapes
Lecithin
Limes
Lychees
Nectarines
Peaches
Pears
Plums
Prunes
Rhubarb
Spinach
Strawberries
Tomato
Wheat Germ

Nutrients

5-HTP
Acetyl-L-Carnitine
Acetylcholine
Aged Garlic
Algae
Alpha-Linolenic Acid
Carnitine
Coenzyme Q10
Cysteine
DHA & DHEA
DNA
Folic Acid
Glutamic Acid
Glutamine
(HGH) Growth Hormone
Histidine
Huperzine
L-Tyrosine
L-Tryptophan
Melatonin
Nicotinic Acid
Nucleic Acids
Oxygen
Phosphatidylcholine (PC)
Phosphatidylserine (PS)
Vitamin E
Vitamin B12

Herbs

Astragalus
Cayenne (hot pepper)
Corn Silk
Evening Primrose Oil
Flaxseed Oil
Fennel
Garlic
Golden Root
Grapeseed Extract
Hemp Seed Oil
Raspberry Leaf
Sage

See Glossary for Definitions and Descriptions of

Amino Acids	Essential Fatty Acids	Nucleic Acids
ATP	Hormones	Peptides
Brewer's Yeast	Lecithin	Prostaglandins
Chelation	Neuropeptides	Soy Tamari
DHA	Neurons	Steroids
EPA	Neurotransmitters	Stevia

Recipes

IQ Elevator

1–2 cups	Pure Water
1 Tbsp	Brewer's Yeast
1 Tbsp	Chlorella, Spirulina, or Blue-Green Algae
2 Tbsp	Wheat Germ
½ cup	Apple Juice
1 Tbsp	Lecithin Granules
1 tsp	Flax, Hemp, or Evening Primrose Oil
½–1 tsp	Vitamin C Powder
Pinch	Stevia

This rich brew of IQ vitamins, essential oils, and nucleic acids will keep you thinking quickly and clearly all day. First 1 cup of water, apple juice, the dry powders and wheat germ, and blend. Stevia is a non-sugar, non-glucose sweetener. It is 300 times sweeter than sugar, so use it sparingly and to your taste. Add only enough water to create your desired smoothie consistency. This drink will be effective even if you are missing one of the ingredients.

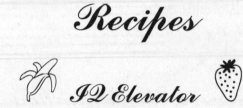

Aluminum Detox

1-2 cups	Grapes
1	Apple, cut and cored
1 cup	Strawberries

These malic acid rich fruits bind aluminum, which is implicated in memory loss and dementia. Juice these fruits in your juicing machine in the amounts listed above or, blend them in a blender. In a blender, add about ½ cup of water or enough to achieve your preferred, thick shake consistency.

Focus & Concentration

2-4 Tbsp	Tahini, raw
1 Tbsp	Spirulina, Chlorella or Blue-Green Algae
1	Apple, cut and cored
1 Tbsp	Lecithin Granules
1 cup	Pure Water

Sesame is one of our best sources of omega-6 fatty acids and coenzyme Q10. Algae are some of our best sources of the nucleic acids RNA and DNA, as well as DHA, the brains most important fatty acid. Blend the tahini (sesame seed paste) first with half the water. Use raw tahini whenever possible. Then add the apple pieces and blend some more adding only enough water to achieve a whirlpool in the blender. Then add the other dry ingredients and enough water to achieve a thick shake consistency. Add more water as required to achieve a whirlpool in the blender and a smoothie consistency.

Mental Tune-Up

½ cup	Apple Juice
2 Tbsp	Tahini, raw
1 Tbsp	Lecithin Granules
2 Tbsp	Wheat Germ
1 Tbsp	Brewer's Yeast
½ cup	Pure Water
1ml	Ginkgo Extract (1 dropperful)

Good morning! You'll be saying that all day if you make this your regular wake up brew. This drink has all the vital ingredients you need for alertness and concentration. Lecithin, wheat germ, and brewer's yeast are our finest plant sources of phosphatidylcholine and acetylcholine. Acetylcholine is the most abundant neurotransmitter in the brain. Ginkgo biloba is an ancient Chinese herb that increases alpha-wave activity in the brain and the number of neuroreceptor sites. Sesame seeds (tahini is sesame seed paste) is one of our best food sources of coenzyme Q10, nicotinic acid, phosphorus, and thiamine, all of which play a role in protecting our neurons from the damage caused by free radicals.

Remember, herbs and nutrients are not drugs. They nourish your neurons in a way that enables higher, long-term functioning. Chemicals may fire your neurotransmitters for a quick jump start, but leave you burned out. Real enhancement takes time. Regular consumption of the good nutrients in this drink and others will accomplish your goals. When you want to think fast, think smart.

Use organic ingredients whenever possible and add them preferably in the order listed. Blend the first 3 ingredients for 15-30 seconds, then add the powders and water and blend again. Finally add ginkgo extract. You may empty the contents of a ginkgo capsule into the blender if the preferred extract is unavailable. This drink will still be powerful even if you do not have all the ingredients.

Attention Spanner

1 cup	Strawberries
1-2 cups	Grapes
1	Apple, cut and cored
2 Tbsp	Ginseng Powder or Extract
To taste	Pure Water

Blend these malic acid fruits together for an energizing, mind expanding experience. They will protect your concentration from robbers like free radicals and toxic metals. Juice the fruits in any order and stir in the ginseng at the end.

Neuron Protector

5 oz	Tomato Juice
3 oz	Spinach Juice
3 oz	Celery Juice
1 oz	Fennel Juice
1 clove	Garlic, juiced
pinch	Cayenne (hot pepper)
1-2 Tbsp	Tamari (Soy Sauce)

Juice these by alternating the spinach, tomatoes, fennel, and celery until done, then add the garlic, tamari, and cayenne (capsicum) red pepper. You may break open a capsule or use the powdered herb. Hot red peppers have numerous health benefits, but they are also one of our finest sources of the IQ elevating vitamin C. Spinach is one of our best sources of coenzyme Q10 which protects neurons from the damage that leads to Alzheimer's disease. You won't be disappointed by this brain nourishing liquid salad.

Anti-Alzheimer

1 cup	Prune Juice

Prunes are our richest source of malic acid, which is a proven remover of aluminum and other toxic metals from the brain. Aluminum toxicity is a factor in Alzheimer's disease. Prunes are dried plums. Whereas plums are difficult to juice, they can be dried and soaked. Their juice fills the soak water suffusing it with its nutritional properties.

Alert & Creative

1-2 cups	Pure Water
2-4 Tbsp	Sunflower Seeds
1	Apple, cut and cored
1 Tbsp	Chlorella, Spirulina, or Blue Green Algae
1 tsp	Flax, Hemp, or Evening Primrose Oil
1 Tbsp	Lecithin Granules
Pinch	Stevia (optional)

The neuropeptides in algae are small enough to pass through the blood-brain barrier giving a quick boost to alertness and concentration. Flax, hemp, and evening primrose oils are superb sources of omega-3 essential fatty acids and particularly Alpha-linolenic acid (LNA), which is the precursor for DHA, the most abundant fat in the brain. Lecithin is our best source of phospholipids, which stimulate intelligence.

Start by blending 1 cup of water and the sunflower seeds until smooth. Add the apple piece by piece and blend. Add the remaining ingredients and only enough water to achieve a thick shake consistency. If you like a nutty, chewy drink, add the sunflowers at the end and only blend for a few seconds. Stevia is a non-sugar sweetener.

Memory Booster

1 bag or tsp	Ginkgo Biloba
1 bag or tsp	Ginseng

Ginkgo is the most famous memory herb and ginseng dramatically improves blood circulation to the brain. Steep these herbs for 5 minutes. *(See "Power Drinks Basics," How to Brew Tea.)*

Anti-Depressive

1 bag or tsp	St. John's Wort
1 bag or tsp	Golden Root

These powerful anti-depressive herbs can be made either with tea bags or loose dry herbs. Steep for 5 minutes. *(See "Power Drinks Basics," How to Brew Tea.)*

Brain Power Drink

by Dr. Dharma Singh Khalsa, M.D.

8 oz	Pineapple Juice
1-2 Tbsp	Green Foods Powder
1-2 Tbsp	Soy Protein Powder

Choose your favorite green foods powder and blend it with soy protein for a delicious breakfast drink. Pineapple juice is a digestive aid, diuretic, and fat burner. Dr. Dharma Singh Khalsa, M.D. is author of *Brain Longevity: The Breakthrough Medical Program That Improves Your Mind and Memory,* and *The Pain Cure: The Proven Medical Program That Helps End Your Chronic Pain.* www.brain-longevity.com

Power Drinks for

Longevity

Foods, Drinks, Vitamins, Herbs and Other Nutrients that Prolong Life

Can We Live Longer?

More and more Americans are celebrating their one-hundredth-year birthdays. But how do we make that century (or more) healthy and functional? The ancient Chinese philosopher Lao Tzu said: "He who is immune is immortal." Basically, we succumb to illness because of a weakened immune system that leaves us more fragile and more vulnerable. But what weakens the immune system? Today, when people can no longer produce in society, they become outcasts. We throw them into nursing homes or the more upscale "adult residential care facilities." Right now, over forty million Americans suffer from some form of arthritis, and seventy seven million aging baby boomers are straining our medical resources. Six hundred and fifty-four billion dollars ($654,000,000,000), or half of our entire health care budget, goes to the treatment of degenerative diseases. After 37 years of fighting our "war against cancer," only now is it starting to turn in our favor. Why? Not because a cure has been found, but because of prevention—better diets, more exercise, less fats, more fiber, more natural foods, fewer pesticides and cigarettes, more self-exams, and more advanced early detection equipment. Yet, out of that $654 billion, less than 5% is spent on prevention! We remain caught in a vicious "3-D" cycle: Disease, Dysfunction, Death. Only if we can improve the quality of our health can we improve the quantity of our lives.

The Three Causes of Aging

Disease shortens life. In 1796 the average lifespan in America was 25 years. In 1900, it was 47. In 1997, it was 82 years. At the beginning of the twentieth century we had diphtheria, meningitis, smallpox, polio and tuberculosis. Today, we are living longer thanks to our conquest of those diseases. But we have a different set of killers—cancer, heart disease, diabetes, stroke, and AIDS. The old diseases caused death relatively quickly. Now, however, in spite of the fact that there are more scientists and more doctors than ever before, we have more "attrition" diseases—arthritis, emphysema, atherosclerosis, chronic fatigue syndrome, candida, diabetes, hypoglycemia, PMS, irritable bowel—diseases that impair the quality of life rather than terminate it.

One of the most widely accepted theories of aging has to do with free radicals. Free radicals are very aggressive chemicals that contain an extra oxygen molecule. Like a pinball machine, they bang into healthy cells and oxidize them. One example of oxidation is rusting metal. So, the more free radicals we generate, the faster we are going to rust. There are two things you can do to fight free radicals. You can change your diet to reduce their occurrence and you can increase your intake of antioxidants. Because antioxidants render free radicals harmless, they are considered a cornerstone of any anti-aging program.

If we can improve the quality of our health,
we will improve the quantity of our life.

Then there is the perpetual biological clock. Basically, cells are willing to subdivide only about fifty times. This is called the "Hayflick limit." As we age, free radicals damage our DNA molecules, causing them to mutate or die. Our bodies repair this damage regularly, but as our cells get older, their capacity to fix things decreases, while the rate of free radical damage increases. This shifting of balance, a turning of the tide, is the essence of aging. It is like a hole in your boat that is getting bigger. At one time you could bail a bucket of water every minute; now you are lucky if you can manage one every hour. It is a losing battle—an increasing rate of damage and a decreasing rate of repair. Genetically speaking, we are drowning in dying cells faster than we can replace them.

Heredity vs. Lifestyle

Vitality in old age may be determined less by genes than by how we live. Retirement is supposed to be the time when we really start to enjoy life. Unfortunately, it is also about the time when people start to experience a more-or-less steady increase in disabilities, culminating in death. What is the point of living longer if we are only going to end up in a nursing home? But, if we could choose healthier lifestyles, the majority of us might reach our ninth decade in relatively good condition.

In one study that tracked 1,741 men and women over 40 years, those who smoked, were overweight, and led sedentary lives began to experience disabilities seven years earlier than the rest of the group. Those who smoked the least, stayed trim, and exercised regularly not only lived longer, but they were less likely to develop disabilities. Even among those who died, the low-risk people experienced shorter periods of disability before dying.[1]

Lifestyle is a choice. It is fully within our control. Make healthy choices right now, no matter what your age. Teenage smokers say: "By the time I get lung cancer, they'll have found a cure." That is a sad excuse and one that has failed to materialize. But if you choose to live healthfully beginning now, it can not only add years to your life, but life to your years.

Diet Suggestions

Eat Less. Eat less and live longer. It's that simple. Since the 1930s, researchers have observed that by reducing the caloric intake of laboratory animals by 30% to 60%, they lived longer and had fewer age-associated diseases like Parkinson's, Alzheimer's, and heart failure. Evidence suggests that caloric restriction reduces free radicals, which damage DNA in the brain, heart, skeleton, and muscle tissues. Many diseases, such as systemic lupus, hypertension, breast cancer, and type-II diabetes occurred much later in life and sometimes not at all.[2]

If caloric restriction is found to have the same benefits in humans as in animals, might people be persuaded to reduce their caloric intake by 30% for an extended period? Can long-term dietary reduction benefit people whose family has a history of early-onset degenerative diseases usually associated with aging?

Americans on the whole are fatter now than at any time in history. Our culture seduces us with a constant stream of high-calorie foods wherever we go. Technology has not helped. Because of modern labor-saving devices, the only exercise many Americans get is pressing on a television remote control. Only about one in five of us get enough exercise to keep our weight down and our health up. Yet, those who do exercise regularly, weigh less and experience less cardiovascular disease, the leading cause of death in America.

Vegetarian Diet. Eat more like a vegetarian if you want to live longer. Epidemiological studies prove that a vegetarian diet increases our chances of living longer with less risk of heart disease, diabetes, and cancers. Saturated, cooked animal fats seem to be the most damaging food we eat, and vegetarians do not consume any.[3] Adam and Eve were the original vegetarians: "Behold I have given you every herb bearing seed which is upon the face of all the earth, and every tree, in which is the fruit of a tree yielding seed; to you it shall be for meat" *(Genesis 1:29)*.

Live Foods. Eat more enzyme-rich, living foods. Enzymes are like a fountain of youth. We manufacture 3,000 of them from the basic enzymes in our diet. All the fabulous nutrients and vitamins we discuss here would be useless without the interaction of these enzymes. But enzymes are fragile things. They have a limited life and must be replaced regularly. Heat destroys them. A diet of cooked, fried, boiled, baked, and irradiated food is devoid of enzymes. In addition, aging reduces our capacity to generate enzymes, and with a weakened immune system, we produce a lesser volume of them.

If you choose to live healthfully, it can add not only years to your life, but life to your years.

Enzymes. Dietary enzymes can relieve many of the symptoms of aging including those of inflammatory diseases such as rheumatoid arthritis. Sixty-seven percent of arthritis patients in one study improved their symptoms on enzyme supplements.[4] Supplements work, but the best sources of these crucial catalysts are freshly squeezed fruit and vegetable juices and baby vegetables such as sprouts. All raw foods contain active enzymes, but juices offer a plethora of enzymes, because they concentrate pounds of produce into one drink.

The enzyme telomerase, for example, may actually control the mechanism behind the so-called biological clock. Each time a cell divides, the telomere section of the chromosome gets slightly shorter. Eventually, it gets too short to replicate and dies. This is the genetic theory of aging. The enzyme telomerase elongates the telomere, and thus can lengthen the lifespan of cells and possibly human life itself.[5]

Foods for Longevity

Bee Pollen is a mixture of plant pollen, plant nectar, and bee saliva. It is like a super, multivitamin and mineral supplement, designed and manufactured in nature's laboratory by some of our hardest workers—bees.

Bee pollen contains an extensive collection of nutrients and offers a long list of benefits that can extend our lives by building the blood, boosting energy, and rejuvenating the body's cells. High in antioxidants, bee pollen counteracts the effects of aging both mentally and physically.

Royal Jelly is another bee food. It contains components that can smooth the wrinkles in aging skin. It is so valuable that it is fed exclusively to the queen bee. It is credited with maintaining the queen's larger size and extending her life. Queen bees live four to five years compared to worker bees, who live approximately 40 days. Imagine what it might do for us! *(For more, see "Bee Products.")*

Sprouts. Alfalfa, radish, broccoli, clover, and soybean sprouts contain concentrated amounts of phytochemicals (plant compounds) that can protect us against disease. The anti-aging benefits of the plant estrogens in these sprouts are similar to those of human estrogen but without the side effects. They increase bone formation and density and prevent bone breakdown (osteoporosis). They are helpful in controlling hot flashes, menopause, and fibrocystic breast tumors. *(For more, see "Alfalfa & Alfalfa Sprouts.")*

Researchers at Johns Hopkins University School of Medicine found substantial amounts of glucosinolates and isothiocyanates, very potent inducers of the phase 2 enzymes that protect cells from mutation, in broccoli sprouts. The sprouts contain 10-100 times more of these enzymes than do the corresponding mature plants.

Sprouts are in the process of rapid growth and tremendous enzyme activity. Proteins, vitamins, minerals, and other plant compounds are multiplying at a ferocious rate. The saponins in alfalfa sprouts, for example, increase by 450% in only 5 days, making these sprouts one of our best sources of this immune boosting compound. Saponins increase the activity of natural killer cells such as T-lymphocytes and interferon. Sprouts also contain an abundance of highly active antioxidants that prevent the destruction of DNA and protect us from the ongoing effects of aging. Since sprouts themselves represent the miracle of birth, it is not inconceivable to find a fountain of youth in them.

Brewer's Yeast. Here is another food made by little friends of nature who do a much better job than our top scientists. If there were awards for nutritional value, brewer's yeast would collect an armful. It is one of the top protein foods on the planet and our finest source of chromium, phosphorus, and potassium. It is the food of choice for most of the B-complex vitamins, including the elusive B12. As a major immune-enhancing food, brewer's yeast protects against diseases that shorten life. Hold onto your skin. Brewer's yeast contains a skin respiratory factor (SRF) that counteracts the aging of skin by bringing more oxygen to the tissues. *(For more, see "Brewer's Yeast.")*

Grapes & Berries. Dark skinned fruits and vegetables may also help you live longer. These foods contain a wealth of bioflavonoids and anthocyanidins, which are superb antioxidants. Found in vascular plants like black currants, blueberries, and grapes, bioflavonoids can protect blood vessels and capillaries from oxidative damage and strengthen connective tissue in the body, which weakens with the passage of time.

Blueberries, black currants, grapes, eggplant, red cabbage, and other dark-skinned fruits and vegetables possess anthocyanidins. Moderate consumption of red wine, because it is made from whole grapes–the skin, seeds and pulp–can also provide anti-aging benefits, including lowered risk of Alzheimer's disease, prevention of atherosclerosis, and reduced risk of age-related macular degeneration.[6]

The seeds of grapes contain the powerful antioxidant oligomeric proanthocyanidin (OPC). Similar to the benefits of berries, grapeseed extract protects us against free radicals that age our vision, and it renews collagen to maintain younger-looking skin.[7] *(For more, see "Grapes.")*

Garlic and aged garlic extract offer many anti-aging benefits, such as improved memory and learning abilities, prevention of atherosclerosis, and lower blood pressure. Animals fed aged garlic extract lived longer than animals fed a placebo.[8] *(For more, see "Garlic.")*

Whey is the liquid that separates from the curds during the manufacture of cheese. Whey protein is absorbed very easily. The body retains a very high percentage of the protein eaten. Whey protein contains a growth factor that, when fed to mice, extended lifespan by 30% over those fed milk protein or standard diets.[9]

Nutrients for Longevity

Vitamins

These vitamins can have very impressive anti-aging benefits, but keep in mind that you can increase their effectiveness by utilizing all their original co-factors and enzymes. Raw fruit and vegetable juices offer concentrated forms of these vitamins since they are contained in whole foods. Without the natural package of enzymes and synergistic cofactors, assimilation of expensive vitamins and minerals may be diminished. Supplements are no substitute for eating right. Supplements are enhanced when taken with freshly squeezed fruit and vegetable juices.

Niacin – Nicotinic Acid – Vitamin B3. Nicotinic acid is a form of niacin, vitamin B3. You are familiar with the infamous nicotine of cigarettes. An oxidation process renders toxic nicotine into nontoxic nicotinic acid, producing a supplement that lowers mortality rates, stimulates the production of growth hormone, and significantly improves memory. But that is not all. Niacin is also great for the heart. It improves blood circulation, lowers cholesterol and reduces hypertension along with the risk of heart attack and stroke.[10] Some of the best sources are bran, hot peppers, peanuts, rice, and wheatgrass.

Vitamin B5 (Pantothenic Acid) is a powerful free radical scavenger. In experiments on animals, B5 extended their average lifespan by 20%. It also promotes the release of human growth hormone when combined with the amino acid arginine.[11] Peanuts, bran, brewer's yeast, chicken liver, beans, nuts, and seeds are the best sources.

Vitamin C and Vitamin E. These vitamins are major antioxidants. As we age, our vitamin C levels decline. Epidemiological studies prove that people who consume 300 mg or more of vitamin C per day live longer. Vitamin C even helps maintain the appearance of our skin by slowing the decline of collagen.[12] Vitamin E also retards skin aging and has demonstrated the ability to extend the life of laboratory animals by preventing the buildup of toxic cell byproducts, which are an intrinsic part of the aging process.[13] Capsicum (hot red peppers), acerola berries, and green leafy vegetables are common foods rich in vitamin C. Nuts and seeds and oils derived from them are the best sources of vitamin E, along with wheat germ and green leafy vegetables.

Antioxidants

There are hundreds of antioxidants. They come in the form of amino acids, bioflavonoids, plant pigments, isoflavonoids, enzymes, minerals, organic acids, herbs, vitamins, and sulfur compounds. Here are a few popular antioxidants. *(Antioxidants are also discussed in "Nature's Finest Healing Foods & Herbs.")*

Beta-Carotene, also known as provitamin A, is probably the best known antioxidant. It is not necessarily the most potent, but it sets the standard against which all other antioxidants are rated. It has the ability to stop common free radicals and those in fats (lipid peroxidation), which may explain why it protects us against cancer, atherosclerosis, heart disease, and stroke. It may also be a critical nutrient for Alzheimer's patients, since they have significantly lower than normal beta-carotene levels.[14] Carrots, apricots, and dark green vegetables are the best food sources of beta-carotene.

Lycopene is a red carotenoid that protects against many age-related diseases, including heart attack and prostate cancer. As an antioxidant, it is still our most effective fighter of singlet oxygen free radicals. In this regard, it is twice as potent as beta-carotene and 100 times stronger than vitamin E.[15] Unlike most other carotenes, however, our body does not convert it to vitamin A. Interestingly, lycopene is more readily available in tomatoes after they are cooked. You can find lycopene in "red" foods such as tomatoes, pink grapefruit, watermelon, and red-skinned grapes. *(For more on lycopene, see "Tomatoes.")*

Glutathione is a sulfur-based, amino acid compound (peptide) whose presence in healthy cells drops by 20-30% as we age. Because it is such an effective antioxidant for the lens tissues in our eyes, it has the ability to arrest cataracts and improve vision.[16] The foods richest in glutathione are tomatoes, spinach, carrots, grapefruit, broccoli, avocado, and apples.

Superoxide Dismutase (SOD) is an antioxidant enzyme manufactured in the body. It is our fifth most abundant enzyme and offers many anti-aging benefits. Tissues hardened by radiation therapy have been partially restored by injecting SOD into the bloodstream. Since SOD concentrates in the lens of the eyes and fights free radicals, it may be an aid in the battle against age-related loss of sight. People afflicted with rheumatoid arthritis and osteoporosis generally exhibit a deficiency of cellular SOD, and they experience a significant reduction of symptoms with SOD supplementation. Even early research on the use of intravenous SOD in Alzheimer's patients is very promising.[17]

Ginkgo, ginseng, green tea, aged garlic extract, and fish oils enhance the body's production of SOD. Also, the body's level of SOD is increased by a reduction in total caloric intake.

Amino Acids

As the building blocks of protein, amino acids have a major responsibility for the growth, maintenance, and repair of our bodies. **Acetyl-L-Carnitine (ALC),** a form of carnitine, declines in the brain, heart, muscles, and blood as we age. ALC keeps our skin looking younger by countering the effects of aging in our subcutaneous tissues. **L-Dopa** is an effective life-extending amino acid with antioxidant properties and the ability to stimulate human growth hormone. Other amino acids that stimulate growth hormone are l-arginine, l-ornithine leucine, and l-glutamine. These are known as secretagogues, nutrients that promote the secretion of growth hormone in the pituitary. **Cysteine** and **NAC (N-Acetyl-Cysteine),** the form of cysteine produced in the body, excels in its ability to halt several types of free radicals, including those that destroy DNA. Since heat destroys cysteine, eat raw nuts, seeds, garlic, onions and broccoli or take cysteine as a supplement in powder, capsule or tablet form.

Nucleic Acids

Nucleic acids are the building blocks of life and found in the nucleus of all living cells. They control the genesis of proteins and heredity. The two main types of nucleic acids are RNA and DNA. The quantity of nucleic acids stored in the brain decreases with age, and their depletion is associated with impaired learning. When rats were injected with RNA and DNA, their average lifespan doubled. Conversely, when nucleic acids were removed from the diet, lifespan decreased.[18] Foods rich in protein, especially blue-green algaes, are the best sources of nucleic acids. Consumers of algae claim an increase in alertness and concentration. *(For more, see "Power Drinks for the Mind.")*

Hormones

Melatonin offers several benefits that could extend life expectancy and defy the natural aging process in all parts of the body. Within the body's cells are universal melatonin receptors that make it easy for cells to behave as if they were younger. Melatonin helps prevent cell death, promotes better sleep for the elderly, and possesses antioxidant properties that protect the DNA content of cells from damage by free radicals.

DHEA (Dehydroepiandrosterone) is an androgen steroid hormone manufactured primarily in the adrenal glands of both men and women. It is the most abundant steroid hormone in the bloodstream. The death rate for people who have naturally high levels of this hormone is lower than for those with reduced levels. Supplements of

DHEA may allow us to hold on to our youth longer by proportionally returning what nature has taken away, bringing such benefits as enhanced short- and long-term memory, free radical scavenging, increased number of neurons in the brain, improved quality of sleep, and fewer wrinkles.[19]

Human Growth Hormone (HGH). As we age, the amount of human growth hormone we produce in the pituitary gland declines. It seems logical that replacing some of the declining human growth hormone with supplements could stop and perhaps reverse the aging process. Mice given injections of HGH lived significantly longer. HGH improves bone density, increases muscle mass, memory, concentration, and sexual drive. In short, it possesses significant life extension potential.[20] HGH is available in micro-dose sublingual or homeopathic formulations.

Secretagogues. HGH is manufactured in the body, and we do not find its equivalent in foods. Similar properties, however, are found in many nutrients that are cofactors for HGH and enhance or stimulate its production, as well as in some plant hormones. *(See "Amino Acids" this chapter.)* These necessary growth cofactors are also contained in foods rich in amino acids, vitamins, and minerals, such as brewer's yeast, algae, grasses, pollen, and other natural protein concentrates. Secretagogues are supplements that contain amino acids, herbs, cellular metabolites, nucleic acids, and other essential cofactors known to play a role in the release of growth hormone.

Pregnenolone. As the precursor of many hormones produced by the brain and sexual system, pregnenolone is very important, since without it, there would be no steroids such as corticosterone, aldosterone, progesterone, testosterone, and estrogen. Pregnenolone production declines markedly as we age and supplemental pregnenolone has the potential to improve many age related complaints including memory, concentration, depression, fatigue, hearing, and wrinkles.[21]

Phytoestrogens are the plant-derived equivalent of human estrogen. While these compounds are not true estrogen, their molecular structures are similar enough to estrogen that they bind to estrogen receptors on cells. When phytoestrogens bind to estrogen receptors, they can stimulate cell growth and have significant hormonal benefits without the harsh side effects of real estrogen. They function as adaptogenic or balancing herbs—i.e. they are useful for problems involving either too little or too much estrogen. Estrogens influence many age-related conditions, such as hot flashes, menopause, estrogen-responsive breast and uterine cancers, osteoporosis, hair loss, and wrinkles.[22] Alfalfa, clover, and soy sprouts are the best dietary source of phytoestrogens.

Fats (Lipids)

Phosphatidylcholine (PC), is a phosphorus-rich, fatty acid. As our cells age, they lose PC and gain cholesterol, making the cells, and us, feel stiff. PC surrounds the myelin sheaths of our brain's neurons that are involved in memory. Ten to 20 grams of PC per day stabilized the memory of patients with Alzheimer's disease.[23] Soy lecithin is the richest food source.

Other Important Nutrients

Coenzyme Q10 is a type of fat-soluble enzyme similar to vitamin E. As an anti-aging nutrient, it has powerful antioxidant properties that retard the death of cells. Nuts, fish, soybeans, spinach, and cruciferous vegetables are good dietary sources. It is also readily available in supplement form.

MSM (Methyl-Sulfonyl-Methane) is a sulfur compound found in the body. It is the active ingredient in DMSO (DimethylSulfoxide). Because our supply of MSM declines as we age, MSM has been recommended to help counter the aging effect of glaucoma, improve the pain and inflammation associated with arthritis and rheumatism, and prevent the loss of collagen in the skin.[24] Dietary sources of MSM are found mostly in raw fruits and vegetables such as broccoli, wheatgrass juice and seaweeds, and in mother's milk.

SAMe (S-Adenosyl-Methionine) is a natural metabolite of the amino acid methionine. It is a potent multi-purpose anti-aging and anti-disease agent. In fact, there is so much scientific literature about its potential health applications that it may be perceived as a panacea, which would cast doubt on its credibility. SAMe maintains mitochondrial function, prevents DNA mutations, restores cellular membranes and enhances a cell's ability to bind hormones. In addition, SAMe has antidepressant action equal to the best FDA approved drugs, protects the liver against the ill effects of alcohol and drugs, and is the daytime equivalent of melatonin. It seems that the natural synthesis of melatonin at night is dependent on the synthesis of SAMe during the day. SAMe is needed for the biochemical reaction that converts serotonin into melatonin.[25] (Serotonin is the neurotransmitter that drugs like Prozac elevate.) SAMe is a prescription drug in some European countries.

Herbs for Longevity

Ginseng has the ability to help many aging human body systems, since it improves the body's ability to use and absorb oxygen. Its antioxidant properties and ginsenosides slow the aging process by increasing alertness, improving concentration, learning ability and memory; increasing testosterone levels and sexual desire; and counteracting the toxic effects of stress. *(For more, see "Ginseng.")*

Ginkgo Biloba is best known for enhancing age-related memory impairment. As a life extension agent, a standardized extract of ginkgo biloba fed to rats significantly increased their lifespan. It reverses the attrition of 5-HT1 receptors in the brain, which normally decreases with age.[26] By improving blood circulation, ginkgo also wards off fatigue, helps retard hearing loss, protects eyesight and fights free radicals. *(For more, see "Ginkgo" and "Power Drinks for the Mind.")*

Green Tea is a powerful antioxidant with numerous benefits for the immune system—protection from cancer, prevention of strokes, and lowered blood pressure. Because of its abundant stores of polyphenols, its antioxidant properties are 20 times that of vitamin E and four times stronger than BHA.[27]

Other Herbs. Chaparral contains a very powerful antioxidant with life extension properties arising from its nordihydroguaiaretic acid (NDGA), polyphenols, quinones, sulfur and zinc. *Paprika* and *rose hips* are rich in the antioxidant lycopene; *gotu-kola* enhances collagen synthesis; and *sarsaparilla* is a good source of phytoestrogens.

How Old Are You, Really?

Aging isn't just the withering of brain cells, arteries, and bones. The older and sicker we get, the more we disengage from society. We stop working, go out less, have less sex, get fewer phone calls, and less mail. We are retreating from life! This is a downward spiral leading to the cessation of activity...*death*. We are aging–and dying–when we stop trying, stop relating, and stop communicating.

Couch potatoes are old at any age. Their muscles, arteries and neurons shrink and shrivel. Yes, a younger person may remember eight items on a grocery list and an older person only four. But with training, the younger person can remember thirty and the older twenty. So the biggest improvement is not a function of age, but effort. The effort of self-improvement, whether in the form of continued learning, socializing, or exercising, leads to better memories, bigger hearts, and stronger limbs.

You don't need a scientist to convince you that exercising, eating a good diet, eating more moderately, and reducing stress helps you live longer and more healthfully. Granted, as we get older we get wobblier. But when a baby learns to walk, we don't count the number of times he falls. Aging, too, is not about how many times we fall, but how many times we get up.

Age is a numbers game. Chronology is not equivalent to biology. The age of our cells is not tied to a clock or calendar. Chronology is a societal charting of time, but our cells age according to divine creation, which we can nourish or starve, shorten or stretch—that's all within our control.

(For more on disease-related anti-aging, see "Menopause," "Liver Problems," "Atherosclerosis," "High Blood Pressure," "Osteoporosis," "Arthritis," "Eye Problems," "Tinnitus," "Prostate," and "Power Drinks-Mind" for info on Alzheimer's and Memory Loss.)

Helpful Foods, Nutrients & Herbs

For more information, see "Nutrient Sources" & "Glossary"

Foods

Acerola Berries
Aged Garlic Extract
Alfalfa Sprouts
Bee Pollen
Black Currants
Blueberries
Berries
Brewer's Yeast
Broccoli Sprouts
Cabbage
Clover Sprouts
Eggplant
Garlic
Grapes
Grape Seed Extract
Fruits (dark skin)
Grapes
Pink Grapefruit
Red Cabbage
Red Grapes
Red Pepper (hot)
Red Wine
Royal Jelly
Soy Sprouts
Sprouts
Tomatoes
Watermelon
Whey
Whey Protein

Nutrients

Antioxidants
Beta-Carotene
Coenzyme Q10
Collagen
Cysteine, NAC
DHEA
Enzymes
Fish Oils
Glutathione
HGH
L-Dopa
Lycopene
Melatonin
MSM
Niacin (B3)
Nucleic Acids
Nicotinic Acid
PC
Phytoestrogens
Pregnenolone
SAMe
SOD
Vitamin B5
Vitamin C
Vitamin E

Herbs

Asiatic Ginseng
Chaparral
Ginkgo Biloba
Gotu-Kola
Green Tea
Paprika
Rose Hips
Sarsaparilla

Recipes

Mental Tune-Up

½ cup	Apple Juice
2 Tbsp	Tahini, raw
1 Tbsp	Lecithin Granules
1 Tbsp	Wheat Germ
1 Tbsp	Brewer's Yeast
½ cup	Pure Water
1ml	Ginkgo Extract (1 dropperful)

Alert, quick thinking epitomizes youthfulness. You'll be saying "good morning" all day when you make this your wake up brew. It has all the vital ingredients needed for alertness and concentration. Lecithin, wheat germ, and brewer's yeast are our finest plant sources of phosphatiydlcholine and acetylcholine. Acetylcholine is the most abundant neurotransmitter in the brain. Ginkgo biloba increases alpha-wave activity in the brain and the number of neuroreceptor sites. Sesame seeds (tahini is sesame butter) is one of our best food sources of coenzyme Q10, nicotinic acid, phosphorus, and thiamine, all of which play a role in protecting our neurons from damage by free radicals.

Remember, herbs and nutrients are not drugs but nourish you in a way that enables higher, long term functioning. Chemicals may fire your neurotransmitters for a quick jump-start, but they will also leave you burned out. Real enhancement takes time. Regular consumption of the good nutrients in this drink and others will help you to think faster, think smarter.

Use organic ingredients whenever possible and, preferably, add them in the order listed. Blend the first 3 ingredients for 15-30 seconds, then add the powders and water and blend again. Finally add ginkgo extract. You may empty the contents of a ginkgo capsule into the blender if the extract is unavailable. (This drink will still work even if you do not have all of the ingredients.)

Collagen Skin Renewal

8 oz	Carrot Juice
1 Tbsp	Wheat or Barley Grass Powder
1 Tbsp	Brewer's Yeast
1 tsp	Royal Jelly
1 tsp	Vitamin C Crystals

This simple recipe is a bonafide collagen and beta-carotene booster. Carrot juice is our most delicious source of beta-carotene, which is our most famous antioxidant. Yeast contains a respiratory factor for the skin (SRF), and is our finest source of PABA, a B vitamin that helps with everything from scleroderma (hardening of the skin) to wrinkles. Wheatgrass contains high amounts of PABA and beta-carotene. Royal jelly is a honey-like liquid that can smooth wrinkles in aging skin. Vitamin C helps maintain the appearance of our skin by slowing the decline of collagen. Stir in the powders slowly but thoroughly.

Capillary Reinforcer

2 oz	Blueberry Juice
3 oz	Red Skinned Grape Juice
4 oz	Pink Grapefruit Juice
1 Tbsp	Bee Pollen

Dark skinned fruits and vegetables contain a wealth of bioflavonoids and anthocyanidins, which are superb antioxidants. Bioflavonoids can protect blood vessels and capillaries from oxidative damage and strengthen connective tissue in the body that otherwise weakens with the passage of time. Juice the seeds of the grapes as well because they contain OPC's, a powerful antioxidant that renews collagen in skin.

DNA Repair

8 oz	Carrot Juice
1 Tbsp	Spirulina Powder

Spirulina and carrots are the two highest dietary sources of provitamin A and beta-carotene. If you want to prevent free radicals from aging your cells, drink this juice daily. Spirulina is also our richest source of the nucleic acids DNA and RNA, which decrease with age. Animals injected with RNA and DNA doubled their longevity.

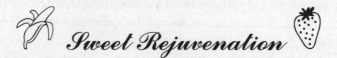

Sweet Rejuvenation

1–2 cups	Pure Water
1	Banana
1 Tbsp	Whey Protein Powder
1 Tbsp	Bee Pollen
1 Tbsp	Lecithin
1 Tbsp	Honey
1 tsp	Vitamin C Crystals
1 tsp	Royal Jelly

Bananas lower blood pressure due to their high potassium content. Whey protein contains a life extension growth factor. Bee pollen is an energy food whose rich nutritional stores promote cell rejuvenation, and royal jelly smooths wrinkles. Vitamin C declines as we age and should be supplemented. Lecithin is our best source of the valuable neurotransmitter nutrient phosphatidylcholine.

Blend the banana and honey in 1 cup of water first, then add the remaining powders. Add additional water and honey only to achieve the desired consistency and sweetness.

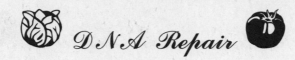

Hormone Regulator

8 oz	Carrot Juice
2 oz	Alfalfa Sprout Juice
1 clove	Garlic, juiced

Carrots are the best known source of beta-carotene, an antioxidant that fights against many diseases of aging including cancer, atherosclerosis, heart disease, and stroke. Alfalfa sprouts are a top source of phytoestrogens, the plant equivalent of human estrogen, which can stimulate cell growth without the harsh side effects of the real hormone. Garlic has several anti-aging benefits, including improved memory and learning and lowered blood pressure.

Wheat Grass Juice

2 oz	Wheatgrass Juice, fresh

Fresh wheatgrass juice is a potent blood purifier that helps transport oxygen to our cells. Along with its capacity to detoxify the liver, it is a superb overall life extension food. To fight aging and disease, we must maintain rich, oxygenated blood, a clear colon, and a fully functioning liver. There are many stories about the rejuvenating powers of wheatgrass. In addition to anecdotal evidence, there is a good amount of research on its therapeutic benefits. *(For more, see "Wheat Grass and Barley Grass," or read: "Wheat Grass, Nature's Finest Medicine," by this author.)*

Wheat grass juice can be purchased at a juice bar. To make your own, grow the grass or buy grown grass and juice it. Be aware that only certain juicer machines will juice its woody fiber. *(See "Juicers, Blenders, & Water Purifiers.")*

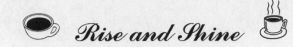

Rise and Shine

1 bag or tsp	Ginseng
1 bag or tsp	Green Tea
1 bag or tsp	Gotu Kola

This can be three separate teas or one mixed tea. Ginseng and green tea stimulate the production of SOD, a major antioxidant. The ginsenosides in ginseng increase alertness and concentration as well as testosterone levels and sexual desire. Green tea lowers blood pressure and prevents strokes and is a stronger antioxidant than vitamin E. *(See "Power Drinks Basics," How to Brew Tea.)*

Disease Protection

4 oz	Tomato Juice
3 oz	Celery Juice
2 oz	Red Cabbage Juice
1 clove	Garlic, juiced

Tomatoes have gotten red-hot press lately because of their high lycopene content and the discovery that this carotenoid reduces the risk of prostate cancer. Red cabbage is also a rich source of anthocyanidins and pro-anthocyanidins, providing anti-aging benefits for Alzheimer's, atherosclerosis, and macular degeneration. Celery lowers blood pressure and garlic stimulates the immune system to the extent that it has been used to fight a variety of cancers.

Medicine Chest

Nutritional Therapies and Delicious Recipes for 115 Different Health Disorders Backed by the Latest Scientific Research

Ailments can fall under many different names. An asthmatic's symptoms may come from allergies; it may bc a form of hay fever; or it could be a chronic bronchitis. Your migraines may be allergies, too. High blood pressure is hypertension, which is hardening of the arteries or atherosclerosis, caused by high cholesterol. The latter is a form of heart disease, which could originate from stress. This book operates under the principles of holistic therapy: there may be many names for a disease, many symptoms, and even many causes, but they all share the same treatment.

Each health disorder listed here includes an explanation of underlying causes, diet suggestions, important foods, herbs, and nutrients that help, and juice, tea, and blended drink recipes using these healthful ingredients. Below is a listing of various ailments and where you can find their conditions described.

The ordinary doctor is interested mostly in the study of disease.
The nature doctor is interested mostly in the study of health.
—Mahatma Gandhi, 1869-1948.

Index of Ailments and Conditions

Acne

Skin Eruptions/Pimples

See also Skin Problems

Do you sometimes find yourself reflecting on your teen-aged years—high school dances or hanging out at the local drive-in? Some reflections you like to remember, but pimples are not one of them.

Acne, also known as "pimples", is one of the not-so-pleasant parts of being a teen. This eruption of the skin occurs in men and women in their teens and even older. It is a visible sign that toxins in the body are fighting for a way out.

When the liver and kidneys fail to flush toxins from the body, the skin is the only other way out. Some areas of the skin, such as the face, offer little resistance. You could also have a minor breakout on the neck, back, and shoulders. When the skin's pores are clogged by overactive sebaceous glands or cosmetics, the toxins must push harder to get out. The result is skin eruptions that are often inflamed and red, and in extreme cases, there is bleeding and scarring.

Causes

Acne stems from both external and internal sources. It may be caused by bacteria that enter the body from outside, such as from dirt and environmental pollution. Internal causes of acne include stress and hormone imbalances (typical in young adults and menstruating women) that result in overactive sebaceous glands. Food allergies and sensitivities can also cause acne.

Protect your skin from external toxins whenever possible and avoid creams and cosmetics that can clog the skin's pores. Internal causes of acne are harder to control. Watch out for dehydration and stress, and stay away from fried, fatty, and processed foods. Wheat, chocolate, and sugar can cause allergic skin reactions.

Diet Suggestions

Eat a high fiber, vegetarian diet, which will help keep the body "clean" internally by improving the liver and kidney functions. Unrefined foods that are high in vitamins, minerals, and complex carbohydrates help detoxify the body, and abundant amounts of water flush away toxins that interfere with healthy, pimple-free skin.

Foods That Help

To keep the skin clean and clear, eat foods high in beta-carotene, such as carrots, sweet potatoes, cantaloupe, squash, spinach, watercress, beet greens, and algae. Foods such as garlic, wheatgrass, plums, and olive oil contain anti-oxidants that help maintain healthy conditions throughout the body, including the skin. Brewer's yeast is the best known source of chromium, a mineral that helps the body maintain normal blood sugar levels and reduces stress, two conditions helpful for healthy skin. The juice of rhubarb soothes the itching and pain associated with acne.

The importance of drinking plenty of pure water cannot be overstated. Adequate hydration flushes away toxins and keeps the skin fresh, clear, and supple.

Nutrients and Herbs That Help

Nutrients and herbs that help acne can be taken internally as supplements or applied topically through steam treatments, tub bathing, and direct application.

Supplements of anti-oxidant vitamins, especially Vitamin A, help prevent and heal acne.[1] Vitamin B6 protects against infection and taking it one week prior to and during menstruation has worked favorably to clear up skin eruptions associated with women's monthly cycles. Folic acid, silicon, and Vitamin E have been known to improve and accelerate the healing of acne. Zinc taken internally and applied topically reduces inflammation caused by acne and is also known to slow the output of the sebaceous glands.[2]

To internally cleanse the body of toxins that can cause acne, use herbs that improve the liver and kidney functions. They include echinacea, red clover, and dandelion root. Taking burdock internally helps nourish the skin and steaming your skin with strawberry leaves, thyme, eucalyptus, and wintergreen is helpful for irritated skin. Sit yourself in a hot tub bath with chamomile, witch hazel, nettles, echinacea, and calendula. Aloe vera, applied directly, cools and calms inflamed skin. Tea tree oil has been known to fight bacteria on the skin and relieves itching associated with acne.

Helpful Foods, Nutrients & Herbs

For more information, see "Nutrient Sources" & "Glossary"

Foods

Chorella	Yellow-Orange Fruits & Vegetables	Potatoes
Garlic	Dark Green Vegetables	Wheat Grass
Onions	Sea Vegetables	Barley Grass
Blue-Green Algae	Spirulina	Brewer's Yeast
		Water

Nutrients

Chromium	Vitamin C	Folic Acid
Vitamin A	Vitamin E	Silicon
Vitamin B6	Beta Carotene	Zinc

Herbs

Tea Tree Oil	Chamomile	Red Clover
Burdock	Calendula	Witch Hazel
Echinacea	Dandelion Root	Aloe Vera

Recipes

Skin and Liver Cleanser

6 oz	Carrot Juice
3 oz	Kale or Collard Greens Juice
1 oz	Wheatgrass Juice
1-2 cloves	Garlic, Juiced

If straight wheatgrass juice is too strong for you, mix it with these other powerful antioxidant vegetables for a wheatgrass cocktail that purges the liver and heals the skin. You can't have healthy looking skin with a clogged liver. Certain vegetable juicers will extract both wheatgrass and carrot juice simultaneously without the need for a second machine. *(See "Juicers, Blenders, & Water Purifiers")*

Skin Rejuvenator

6 oz	Carrot Juice
2 oz	Aloe Vera Juice
1 Tbsp	Blue-Green or other Algae Powder
2 Tbsp	Wheat Grass Powder
1 Tbsp	Brewer's Yeast

This simple recipe is a bonafide beta-carotene booster. Make your carrot juice and add your favorite brand of aloe vera juice. You can also grow the aloe vera plant at home and use its juice directly on the skin. Stir in the algae, wheatgrass, and yeast powders. Yeast is our finest source of chromium, the mineral your body needs to maintain normal blood sugar levels and reduce stress.

Liver Detox Tea

1 bag or tsp	Echinacea
1 bag or tsp	Red Clover
1 bag or tsp	Dandelion Root

Use a teaspoon of loose tea or buy tea bags. These three herbs are known for their liver purging abilities. Liver performance is crucial for healthy skin. Make a big pot and drink daily. Add honey or your favorite sweetener if you wish. However, avoid adding milk. Dairy slows down detoxification. Be sure to drink plenty of pure water and occasionally get a liver massage.

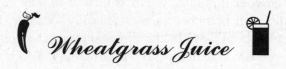

Wheatgrass Juice

2 oz	Wheatgrass Juice, fresh

Fresh squeezed wheatgrass juice is one of the best liver detoxifiers you can find and is purging to the colon, our largest internal organ, whose condition is closely tied to the health of the skin. Wheatgrass is a major blood purifier, and clean blood makes clean skin.

Wheatgrass juice can be purchased at a juice bar. To make your own, grow the grass or buy grown grass and juice it. Be aware that only certain juicer machines will juice its woody fiber. *(See "Juicers, Blenders, & Water Purifiers")*

Allergies

and Hay Fever

See also Cold & Flu

Itching? Sneezing? Wheezing? Is it a cold? Maybe not! You may be having an allergy attack. Allergies are overreactions of your immune system to allergens, substances that register as an "intruder" in your body. The immune system is alerted when foreign substances, such as bacteria, viruses, and toxins enter your body or contact the skin. Most of the time, your body just adapts to allergens, but if it tries to reject them, your immune system works overtime and may cause an allergic reaction. When your immune system is unable to stay on top of this influx of toxins, your body becomes chronically sensitive. Like a tired boxer, you get knocked down by the slightest punch, whereas when you are vigorous, you can take many hits with impunity. This is why allergic people are sensitive to a wide range of impurities.

The body fights invasion by releasing an excess of histamine, an inhibitory neurotransmitter that is responsible for several different forms of discomfort including skin rashes, runny nose, congestion, and itchy eyes, as well as more severe, life-threatening reactions.

Causes

The frequency and intensity of allergic reactions vary greatly among individuals. Common allergy triggers include dust, mold, pollen, latex, chemicals, pets, medication, and many food sources such as alcoholic beverages, wine, beer, bee pollen, cheese, chocolate, coffee, nuts, caffeine, dairy products, wheat, and shellfish. The widespread "hay fever" during springtime is a reaction to plant grass and flower pollens.

Allergic reactions can be minimized and often prevented by avoiding identified allergens. Equally important, one of the best forms of protection against allergic reactions is a strong immune system. Therefore avoid foods such as sugar, refined foods, alcohol, tobacco and stress, and behaviors that weaken your defense.

Diet Suggestions

Generally, if a substance has registered in the body as a toxin, a detoxification diet will help remove some or all of the allergy-causing toxins. Whether the toxins are food, pets, chemicals, or other environmental irritants, a juice and water detoxification diet purifies and nourishes your system while providing allergy relief. Vegetable juices are preferred over fruit juices because vegetables have a lower sugar content.

More specific, because many allergies are food-related or exacerbated by certain foods, diet is an obvious catalyst for preventing allergic reactions. Try to identify foods that trigger an allergic reaction and avoid them.

Foods That Help

The key to managing allergies is in controlling the amount of histamine that is released into the body. Quercetin, a class of water-soluble plant pigments called bioflavonoids, is a natural antihistamine. Foods rich in quercetin include onions, apples, and black tea, while leafy green vegetables and beans are secondary sources of this helpful bioflavoniod.

Vitamin C is also a natural antihistamine. Ironically, pharmaceutical antihistamines, which are often prescribed as a traditional remedy for allergy relief, use up your body's reserve of vitamin C. If allergy sufferers turn first to food sources of antihistamines such as vegetable and fruit juices, not only can they receive relief but also preserve precious supplies of immunity-building vitamin C.

Flaxseed oil is rich in vitamins C, B1, and E and helps relieve some allergies while offering increased stamina and energy.

It is essential to drink enough water and juices to alleviate and prevent allergies. Dehydration is considered to be an underlying cause of allergies. Also, many wheatgrass users report that their allergies have been alleviated. (Although many are allergic to wheat, wheatgrass juice does not carry the allergic properties of the grain.)

Nutrients and Herbs That Help

Vitamin C and quercetin when taken together help alleviate allergic symptoms. Each acts as a natural antihistamine. Additionally, quercetin enhances vitamin C, and also acts as an anti-inflammatory agent. Vitamin E also works to reduce the inflammatory symptoms of histamines.

Certain herbs, such as aloe vera, feverfew, and nettle leaf, discourage the excess release of histamine. Ginkgo biloba helps build your immune system, while Vitamin B6 has been known to provide allergy relief.

Helpful Foods, Nutrients & Herbs

For more information, see "Nutrient Sources" & "Glossary"

Foods

Onions	Strawberries	Wheat Grass
Apples	Citrus Fruits	Flaxseed Oil
Leafy Green Vegetables	Cantaloupe	Water
Beans	Barley Grass	

Nutrients

Vitamin B1	Vitamin C	Quercetin
Vitamin B6	Vitamin E	

Herbs

Aloe Vera	Paprika	Hawthorne
Fever Few	Rosehips	Parsley
Chili (Cayenne)	Ginkgo Biloba	Black Tea
Passion Flower	Nettle	

Recipes

Quercetaloupe

½	Cantaloupe

So delicious. So easy! Cantaloupe is a treasure trove of the anti-allergy nutrient quercetin. Just cut a fresh cantaloupe melon in half and clean out the seeds. Scoop out balls from ½ the melon and add them a few at a time into the blender. If you add too many, you won't be able to purée them without adding extra water, and we don't want to do that.

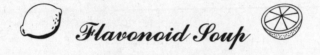

Flavonoid Soup

1	Orange
1	Grapefruit
1	Lemon
½–1 tsp	Flaxseed Oil

Juice these fabulously healthy citrus fruits for their vitamin C, quercetin, and bioflavonoids. What a delicious way to keep the allergies under control. Make sure to scrape out the white pulpy part of these fruits, where most of the bioflavonoids reside. This is a great place to add flaxseed oil to your diet, which helps some allergies.

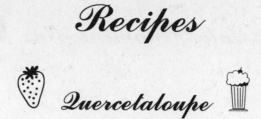

Anti-Histamine Plus

8 oz	Carrot Juice
1 oz	Wheatgrass Juice
1 oz	Aloe Vera Juice

What a heavenly way to regulate your histamine level. If you are new to wheatgrass juice, start with 1 ounce and build your way up to 2-3 ounces per drink. Select whole leaf aloe vera juice. Aloe vera can vary in taste, so shop for the best tasting brand.

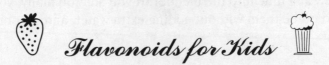

Flavonoids for Kids

1	Apple, cut and cored
4-8	Strawberries
½ tsp	Vitamin C Powder
1 Tbsp	Bee Pollen
1 + cup	Pure Water
1 tsp	Honey (optional)

Always strive to buy organic fruits and vegetables. Allergically sensitive people may react to chlorine in water and pesticides in produce. If you are allergic to strawberries, substitute another berry.

First core and quarter the apples, eliminating the seeds. Blend it with half the water. Add the remaining ingredients and enough water to achieve the desired consistency.

Anemia

See also Heart Disease, Fatigue, Pregnancy

Anemia is a blood-related condition. When the blood contains too few red blood cells, or lacks the capacity to carry enough oxygen throughout the body, a person is said to be anemic. Cells need oxygen to survive, which is why an anemic person often feels tired and weak.

Anemia may be a symptom of several different problems, but the common condition results from one of three basic causes: acute or chronic blood loss, excessive destruction of red blood cells, or a deficiency of vital nutrients such as iron, vitamin B12, or folic acid.

Causes

Chronic blood loss can stem from a variety of conditions, such as cancer, menstruation, hemorrhoids, or peptic ulcers, any of which can result in anemia. More often, anemia is brought on by a deficiency of nutrients, either through neglect or conditions such as pregnancy or diabetes, which both require extra nutrients.

Because iron is necessary for the development of healthy red blood cells (the cells that carry oxygen to tissues throughout the body), and because folic acid is necessary for cell reproduction, a diet deficient in these nutrients can cause anemia. Too much alcohol and salt can hinder healthy blood building and should be avoided. Also beware of excessive caffeine and calcium supplements, which can interfere with the absorption of iron.

Diet Suggestions

A diet rich in vitamins, iron, and folic acid is often recommended for alleviating anemic conditions. Eating a variety of whole, unrefined foods and a good supply of raw foods and protein will help supply the nutrients needed to maintain healthy red blood cells. Include aerobic exercise in your lifestyle to increase your ability to assimilate oxygen, which enriches the blood.

Foods That Help

To help increase the number of oxygen-rich cells in our bodies, be sure to consume foods rich in vitamin B12 and iron: kelp, wheat and barley grass, rice bran, brewer's yeast, wheat bran, bee pollen, soy foods, yogurt, alfalfa sprouts, algaes, and liver (beef).

Chlorophyll-rich drinks made from grasses, algaes, alfalfa, parsley, watercress, and spinach are valuable for people suffering from anemia. Chlorophyll is the "blood" of plants. Its structure is similar to hemin, a component of the hemoglobin in blood that carries oxygen. The chlorophyll molecule is bound by magnesium, while hemin is bound by iron. Anemic patients are able to build iron-rich blood simply by increasing their intake of chlorophyll.[1] Getting kids to drink green drinks is also important, because children are vulnerable to anemia during periods of rapid growth and when they give in to poor eating habits.

Sources of folic acid are especially important for healthy prenatal development. These include brewer's yeast (the highest), wheat germ, soy foods, bee pollen, grasses, algaes, wheat bran, walnuts, spinach, kale, legumes, beef liver, and beets.

Nutrients and Herbs That Help

Iron, folic acid, and vitamin B12 are vital nutrients to the process of producing healthy blood. Vegetarians must make an extra effort to eat foods rich in B12, since it is not common in fruits, vegetables, grains, and beans. However, it is a myth that this vitamin is unavailable to vegetarians. Beef liver is the animal food richest in B12 (80mcg/100grams), while the richest plant food is spirulina (218mcg/100grams). Supplements of vitamin B12 in a sub-lingual form are also available. Vitamin C increases iron absorption slightly, and taking vitamin A with iron helps treat iron deficiency, since vitamin A helps the body utilize the iron stored in the liver.

L-Carnitine has helped patients who suffer from anemia while undergoing dialysis treatment, which indicates that it may help other types of anemia as well.[2] The Chinese herb rehmannia, a general tonic for blood-building, increases the number of red blood cells in the bone marrow.[3] It is available as a root herb, a tincture, or in capsules. The antioxidant properties of vitamin E have been proven to protect red blood cells from the toxic effects of free radicals.[4] The herb gentian stimulates hydrochloric acid in the stomach, which is especially important for the elderly and others with a weakened digestive system. Hydrochloric acid supplements may also be helpful.

Helpful Foods, Nutrients & Herbs

For more information, see "Nutrient Sources" & "Glossary"

Foods

Brewer's Yeast
Wheat Germ
Liver - Beef
Tofu, Tempeh
Bee Pollen
Kelp
Wheat Grass
Barley Grass
Spirulina
Chlorella
Blue-Green Algae
Bran
Kidney Beans
Mung Bean Sprouts
Lima Beans
Alfalfa Sprouts
Dried Fruits
Molasses
Sesame & Flaxseeds
Hot Peppers
Leafy Green Vegetables

Nutrients

Iron
Vitamin B12
Folic Acid
Hydrochloric Acid
L-Carnitine
Vitamin E
Vitamin C

Herbs

Dandelion Root
Gentian
Yellow Dock
Alfalfa
Rehmannia Root
Parsley
Ginseng
Burdock Root
Comfrey Root
Dong Quai

Recipes

Chlorophyll Cocktail

6 oz	Celery Juice
2 oz	Kale or Collard Greens Juice
2 oz	Alfalfa Sprouts Juice
2 oz	Spinach Juice
1 oz	Wheatgrass Juice
1 tsp	Spirulina or Chlorella Powder

It doesn't get any greener than this! This drink contains our highest dietary sources of chlorophyll, arguably the most effective nutrient for treating anemia. Chlorella, blue-green algae, spirulina, alfalfa, and the grasses top the list with incredible amounts of this "blood" of plants—liquid sunshine distilled into food through photosynthesis. These algaes are also our finest sources of vitamin B12. Spinach and kale are great sources of folic acid. If you lack one or two of the ingredients, this drink will still be effective.

Iron Infusion

1-2 cups	Pure Water
2 Tbsp	Rice, Oat, or Wheat Bran
2 Tbsp	Tahini (ground sesame seeds)
1 small	Apple, cut and cored (substitute: Banana)
1 Tbsp	Wheat or Barley Grass Powder
1 Tbsp	Brewer's Yeast
1 Tbsp	Bee Pollen
1 Tbsp	Pumpkin Seed
Pinch	Stevia

Here, in one delectable potion, are the best dietary sources of iron. The grasses top the list *(see "Nutrient Sources"),* while brewer's yeast is our finest source of folic acid, another important nutrient for treating anemia. The powdered grasses are available in any health food store. Tahini is sesame seed paste. Try to obtain raw, organic tahini whenever possible.

Begin with 1 cup of water in your blender and slowly add the ingredients in the order listed. Choose apple or banana, your preference. Since both are thickeners, you may need to add additional water to achieve a whirlpool in the blender and your desired consistency.

Folic Fruity

1 cup	Soy Milk, vanilla flavor
½	Papaya (substitute: Banana or Apple)
1 Tbsp	Brewer's Yeast
2 Tbsp	Wheat Germ
1 Tbsp	Bee Pollen
1 Tbsp	Wheat or Barley Grass Powder

Since folic acid can help prevent the megaloblastic form of anemia, you should make sure it is in your diet. Here is a fruity smoothie made with our best sources of folic acid. Brewer's yeast, the number one source, also contains the all-important vitamin B12, and soy milk along with wheat grass are excellent sources of iron.

Choose a good tasting soy milk; clean the seeds out of the ripe (pink) papaya, and blend. If you cannot find a papaya, substitute a small apple or banana. Add the remaining ingredients slowly, blending in each one in turn.

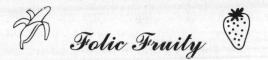

Arthritis

Osteoarthritis, Rheumatoid Arthritis, Gout

Arthritis is the collective name of several diseases that affect the joints of the body. All forms of arthritis cause joint stiffness, pain, and swelling. Osteoarthritis, the most common form of arthritis, occurs when the cartilage cushioning of the joints has worn down. Pain resulting from loss of cartilage occurs when bones touch bones, usually in weight-bearing joints such as the ankles, knees, and hips but also in the spine and neck and in fingers, wrists, and elbows.

When a person's immune system attacks its own body, it may result in rheumatoid arthritis, a chronic inflammatory condition of the joints. When the spaces between the bones are not lubricated, the area becomes inflamed and sometimes extra fluid leaks into the joints causing swelling. Although the joints are its main target, arthritis can affect the whole body.

Gout is a form of arthritis that occurs when excess uric acid is not eliminated from the body through urination. The uric acid crystallizes and eventually settles in the joints, causing swelling and pain.

Causes

Osteoarthritis and rheumatoid arthritis can be caused by aging, injury, or overuse of the joints. Additionally, much research points to food allergies and imbalances caused by environmental toxins as sources of all types of arthritis.[1] Determining which allergies are triggering painful joint reactions and eliminating the culprits can reverse some forms of arthritis. Highly acidic foods and pork seem to provoke arthritis.

Gout appears to be related to animal food sources. Avoiding meat and dairy may reduce the excessive uric acid that triggers this type of arthritis.

Diet Suggestions

A vegetarian diet of complex carbohydrates, fresh fruits and vegetables, whole grains, and small portions of protein can help eliminate the causes of arthritis as well as soothe some of the symptoms. Additionally, a diet free of chemicals, sugar, eggs, and processed food can eliminate possible allergic reactions that aggravate some forms of arthritis. Fat, especially animal fat, can also lead to auto-immune reactions and gout. A low fat diet is recommended for anyone who suffers from rheumatoid arthritis and gout. A high intake of antioxidants is also known to slow down the deterioration rate of joints.

Foods That Help

Foods that contain copper are readily available sources of relief. Copper helps maintain healthy connective tissues and collagen fibers. In fact, wearing a copper bracelet is often used as a source of relief from rheumatoid arthritis. Legumes (barley, lentils, soya beans, and split peas), mushrooms, and nuts (almonds, brazil nuts, hazelnuts, pecans, pistachio, walnuts, and pine nuts) contain copper in highly usable and delicious forms.

Plums, tempeh, wheat grass, dark green and orange-yellow vegetables, wheat germ oil, nuts, seeds, vegetable oils, whole grains, and green tea possess valuable antioxidant properties for counteracting degeneration and inflammation of body tissues. Omega-3 fatty acids in fish oil, especially salmon (and in flaxseed oil for the vegetarian) also work as anti-inflammatory factors.

Because alfalfa works as a blood purifier, eating or juicing with alfalfa, alfalfa sprouts, and other foods high in chlorophyll helps eliminate the excessive uric acid that causes gout.

Nutrients and Herbs That Help

Pain relief and anti-inflammatory agents are found in herbs such as turmeric, ginger, sarsaparilla, and evening primrose oil. The herb bosweilla also acts as an anti-inflammatory and has qualities that stimulate tissue repair by increasing circulation to the joints. Extensive scientific research affirms the benefits of glucosamine sulfate, the amino sugar of glucose that our body manufactures in the intestinal tract. It is a necessary component for building cartilage. As a dietary supplement, the usual dosage is 1500-2000mg/day.[2]

Anti-oxidants found in Vitamins A, C & E and grapeseed extract work to strengthen the whole body while specifically targeting inflammation.

Helpful Foods, Nutrients & Herbs

For more information, see "Nutrient Sources" & "Glossary"

Foods

Legumes	Broccoli	Almonds, Pecans
Whole Grains	Plums	Salmon
Alfalfa		

Nutrients

Copper	Vitamin C	Boron
Vitamin A	Vitamin E	Glucosamine Sulfate

Herbs

Tumeric	Sarsaparilla	Boswellia
Ginger	Evening Primrose Oil	Wheat Grass
Comfrey	Flaxseed Oil	Barley Grass
Chamomile		

Recipes

Green & Mellow Teas

1 bag or tsp	Green Tea
1 bag or tsp	Chamomile
1 bag or tsp	Comfrey

These are 2 separate teas. Green tea is known to be a powerful antioxidant and immune system booster. Both are desirable qualities for counteracting degeneration and inflammation of body tissues. Chamomile is known for its anti-inflammatory properties and comfrey knits bones due to its high allantoin content. *(See "Power Drinks Basics—How to Brew Tea")*

Blood Purifier

6 oz	Celery Juice
1 oz	Wheatgrass Juice
1 oz	Spinach Juice
1 oz	Cabbage Juice
1 oz	Alfalfa Sprouts Juice
1 tsp	Spirulina or Chlorella Powder

This fresh, organic green vegetable juice is an unsurpassed source of chlorophyll, one of the essential nutrients on the planet, required by animals and plants alike. Alfalfa, wheatgrass, chlorella, and spirulina are the top sources of chlorophyll, which reduces the excessive uric acid that crystallizes in our joints. Chlorophyll is similar to hemoglobin, and drinking these juices is like having a blood transfusion. Good blood is the solution to degenerative diseases such as arthritis, because blood nourishes and cleanses the cells that make up our bones and tissues.

Immune Strengthener

6-10	Almonds
5	Pecans or Walnuts
2 Tbsp	Wheat Grass or Barley Grass Powder
2 Tbsp	Sesame Seeds
1 tsp	Flaxseed Oil
pinch	Stevia
1-2 Cups	Pure Water

Blend the sesame seeds in a dry blender until puréed into a meal. Then add half the water and blend to a smooth paste. Add the wheat grass or barley grass powder along with the stevia. Stevia is a sweet herb that is not a sugar *(see Glossary).* Mix in the flax oil and nuts last. You may choose to use only one kind of nut. Add more water to achieve a thick shake consistency. For best digestion, almonds should be pre-soaked for several hours to soften them. If you like a crunchy, chewy drink, add the almonds and pecans at the end, blending only to a chop. Otherwise, blend them thoroughly.

Flaxseed oil has anti-inflammatory properties, and almonds and pecans are high in oils as well as copper, an essential mineral for healthy joints.

Asthma

and Bronchitis

See also Allergies, Cold & Flu

It's a beautiful spring day. Step outside and take a deep breath of fresh air laden with the scent of flowers and new-mown grass. Isn't it wonderful? Not if you suffer from asthma or bronchitis. You'll wheeze and fight to get air in and out of your lungs while your bronchial passages go into spasms. Then you'll cough as your body tries to expel excess mucus.

Asthma is a disorder of the respiratory system that affects the lungs and airways and makes breathing difficult. Bronchitis, another disorder that interferes with proper breathing, is an inflammation of the bronchial tubes in particular, the larger passages of the lungs that deliver oxygen to the body.

Causes

A variety of factors can lead to spasms of the airways to the lungs, cause swelling in the airways, and produce excess mucus, all of which restrict the smooth flow of air in and out of the lungs.

Because allergies are cited as a common cause of asthma, the disease is considered a disorder of the immune system. Although there is no cure for asthma, it can be controlled with proper treatment.

Typical causes of asthma and bronchitis include air pollution, smoking, second-hand smoke, viral infection, food allergies, food additives, and chemicals. The lungs and airways over-react to these triggers and become inflamed and clogged.

To help avert an attack, those who are prone to asthma should identify their own unique group of triggers and avoid or minimize exposure to them. Asthma and bronchitis can generally be controlled by 1) minimizing exposure to environmental pollution including dust and mold; 2) identifying and avoiding problematic foods; 3) eliminating chemicals and food additives such as sulfites in dried fruits, food coloring, MSG, aspartame, calcium and potassium benzoate, and tartrazine; and 4) strengthening the immune system with proper rest, exercise, and nutrition.

Diet Suggestions

Since obesity increases the risk of asthma, weight reduction is a good first step. Also, an allergy elimination diet is recommended, since many asthma symptoms come from reactions to foods. Fasting is a good way to eliminate offensive foods from your system and relax the body's irritated and inflamed mucous membranes. And finally because chronic dehydration may be an underlying cause, drink lots of water.

A diet rich in organically grown, whole, unprocessed foods provides vital nutrients without detrimental additives and chemicals. A vegan diet helps many asthma sufferers by eliminating dairy and animal products. A diet of raw foods also eliminates dairy and animal products, plus it prevents the alteration of foods by heat, which denatures the quality of many nutrients. Diets rich in hot peppers are beneficial, and vegetable juices high in beta-carotene and vitamin C are good for rebuilding a depressed immune system.

Foods That Help

Oily fish is our best source of EPA and DHA oils, which along with evening primrose oil (a plant oil) reduces the symptoms of bronchitis and asthma. These oils contain anti-inflammatory properties that widen the air passages.[1]

According to Chinese medicine, the colon and lungs are interrelated. Diets high in chlorophyll promote detoxification of the liver and colon. Such cleansing foods include fresh squeezed wheatgrass, alfalfa sprouts, parsley, and celery juice.

Radishes, horseradish, ginger, and cayenne pepper all heat up the respiratory system and help break up congestion in the lungs. Moderate amounts of garlic and onions have been known to help relax bronchial muscles and reduce the incidence of bronchial spasms.

If you are a coffee lover, you are going to love this. Caffeine expands the bronchial tubes, making it easier for asthmatics to breathe.[2]

Nutrients and Herbs That Help

Herbs such as dong quai, ginkgo biloba, marshmallow, mullein, licorice, and ephedra have a longstanding reputation for treating respiratory ailments. In Europe, licorice is a standard treatment for coughs, sinusitis, and bronchitis. Ephedrine, an alkaloid extracted from the herb ephedra (Chinese ma huang), is an approved over-the-counter remedy for reducing bronchial tightness. Because some of these herbs are powerful, please consult your health care professional to assure safe management of your therapy.

Magnesium is the mineral of choice for treating spasms of the bronchial passages. Given intravenously, it can actually relieve acute attacks.[3] Vitamin C reduces the level of histamine in the blood, which is high in asthma patients.[4] Very high amounts of vitamin B12 supplements (1,500 mcg per day) may desensitize an allergic reaction to sulfites, the yellow dye in dried fruits.[5] Vitamin B6 (pyridoxine), in amounts of 100 mg per day, decreases the frequency and severity of wheezing.[6] The amino acid cysteine, especially N-Acetyl-Cysteine (NAC), helps bronchitis sufferers by hydrating the mucous membranes that clog the bronchioles.[7]

Helpful Foods, Nutrients & Herbs

For more information, see "Nutrient Sources" & "Glossary"

Foods

Apricots	Reishi Mushrooms	Caffeine Drinks
Garlic & Onions	Plantain Seeds	Oily Fish
Pure Water	Royal Jelly	Evening Primrose Oil

Nutrients

Vitamin B6	Vitamin C	PABA
Vitamin B12	Vitamin D3	Magnesium
NAC	Coenzyme Q10	Calcium

Herbs

Ephedra/Ephedrine	Dong Quai	Licorice
Marshmallow	Ginkgo Biloba	Mullein
Passion Flower	Cayenne/Chili	Skullcap

Recipes

Open Air Tea

1 Tbsp	Licorice Bark
½ tsp	Vitamin C Crystals
1 ml	Ginkgo Extract (1 dropperful)

Licorice is one of the best respiratory toners in the herbal pharmacopeia. Vitamin C reduces the level of histamine in the blood, and ginkgo biloba inhibits the activity of eosinophils, both of which are high in asthma patients. If you prefer a sweeter flavor for this tea, use honey or your favorite sweetener.

Lung Relaxer

5 oz	Celery Juice
2 oz	Kale or Collard Greens Juice
2 oz	Alfalfa Sprouts or Parsley Juice
1 clove	Garlic, juiced
1 oz	Lemon Juice
1 tsp	Spirulina Powder (optional)

Diets high in chlorophyll promote detoxification of the liver and colon. Optimum functioning of these two vital organs are crucial to any asthma treatment program. These foods are also some of the highest dietary sources of calcium and magnesium, minerals necessary for the health and balance of the nervous system. A healthy nervous system reduces stress and constriction in the lungs. Magnesium and garlic both alleviate bronchial spasms. This all-green chlorophyll cocktail will have a powerful quieting effect on your respiratory system. Make sure you sit down and sip it slowly.

Bronchial Opener

4 Tbsp	Tahini
½ cup	Apple Juice
2 Tbsp	Wheat, Oat, or Rice Bran
1 Tbsp	Brewer's Yeast
1 Tbsp	Bee Pollen (substitute: Royal Jelly)
1 cup	Pure Water

Bran is one of our best sources of magnesium, while bee pollen is very rich in calcium. Brewer's yeast contains lots of both minerals. Brewer's yeast is our best source of the asthma friendly vitamin B6 (pyridoxine), and B12.

Purchase a soy milk brand whose taste you like, since it will dominate the flavor of this drink. Bee pollen adds some sweetness. If you want to sweeten it more, substitute with royal jelly, another honey-like bee product, or just honey. Add the ingredients in the order listed, blending each in turn. Add only enough water to achieve the desired consistency. For best digestion, almonds should be pre-soaked for several hours to soften them. If you like a crunchy, chewy drink, add the almonds and pecans at the end and blend on the chop setting. Otherwise, blend them thoroughly.

Cancer

See also "Skin Cancer," "Colon Problems," "Liver Problems" and the various individual foods and herbs in this book for more details about their cancer protective abilities.

Cancer is arguably a patient's greatest worry when visiting the doctor. It is everyone's worst nightmare. It changes the lives of its victims and, in some cases, ends them. In her book, *Cancer Doesn't Scare Me Anymore*, Loraine Day makes the case for cancer as a teacher and a wake-up call. Most cancer survivors–and there are many–affirm that cancer changed their lives for the better.

Cancer is not a single disease, but a group of many diseases with a common characteristic: uncontrolled, invasive cell growth at the expense of normal cell growth. Various factors transform healthy cells into cancerous cells that wreak havoc over orderly cell growth.

Cancer is classified as an ailment of the immune system that can manifest in several forms with varying consequences. Let's get some terms straight. Carcinoma is a tumor that originates on the skin or in glandular tissue, while sarcoma is a type of cancer that affects the connective and supportive tissues. Skin cancers are called melanomas, while lymphoma and leukemia affect the lymphatic systems and blood-forming organs, respectively.

Although it is one of the most dreaded diseases, cancer is not inevitably fatal. Today, more and more screening tests are readily available to detect cancerous cells in early stages. Early detection and treatment combined with a healthful diet enhance the prospects for preventing and conquering this malevolent disease.

Causes

There are more doctors and scientists alive in the world today then there were 100 years ago, yet we have more cancers. What has changed? Arguably, it is our diet of mass-market, processed foods. We take good whole foods such as grains, remove the germ (because it's perishable), remove the bran, bleach out the uneven color, and add synthetic vitamins to replace the ones removed, all in an effort to achieve a longer shelf life for the product. Have we exchanged shelf life for human life? The Standard American Diet (SAD) today is floured, frozen, boiled, broiled, canned, sugared, preserved, packaged, and laden with pesticides. Is it no wonder we are sick?

This is why we have immunological weaknesses and nutritional deficiencies. We may even pass these on as genetic tendencies. Added to this is our over stressed lifestyles, polluted air and water, and unhealthy work environments. If you work in a plastics factory and breathe in polyurethane fumes month after month, year after year, is it such a surprise that you might develop liver cancer? Shouldn't you have quit after your first warning—when you contracted emphysema? Our body may provide a barrier, but it is not a cement wall. Pollutants make it into our blood and our cells. Ultimately, when our cells become compromised, they misfire and go haywire, mutating and growing abnormally. Over time, the cells in these "dead zones" start to darken, choking on bacteria, yeast, fungi, and toxins. They cannot get enough oxygen. You have become a victim cancer.

Diet Suggestions

We can control where we work. We can control our lifestyles, and most important of all, we can determine our own diets. Choose, for example, not to eat pesticides with your salad. Avoid food additives such as preservatives, colors, nitrates, nitrites, and MSG. Be suspicious of artificial foods such as olefin, cyclamates, and saccharin and food processed by barbecuing, smoking, frying, irradiation, as well as the use of overheated oils and genetically modified crops. Such methods should be replaced by methods that preserve nutrients, such as steaming, broiling, and baking, and by eating lots of raw, organic foods.

The National Cancer Institute and National Institutes of Health recommend eating 5 fruits and vegetables each day. They now realize that raw foods are the best sources of phytochemicals—natural plant compounds that enhance our immune system and inhibit cancer. In other words, even if you are not a vegetarian, you should eat like one.

Vegetarians generally have a lower risk of contracting cancer. In a study published in the *New England Journal of Medicine*, vegetarian women had a 46% lower risk for contracting breast cancer than other females.[1]

Whether we like it or not, many types of cancers are treated with chemotherapy. These are highly toxic drugs that thrash our immune system and cause nausea, hair loss, weight loss, and, ironically, even cancer. The best way to bolster a weakened immune system is through a low-fat diet that is rich in antioxidants, unprocessed whole foods with no additives, soy products, and pesticide-free fresh vegetables. Fresh squeezed juices supply those nutrients in a readily absorbed form, with all their botanical co-factors in place. Also, don't forget to drink lots of pure water daily and enjoy phytochemical rich teas like green tea.

Foods That Help

Since fresh, organic fruits and vegetables are the best anti-cancer foods, strive to buy from the local farm or take up gardening. It doesn't get any better than eating food fresh from your own garden. If you live in a city, or don't have a green thumb, consider indoor gardening with sprouted vegetables. Sprouts usually have a growing cycle of about one week, and there is no messy soil. Since sprouts are baby vegetables, they contain concentrated amounts of nutrients and phytochemicals. Broccoli sprouts represent the highest known source of the potent phytochemical sulforaphane, which stimulates the production powerful cancer killing enzymes. While all cruciferous vegetables such as cabbage, broccoli, radishes, and cauliflower are important, their sprouts contain 20-50 times more sulforaphane than the mature vegetables.[2] Alfalfa sprouts are one of the finest dietary sources of canavanine, an amino acid analog that can prevent the growth of pancreatic, colon, and leukemia cancers.[3] *(See "Broccoli" and "Alfalfa," for more information.)*

Legumes and soy products such as tofu, miso and soy milk are good sources of anti-cancer agents as well as protein. Blue-green algae foods such as spirulina and chlorella, are the planet's richest sources of protein loaded with genetic material RNA and DNA to bolster our immunity. *(See "Algae.")*

Fruits such as apples, red grapes, grapefruit, and lemons all have cancer preventative properties, and strawberries protect against the potent carcinogen nitrosamines. Even the lowly fig can shrink tumors.[4] The list goes on. *(See the various individual foods and herbs in this book for more details about their cancer protective abilities.)*

Nutrients and Herbs That Help

Antioxidants are some of our best cancer fighters. They protect us from the free radical scavengers that turn our cells malignant and age our bodies. Some antioxidants even reduce the toxicity of chemotherapy drugs. Some of our most popular antioxidants include vitamins A, C and E, beta carotene, selenium, coenzyme Q10, bioflavonoids, and grapeseed extract to name a few. Coenzyme Q10 actually increases the life expectancy of patients by five to 15 years for various forms of cancer.[5]

Vitamin C also reduces the pain associated with some cancers and can minimize the toxic side-effects of chemotherapy. The fat soluble forms of Vitamin C are much more effective than the water-soluble forms. Shark cartilage, as well as vitamin E, cuts off the blood supply to cancerous cells in some tumors, giving the immune system a better chance to destroy the smaller tumor mass.

Many herbs act to prevent and control cancer-cell activity. Essiac tea, a mixture of sheep sorrel and other herbs, is purported to completely eliminate some types of cancer and has gained a devoted following. Wheatgrass juice is used by several cancer clinics for its ability to rejuvenate the liver, detoxify the colon, and cleanse the blood and lymph systems. Garlic and echinacea both fight tumors and enhance immunity. Ginger helps tame the nausea associated with chemotherapy, and green tea shows potential in the treatment of breast and prostate cancers.[6] Some of the other herbs known for their anti-cancer benefits include ginseng, red clover, and rosemary.

If you have cancer, don't give up. Fight. Our 75 trillion cells change every few months, so we are constantly remaking ourselves. You are not a statistic and cancer is not automatically fatal. When things get tough, you must get tougher. Lance Armstrong, the USA Olympic cycling champion, said it best when he learned he had testicular cancer: "With my fitness level, my drive and desire, I'm not going to lose. I can't lose." He didn't and he went on to win the Olympics.

Helpful Foods, Nutrients & Herbs

For more information, see "Nutrient Sources" & "Glossary"

Foods

Broccoli
Broccoli Sprouts
Alfalfa Sprouts
Cabbage
Cauliflower
Kale
Turnip
Radishes
Soy Products
Legumes
Algae
Figs
Grapefruit
Red Grapes
Strawberries
Apples
Pure Water
Lemons

Nutrients

Coenzyme Q10
Vitamin A
Vitamin B2
Vitamin C
Vitamin E
Shark Cartilage
Selenium
Boron
Magnesium
Calcium

Herbs

Ginger
Echinacea
Garlic
Ginseng
Red Clover
Rosemary
Green Tea
Essiac Tea

Recipes

Green Tea

1 bag or tsp Green Tea

Green tea is a powerful antioxidant and immune system enhancing herb with known benefits for cancer. It is particularly effective in counteracting the degeneration of body tissues. *(For more, see "Green Tea.")* When using loose tea, steep for 3 minutes before drinking.

Wheatgrass Juice

2 oz	Wheatgrass Juice

Fresh wheatgrass juice is a very potent blood purifier and helps transport oxygen to our cells. In larger amounts, it acts as a laxative to clear the bowel. This, along with its capacity to detoxify the liver, make it a superb overall cancer treatment. Beating any disease requires good blood, plenty of oxygen, a clear colon, and a fully functioning liver. There are many cancer stories about wheatgrass saving people's lives, and, in addition to anecdotal evidence, there is a good amount of research on its therapeutic benefits. *(See also "Wheatgrass and Barley Grass")*

Green Healer

5 oz	Celery Juice
2 oz	Kale or Collard Greens Juice
2 oz	Alfalfa Sprouts Juice
2 oz	Spinach Juice
1 oz	Wheatgrass Juice
1 tsp	Spirulina or Chlorella Powder

Green is the color of healing and it doesn't get any greener than this. This drink contains our highest dietary sources of chlorophyll, the most effective nutrient for purifying the bloodstream. Chlorella, blue-green algae, spirulina, alfalfa, and the grasses top the list with incredible amounts of this "blood" of plants, the distilled, liquid sunshine of photosynthesis. The algaes are also our finest source of vitamin B12, which will boost any immune system. Spinach is one of our best sources of coenzyme Q10, which increases life expectancy for several types of cancers. If you can make this juice with only part of the ingredients, it will still be effective.

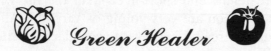

Cold & Flu

Cough, Sore Throat, Sinusitis, Congestion

See also Asthma & Bronchitis, Allergies, Ear Infections

Coughing, sneezing, wheezing, aching all over? Whether you feel a cold gradually creeping up on you or are stopped in your tracks by influenza (the flu), the discomfort of a runny nose, sore throat, cough, congestion, fever, chills, digestive distress, inflamed sinuses, or head and body aches is usually part of the package.

Both the common cold and the flu involve the respiratory tract and are highly contagious, yet the common cold is an infection that is usually less threatening and short-lived than the flu, which can hit harder, especially if you are very young or very old. All cold or flu symptoms should be treated to prevent secondary infection and prolonged misery and to reduce the chances of infecting someone else.

Causes

Let's face it. We live in a world where bacteria and viruses outnumber people. We're surrounded. These microbes can cause respiratory illnesses, and our immune system is our shield. When our shields are down, these intruders break in and make us feel miserable.

A sore throat can be the result of many things: a cold, allergies, tonsilitis, chronic fatigue syndrome, environmental pollutants, and even Lyme disease. Although bothersome, some coughing is good for us since it expels the mucus and other foreign material that makes us cough. But a dry or prolonged cough could indicate bronchitis, pleurisy, asthma, or tuberculosis, each of which require a different treatment.

Mucus blocks our nasal passages, causing congestion. Allergies, hay fever, candida albicans, and even vitamin A deficiency or swimming in chlorinated water can cause sinusitis (inflamed sinuses). Sinusitis, in turn, can cause bad breath (halitosis), earache, ringing in the ears, and loss of smell.

Diet Suggestions

A strong immune system is the best defense against cold, flu, and all of its annoying symptoms. Fortify your body with easy-to-digest fresh fruits and vegetables, which are rich in vitamin C, and avoid dairy products, which stimulate the production of mucus. Lots of fluids, especially pure water, clear broth, vegetable and citrus fruit juices, and herbal teas, help calm a fever, break up mucus, and clear our bodies of toxins.

Foods That Help

Indeed, hot chicken soup tops the list of remedies for clearing mucus and relieving congestion caused by the common cold, flu, and sinusitis. (Vegetarians can drink hot vegetable broth.) Also at the top of the list is anything containing vitamin C. The finest sources of vitamin C are acerola cherries, hot red peppers, guava, black currants, kale, parsley, collards, and broccoli. Truth be told, the ever famous orange juice has a mere 50mg/100g of vitamin C, while sweet red peppers contain over 200mg *(see Nutrient Sources)*. Nevertheless, the white pith of citrus fruits contains bioflavonoids, which work with vitamin C to fight infection and break down mucus. Blackberry and grapefruit juices are used treat coughs and sore throats. Hot red peppers and spirulina are our best sources of the valuable immune supporter provitamin A, along with (in order) carrots, apricots, kale, collards, sweet potatoes, parsley, and spinach. Elderberry has remarkable properties that actually stop the flu virus from replicating and the lentinan content of the shiitake mushroom stimulates the production of the valuable immune protein interferon.[1]

Propolis, a mixture of the flora components gathered by bees, relieves sore throats and sinusitis, and prevents tonsillitis. It is rich in antioxidants and antibiotics that fight the viruses that cause the common cold.[2] Garlic's antiviral and antibacterial properties work to break down mucus in the sinuses. Garlic can help repel the initial infection and relieve many of the symptoms of the flu. Fenugreek and mustard seeds are folk remedies known to lessen some symptoms of the common cold.

Nutrients and Herbs That Help

Vitamin C is good for stimulating white blood cells, which helps you feel better quickly. Sucking on zinc lozenges is a proven remedy for sore throat and is capable of speeding up the recovery time from a cold.[3] Vitamin A boosts immunity to viruses that cause colds, and vitamin E helps protect the lungs against influenza.[4]

Echinacea, goldenseal, ginseng, astragalus, and schisandra are herbs that strengthen the immune system and fight off new infections.

Herbal remedies for the common cold are bayberry, blue vervain, catnip, chamomile, chickweed, feverfew, gentian, ginger, hyssop, licorice root, and St. John's wort. If fever is one of your symptoms, try lemon balm or lemon grass. Sinusitis is helped by alfalfa, black cohosh, olive leaf, and tea made with eyebright, goldenrod, or lavender.

For the flu, try aloe vera juice, astragalus, blue vervain, boneset, catnip, echinacea, goldenseal, skullcap, and tea made with lemon balm or linden flower. Green tea is also known to suppress the influenza viruses.[5]

Whether your sore throat is caused by viruses, bacteria, allergies, or pollutants, one thing for sure: you need soothing relief. Bayberry, black walnut, gotu kola, hawthorn berries, licorice, sage tea, and slippery elm help calm inflamed throats.

Many over-the-counter cough medicines contain chloroform, a cancer-causing agent. With so many herbs that can relieve coughs, there is no reason to subject your body to carcinogens contained in over-the counter cough medicines. Instead try a tea made with aniseed, comfrey, chickweed, licorice, or thyme. Other herbal remedies for coughs include slippery elm, mullein, black cohosh, blue vervain, red clover, and schisandra.

Herbs that act as decongestants and clear the sinuses include chili (cayenne), horseradish, ginger, and peppermint tea. Herbal steam treatments using lavender oil, tea tree oil, or eucalyptus relieve head congestion as well as stress that can weaken an immune system.

Gargling is another method that relieves sore throats, sinusitis, and the flu. Try gargling with a mixture of water and any of the following ingredients: apple cider vinegar, grapefruit seed extract, salt, marshmallow root, myrrh, or tea tree oil.[6]

Helpful Foods, Nutrients & Herbs

For more information, see "Nutrient Sources" & "Glossary"

Foods

Chicken Soup
Vegetable Broth
Lemon
Grapefruit
Acerola Cherries
Pineapple
Melons
Cabbage
Broccoli
Spinach
Blackberry Juice
Elderberry
Shiitake Mushrooms
Propolis
Red Peppers
Collards
Apricots
Kale
Carrots

Nutrients

Vitamin A
Grapefruit Seed Extract
Vitamin C
Vitamin E
Zinc
Cider Vinegar

Herbs

Garlic
Echinacea
Goldenseal
Ginseng
Astragalus
Bayberry
Ginger
Hyssop
Licorice Root
St. John's Wort
Lemon Grass
Olive Leaf
Aloe Vera Juice
Green Tea
Black Walnut
Hawthorn Berries
Slippery Elm
Aniseed
Comfrey
Thyme
Red Clover
Cayenne - Chili
Horseradish
Peppermint
Tea Tree Oil
Eucalyptus
Myrrh

Recipes

Vitamin A & C Potion

6 oz	Carrot Juice
1 oz	Red Pepper Juice, sweet
1 oz	Spinach Juice
1 oz	Collard Greens Juice
1 oz	Kale Juice
1 tsp	Spirulina or other Algae Powder

Vitamins A and C are the fundamental cold and flu fighters, and these foods are our richest sources of them. To see just how fantastic these sources are, refer to *"Nutrient Sources."* Experience how their freshness and living enzymes help to rebuild your immunity. Sip this juice slowly. It is not a cocktail, but a potent botanical medicine.

Decongest Teas

1 bag or ¼ inch	Ginger
1 bag or Tbsp	Licorice
1 bag or Tbsp	Peppermint

These are 3 separate teas. Ginger gets the blood circulating, warms you up, and reduces inflammation. Fresh ginger tea can be made by grating a ¼ inch piece into 1–1½ cups of water. Steep for about 15 minutes. Make enough so that you can refrigerate the left-over tea and quickly warm it up later.

Licorice is one of the best cough and bronchitis healers in the entire herbal pharmacopoeia. Fresh licorice tea can be made from natural licorice sticks (bark) by steeping a 2 inch piece in 1–1½ cups of water for about 15 minutes. Peppermint clears the respiratory passages and sinuses. Be sure to breathe in the healing aroma before sipping.

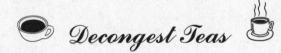

Citrus Flu Tonic

1	Grapefruit, juiced
2	Oranges, juiced
1	Lemon, juiced
1 tsp	Orange Rind Juice
1/4 inch	Ginger Root, minced
2 ml	Echinacea Liquid Extract (2 dropperfuls)
1 tsp	Royal Jelly

Cut the grapefruit and orange into eighths, but only after you scrape, scrape, scrape the pulp from inside the rind. Therein rests the miracle flavonoids and their magical curative powers. Buy organic fruits so you can include a bit of rind with its potent essential oils without the pesticides. Remove as many seeds as possible. Mince the fresh ginger and blend all ingredients until smooth. Royal jelly takes the edge off of the acidic flavor and, as a cousin to bee propolis, adds its own antibacterial capacity to suppress staphylococcus and streptococcus.[7] But you could substitute with honey. A morning drink.

Colic

See also Indigestion, Colon Problems, Nausea, and Diarrhea

Sometimes an otherwise healthy baby cries excessively for long periods of time for no apparent reason. The message may be that the baby is suffering discomfort in the abdomen because of intestinal distress. Colic is characterized by frequent attacks of abdominal pain in periodic waves and is generally experienced by newborn to three-month old infants. People other than infants experience colic, too. Unlike infant colic, when colic occurs in adults and children, it is often a symptom of disease or a more serious disorder.

Causes

Pinpointing the causes of infant colic is difficult, but it is commonly attributed to lactose intolerance and allergic reactions to formula or breast milk. A colicky baby might be sensitive to iron or certain foods in the breast-feeding mother's diet. Certain foods give babies gas or cause them to be constipated or experience diarrhea, just as they do children and adults. Another explanation for colic in infants is the immature development of their organs, which may explain why we seldom hear about colic in babies older than three months.

We naturally associate colic with babies, but all ages are susceptible when colic is caused by constipation or by an obstruction or irritation of the intestines or gall bladder. Adult colic is usually caused by gall stones, kidney stones, or appendicitis, while lead or zinc poisoning can cause both infant and adult colic.

Diet Suggestions

Colicky children and adults and breast-feeding mothers should try giving up dairy products and chocolate. Instead eat non-dairy foods rich in calcium and take calcium supplements. Avoid cruciferous vegetables (those in the cabbage family) to minimize discomfort caused by gas-producing foods. If the lactating mother avoids cruciferous vegetables, the breast-fed infant also avoids the possibility of gas that might cause colic. Drink lots of water and, of course, avoid alcohol, caffeine, and tobacco.

Foods That Help

Infants consume either infant formula or breast milk, diets that are obviously limited. However, a colicky baby may become less colicky drinking a soy-based formula instead of a formula made with cow's milk. Other alternatives to dairy that are available in natural food stores are rice, oat, and almond milks. For children and adults, colic relief can come from a diet that includes extra drinking water (2-3 quarts/day), bran from wheat, rice, or oats, and limiting animal fats. Chewing coriander and fennel seeds and eating onions are thought to relieve colic. Lactating mothers can get extra calcium from dark leafy vegetables, algae, tofu, sardines and salmon, all good substitutes for sometimes troublesome dairy products.

Helpful Foods, Nutrients & Herbs

For more information, see "Nutrient Sources" & "Glossary"

Foods

Soy-based Infant Formula
Rice or Oat 'Milk'
Wheat or Oat Bran
Barley
Coriander Seeds
Fennel Seeds
Onions
Tofu
Dark, Leafy Green Vegetables
Sardines
Salmon

Nutrients

Calcium

Herbs

Blue Cohosh
Cashew Leaf
Catnip
Chamomile
Ginger
Peppermint
Dill
Juniper Berries
Passion Flower

Nutrients and Herbs That Help

Taking calcium supplements instead of eating dairy products helps mothers and their breast-fed babies. Herbal teas can be calming and bring relief. Grandma's remedies included blue cohosh and catnip. Tea made with chamomile, ginger, and peppermint are known to calm the digestive track and ease the discomfort of colic. Dill, juniper berries, and passion flower tea have similar characteristics. Exercise caution when giving babies weak herbal teas either directly as a drink or indirectly through the mother's milk.

Recipes

Child & Adult Colic Teas

1 bag or tsp	Catnip
1 bag or tsp	Chamomile
1 bag or tsp	Peppermint
1 bag or ½ inch	Ginger Root
1 bag or tsp	Fennel Seeds, or
1 bag or tsp	Coriander Seeds, or
1 bag or tsp	Dill Seeds

To prepare the children's teas, steep a single tea bag for 5 minutes. Make sure the tea is warm and clear of sediment. Feed it to the infant warm using a dropper. Use only one tea at a time. Try to feed the infant 2-3 ounces. Older children should drink a full cup of hot tea and place a hot water bottle on their tummies.

For the adult, tea, fresh seeds, and herbs are always preferred over tea bags whenever possible. When using fresh ginger, grate a ¼-inch piece into 1–1½ cups of water. Steep the seeds and ginger root for about 15 minutes. Make enough so that you can refrigerate the leftover tea and quickly warm it up later. Either fennel, coriander, or dill seeds can be used alone with ginger in this recipe or all together. You can even steep the 3 seeds as a separate tea without ginger.

Stomach Greens

6 oz	Celery Juice
1 oz	Kale or Collard Greens Juice
1 oz	Spinach Juice
1 oz	Alfalfa Sprouts Juice
1 oz	Lemon Juice

In color therapy, green is the color that soothes and calms. So, it is no wonder that this green juice is also an excellent source of calcium, the mineral most important to a calm nervous system. This fresh, organic green vegetable juice is also soothing to the entire digestive tract while being nourishing and quieting. Sip this juice slowly. It is like medicine. Take your medicine and relax.

Colic Smoothie

½	Banana, yellow
1 small	Apple, cored and cut
2 Tbsp	Oat Bran
1+ cup	Soy, Rice, or Oat Milk

Let's face it, bananas smooth things out. Apples have many benefits for the whole digestive tract because of their high pectin content. Soy, rice, and oat milks make very balancing and soothing drinks. They are also easier to digest than milk and thus preferred for an upset stomach or when there is a possibility of lactose intolerance (milk sensitivity).

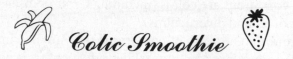

Colon Problems

Crohn's Disease, Irritable Bowel, Colitis, Diverticulitis

See also Constipation, Colic, Indigestion, Diarrhea, Parasites & Candida, Ulcers, Stress

As you might recall from high school biology, the colon, also known as the large intestine, is the final section of the digestive tract. The colon's job is to facilitate the absorption of water into the bloodstream and eliminate undigested food—a seemingly simple job description. Several conditions, however, can interfere with the smooth delivery of the stool from the small intestine to the rectum. Three such conditions are colitis (including Crohn's disease), irritable bowel syndrome, and diverticulitis.

Colitis refers to a group of conditions that involve inflammation of the small and/or large intestine. Ulcerative colitis is an inflammatory disease of the inner lining of the colon and rectum. Ulcerative colitis and Crohn's disease are similar in that both are forms of colitis and distinguished by an inflamed intestine. Crohn's disease, however, causes an inflammation that extends into the deeper layers of the small or large intestinal wall where it can cause more severe consequences.

Because inflammation causes the colon to empty more frequently, the most common symptom of both ulcerative colitis and Crohn's disease is diarrhea, sometimes severe and accompanied by abdominal cramps. Blood may also appear in the stools, especially with ulcerative colitis. Fever, fatigue, loss of appetite, and weight loss may accompany these symptoms. Sometimes, both ulcerative colitis and Crohn's disease patients experience constipation.

Diverticulitis is another colon condition that involves inflammation. Diverticula are small pocket-like outgrowths in the weaker portions of the colon walls. Initially harmless, the pockets become receptacles of undigested food and other irritants and can become infected. Constipation and diarrhea are symptoms of diverticulitis.

Unlike other colon problems, there is no intestinal inflammation associated with irritable bowel syndrome. Abnormal muscular contractions in the colon give irritable bowel syndrome its more common name, spastic colon. Spastic colon is characterized by bloating, gas, abdominal pain, and alternating diarrhea and constipation. Fever or bleeding are normally not characteristic of irritable bowel syndrome, but backaches and fatigue are common symptoms.

Causes

Food allergies and sensitivities and poor diets are highly suspicious causes of colon problems. Wheat and cow's milk are particularly troublesome allergens. Stress is also likely to initiate or aggravate colon problems, and an immune system disorder may be responsible for Crohn's disease. Infected debris caught in the pockets in the intestinal wall is the cause of diverticulitis.

Bacteria and parasites are also common causes of colon problems. Because the colon is filled with bacteria–both good and not so good–many colon problems are directly or indirectly caused by bacteria. Ironically, colitis can be caused by a cure for bacterial infection. Antibiotics taken to fight intestinal infections often kill the good bacteria while allowing the growth of more harmful bacteria.

Diet Suggestions

Increased fiber and lots of water are our passports to better colon health. To restore health and energy, eat a low-sugar, low-fat, vegetarian diet, rich in high-fiber grains, fruits, and vegetables. And to avoid aggravating the colon, eliminate most dairy products, sugar, caffeine, alcohol and baker's yeast.

Drinking lots of water is important, especially if you are increasing your fiber intake. But drink your water between meals. Liquids dilute digestive juices, which are responsible for transforming the food we eat into usable energy. Food that is not completely digested robs us of nutrients and can further annoy an irritated colon.

Of special note: Sufferers of diverticulitis should avoid eating nuts, seeds, and seedy fruits or vegetables, parts of which could get trapped and increase discomfort.

Foods That Help

Colon problems can make you feel bloated, uneasy, and fatigued. Eat comfort foods to nourish the body as well as calm the mind. Simply prepared vegetables, brown rice, oatmeal, and barley provide nutrients and fiber while working gently to treat either diarrhea or constipation, the two common symptoms of colon disorders.

Yoghurt with acidophilus is another good choice for calming and healing the colon. Yoghurt is especially helpful for treating problems caused by bacteria and parasites, and it can be blended with drinks for a satisfying tonic. Those on a dairyless diet can take rejuvelac, or other acidophilus-rich dairy alternatives (see recipes). Fennel is a nice addition for two reasons: it has a light anise flavor and fights detrimental bacteria.

Choose foods that replenish the nutrients lost through diarrhea yet are also gentle on the digestive tract. Algae, bananas, sweet potato, pumpkin, carrot, watercress, parsley, and spinach are soothing as well as high in iron, folic acid, and vitamins A and B12. Salmon and fish oils are good sources of vitamin D. If you suffer from colitis, try eating or juicing with papaya. Because papaya improves the digestion of dietary proteins, it is helpful for Crohn's disease patients.

Nutrients and Herbs That Help

If you have a problem with alternating diarrhea and constipation, try adding psyllium or flaxseeds to your diet to regulate bowel activity. This additional fiber with bulk-forming properties can move waste through the intestines to relieve constipation or, conversely, to absorb excess fluids and carry away the toxins that cause diarrhea.

Nutritional deficiency is common in Crohn's disease patients, because the body loses some of its ability to absorb nutrients from food. In particular, add supplements of vitamin D, zinc, folic acid, vitamin B12, and iron.[1] Vitamin A is also needed for the growth and repair of the cells that line both the small and large intestines.[2] Fish oils provide nutrients and encourage anti-inflammatory activity.

Chamomile tea is the herb of choice because of its many beneficial properties; it alleviates colitis, relieves gas and cramping, and cleanses the colon. Ginger and licorice root are also good colon cleaners. Other herbs with calming characteristics include dandelion, feverfew, red clover, yarrow, fennel, and cat's claw. Peppermint oil is especially helpful for calming colon spasms.

Helpful Foods, Nutrients & Herbs

For more information, see "Nutrient Sources" & "Glossary"

Foods

Brown Rice
Oatmeal, Oat Bran
Barley
Algae
Bananas
Cabbage
Sweet Potato
Pumpkin
Carrot
Watercress
Parsley
Spinach
Salmon
Yoghurt
Fennel
Papaya

Nutrients

Psyllium Seed
Flaxseed
Fish Oils
Zinc
Folic Acid
Vitamin A
Vitamin B12
Vitamin D
Iron

Herbs

Chamomile
Ginger
Licorice Root
Dandelion
Feverfew
Red Clover
Yarrow
Fennel Seed
Peppermint Oil
Cat's Claw
Wheatgrass
Barley Grass

Recipes

Rejuvelac - Nondairy Acidophilus

½ cup	Soft Wheat Berries
6–7 cups	Pure Water
	Makes approximately 2 quarts

This is homemade liquid acidophilus. While you can buy liquid acidophilus or powdered probiotics, it is always better and more economical when it is home-made. You may feel like you are brewing something here, and you are—good health! To get the full recipe for brewing rejuvelac, *see page 203. (For the full story on the many benefits of rejuvelac, read "Sproutman's Kitchen Garden Cookbook" by this author.)*

Colon Cleanser

2 Tbsp	Flaxseed
½	Banana, yellow
½	Papaya, ripe
2 Tbsp	Wheat or Barley Grass Powder
2 Tbsp	Rejuvelac or Acidophilus
1–2 cups	Pure Water

Put the dry flaxseeds in the blender and blend into a meal. Next add 1 cup of water and blend thoroughly. Add the papaya, banana and wheat or barley grass. Rejuvelac is a home-made, non-dairy acidophilus (see recipe above). If unavailable, use store-bought liquid acidophilus or probiotic powder. Acidophilus is also available in capsules. Either way, be sure this valuable aid is in your daily diet.

Intestinal Teas

1 bag or ¼ inch	Ginger Root
1 tsp	Honey
1 bag or tsp	Chamomile
1 bag or tsp	Peppermint

These are 2 separate teas. Fresh ginger is always best. Just grate a ¼ inch piece into 1–1½ cups of water. Steep for about 15 minutes. Make enough so that you can refrigerate the leftover tea and quickly warm it up later. Chamomile and peppermint are leaf teas that steep for just a few minutes. They soothe colitis, relieve gas and cramping. Drink these teas hot. Heat can be beneficial to healing because it increases circulation to the digestive tract.

Colon Tissue Repair

6 oz	Celery Juice
1 oz	Wheatgrass Juice
1 oz	Spinach Juice
1 oz	Cabbage Juice
1 oz	Parsley or Alfalfa Sprouts Juice

Fresh, organic green vegetable juice is one of the fastest ways to stimulate tissue healing. Colon problems all involve irritated or inflamed tissues. There is a great deal of research that demonstrates the ability of raw cabbage and wheat/barley grass to heal stomach ulcers and irritated tissues. This green juice will wash your entire intestinal tract with living enzymes. It is calming, healing, cleansing, and nourishing.

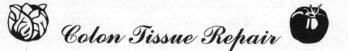

Constipation

See also Colon Problems, Colic, Hemorrhoids, Diarrhea, Ulcers, & Indigestion

What is the first thing that comes to mind? Prunes! Prunes or prune juice, the butt of many jokes, have been consumed typically to relieve constipation, a condition that results when the food we eat doesn't want to exit our lower gastrointestinal tract within a reasonable amount of time.

Most people experience an occasional bout of constipation that is easily corrected by diet and the passage of time. Others are not so fortunate and have to take measures to relieve the discomfort.

Most often, constipation is a result of another intestinal tract condition, such as irritable bowel, diverticulitis, candida, or a more general condition such as dehydration. Constipation can also be the hidden cause behind a myriad of health problems such as bloating, indigestion, colic, halitosis, hemorrhoids, anemia, nausea, depression, insomnia, vertigo, and, paradoxically, diarrhea.

Causes

Poor diet, inadequate exercise, too much iron, overuse of laxatives, and not enough fiber, water, or exercise can all lead to constipation. Processed foods and animal fats lack enough fiber and bulk to move the food through the system effectively. On top of this, we drink too little water. Altogether, this combination is the American recipe for constipation.

Other causes of constipation include pregnancy and some pharmaceutical drugs. Pregnant women can become constipated because of hormonal changes and a growing baby that presses against the intestines. One side effect of some medications is constipation, often exacerbated by dehydration, which is yet another side effect of certain medications. Less frequently, constipation may be caused by abnormalities or obstructions of the digestive system. You should check with your doctor if you experience prolonged constipation and pain.

Often laxatives, intended to relieve constipation, can open the dam temporarily, but overuse can actually increase constipation, because the digestive tract becomes "lazy" and begins to rely on laxatives to do what should occur naturally.

Diet Suggestions

Diet is the best approach to preventing constipation. Drink plenty of fluids and eat unprocessed foods, preferably from plant sources. These strategies stimulate the intestinal muscles leading to more frequent eliminations. A diet rich in fiber from whole grains, bran, and seeds helps move the intestine's contents on its journey. Be sure your diet includes lots of friendly bacteria, also known as probiotics, lactobacillus, acidophilus, bifidus, bulgaricus, and so on. These have wide-reaching health benefits, since they help maintain the proper balance of flora in the intestinal terrain. Natural dairy yoghurts and clabbered milk products are traditional sources and so are non-dairy products such as nut and seed yoghurts, rejuvelac, sauerkraut, sour dough breads, amazake rice drinks, umeboshi (salty plum), and soy foods such as miso, tamari and tempeh. You should include magnesium-rich foods in your diet, because this mineral has properties that keep the intestines hydrated and also help intestinal muscles to contract (push). Magnesium oxide supplements are very effective.

It is often an unmentionable subject, but let's face it: The human intestinal tract is a plumbing system. What happens when the plumbing in your house backs up? A cesspool! A detoxification diet is very helpful for relieving long-term constipation and for cleansing the body of toxins that accumulate in the retained stools.

Foods That Help

Lots of raw fruits and vegetables, including the venerable prune, relieve and prevent constipation by providing water and fiber for bulk. Juicing provides liquid for hydration, minerals for intestinal contraction, and enzymes for nourishment and detoxification. Juicing with apples and chlorophyll-rich, leafy green vegetables and sprouts, aid digestion and help prevent constipation. Beetroot and cabbage juice alleviate constipation, and carrots help soften the stool, making it easier for it to absorb water and move. Apples are a good ingredient in juices for relieving constipation, because they give a light natural sweetness that balances the stronger tasting vegetable juices. They also contain pectin, a thickening agent used in food processing, and sorbitol, a sugar with natural laxative properties.

Wheat, rice, and oat brans, whole grains, legumes, and seeds, all add bulk, fiber, and nutrition to a diet designed to prevent and relieve constipation. The husks of psyllium seeds offer proven relief by adding bulk to stools.[1] It is the primary ingredient in the best-selling drug store constipation remedy. Flaxseed achieves the same results but is milder and it protects us from colon and other cancers.[2] Your diet should also include magnesium-rich foods such as figs, apricots, lemons, apples, wheat grass, alfalfa, legumes, nuts, kelp, sunflower seeds, sesame seeds, spinach, and brewer's yeast. Many of these foods have additional therapeutic properties that are advantageous for our general well-being as well as relieving constipation.

Drinking herbal teas is an effective way to increase fluid intake while delivering natural laxatives that relieve constipation. Teas made from nettle, raspberry leaf, and chickweed have been used to relieve constipation. Drink green tea, but avoid too much black tea, since it contains tannin, a known cause of constipation.

Nutrients and Herbs That Help

Laxatives are used to stimulate intestinal action or to provide water-absorbing bulk to stimulate intestinal action. The laxative properties of certain herbs serve both purposes. The next time you are at the drugstore, read the labels on over-the-counter laxatives; many contain the herbs we mention. Some drugstore laxatives, however, also contain ingredients that can deplete the body of essential vitamins and minerals. Even all-natural, herbal remedies can have very strong effects, so use all laxatives sparingly and cautiously.

The more mild herbal laxatives that stimulate your intestines include fo-ti, dandelion, and cascara sagrada. Senna is a stronger herbal stimulant, which boosts peristaltic motion by causing the intestinal wall to expel it. Although it is a natural herb, its action is that of a chemical irritant, so consider your alternatives.

Another aid for constipation is castor oil. The mere mention of the word caused our grandparents to flee from their mother's arms. Castor oil lubricates the intestinal walls, allowing the stool to pass more easily through the colon. It relieves congestion so effectively that it is often used to induce overdue pregnancies.

Take additional vitamin C to help move stools through your system more quickly. And vitamin B5 helps to establish more consistent rhythmic action within the intestine walls. Take FOS (fructo-oligosaccharides) to nourish the production of friendly bacteria (lactobacillus).

Helpful Foods, Nutrients & Herbs

For more information, see "Nutrient Sources" & "Glossary"

Foods

Water	Watermelon	Wheat Grass
Apples	Barley	Alfalfa
Prunes & Apricots	Oat & Wheat Bran	Leafy Green Vegetables
Grapefruits, Lemons	Psyllium & Flaxseed	Legumes
Figs, Plums	Sunflower & Sesame Seeds	Nuts
Umeboshi		Kelp
Amazake Rice Drinks		

Nutrients

Magnesium	Olive Oil	Vitamin C
Chlorophyll	Brewer's Yeast	FOS
Castor Oil	Vitamin B5	

Herbs

Cascara Sagrada	Raspberry Leaf Tea	Fo-ti
Chickweed Tea	Green Tea	Senna
Nettle Tea	Dandelion	

Recipes

Rejuvelac - Nondairy Acidophilus

½ cup	Soft Wheat Berries
6–7 cups	Pure Water
	Makes approximately 2 quarts

This is homemade liquid acidophilus. You may feel like you are brewing something here, and you are—good health! First, you will need a half gallon jar, and a sprout bag or sprouting jar. (The author is the inventor of the *Flax Sprout Bag,* see *"Resources."*) Although rejuvelac can be made with unsprouted grain, sprouting the wheat brings a wealth of vitamins and enzymes to the water. While you can use common hard wheat, the sweeter soft wheat is preferred. *(For the full rejuvelac recipe, see "Indigestion.")*

Meyerowitz Water Cleanse

1 Liter	Pure Water. Drink in 20 minutes

This is the author's daily constitutional drink. When it comes to constipation, water is the ultimate solution. Unfortunately, we don't drink enough of it. Water is the river of life. Sometimes, a dam happens, but a good rain washes it away. Take a tip from nature and wash your troubles away. Always drink the purest water you can find. Get rid of the microwave and put a distiller or water purifying filter in its place. Timing is everything in this recipe. This much water (a little more than a quart), flushes the intestinal tract from top to bottom. It is an inexpensive self-help tool that keeps the plumbing clear, the body hydrated and all things running smoothly. Water is one of our top three fundamental healers (along with oxygen and exercise). Don't neglect it.

Basic Nut And Seed Yoghurt

1 cup	Cashews
1 cup	Pure Water

The instructions for making nut and seed yoghurt are simple, but the technique of refining a batch to taste just the way you want it is akin to that of making a fine wine. It is an art for which experience is the best teacher. Although, this recipe works for a variety of nuts and seeds, it is best to start with sunflower seeds, cashews, or almonds. This recipe uses the voluptuous, milky colored cashew.

Blend the cashews with pure water until smooth. If you achieve the consistency of heavy cream, you have successfully added the proper water-to-nuts ratio. Pour into a pint jar and cover with a cheese cloth, towel, napkin, or other loose fitting cover allowing for air transfer. Set jar in a warm place where the yoghurt temperature can heat up to 90°-100° F. It is done when the taste is tart or sour, approximately 6 to 8 hours. (For more about nut and seed yoghurts, see *"Power Drinks Basics"* or read *Sproutman's Kitchen Garden Cookbook* by this author.)

Slippery Road

2 Tbsp	Flaxseed
1	Apple, cut and cored
½	Papaya or Banana
2 Tbsp	Rejuvelac, or liquid/powdered Acidophilus
1–2 cups	Pure Water

Put the dry flaxseeds in the blender and blend into a meal. Then add 1 cup of water and blend thoroughly. Next, add the papaya or banana and chopped apple. Rejuvelac is a home-made, non-dairy acidophilus (see recipe above). Alternatively, add store bought liquid acidophilus or other probiotic powder. Acidophilus is available as a powder and in capsules. Be sure to make it a part of your daily diet.

Let this mixture sit in the blender for 10 minutes prior to drinking. This allows time for the flaxseed to absorb its water before you take it. Add one cup of water to start. Add more water, if it becomes too viscous, and blend to a thick shake consistency.

Rapid Transit

1–2 cups	Pure Water
2 Tbsp	Oat, Wheat, or Rice Bran
½	Apple, cut and cored
2 Tbsp	Wheatgrass or Barley Grass Powder
2 Tbsp	Acidophilus liquid, or 1 Tbsp Powder
2 Tbsp	Sunflower Seeds
Pinch	Stevia (optional)

Gotta keep things moving! Let's face it, everything has a schedule, even our insides. If you have ever had to call your plumber because of a clogged pipe, then you know just how much trouble this kind of thing can be. Nobody likes a cesspool. So, let's get with the program and have one of these energizing and cleansing drinks every morning. After all, the best way to get up and go, is to get up and GO!

Blend the bran, water and apple. Oat bran is finer than wheat bran and smoother on the intestines, although the latter is a good substitute. Let the bran sit in the blender and absorb the water for 10 minutes before drinking. It should be the consistency of a thick shake. Wheatgrass and barley grass powder add soothing chlorophyll to the intestinal walls, and they detoxify the liver. If you like to chew, add the sunflower seeds last and stir rather than blend them in.

Depression

See also Stress, Fatigue, Power Drinks for the Mind

People are such emotionally fragile beings. It doesn't take much to bring on feelings of sadness or unhappiness. True depression, however, assumes many forms with an equal variety of causes. The first step is to identify the type of depression you have and its cause. Once you do, using the right nutrition, diet, and herbs will help.

Endogenous depression is brought on by chemical imbalances and accounts for about 40% of all cases of depression. Clinical depression is described as feelings that overwhelm and prevent you from performing daily functions. Typical symptoms include a change in appetite or sleep patterns, fatigue, loss of interest in common activities, guilt, excessive worry, lack of focus, and suicidal thoughts. Manic depression, also called bi-polar disorder, is marked by alternating episodes of mania and depression that is equally debilitating.

Minor depression may be less disturbing, but it still interferes with normal life functions. Symptoms include pessimism, self-imposed isolation, low self-esteem and lack of confidence, fatigue, excessive anger, lamenting the past, lack of concentration, and impaired decision-making ability.

Reactive depression is the most common and easily explained, because it is an event-driven response. The death of a loved one, a serious illness or accident, or a diagnosis of serious disease are triggers. Depression related to giving birth and pre-menstruation are somewhat similar types of depression tied to a recognizable event.

Depression can block creativity and cause fatigue, loss of appetite, insomnia, high blood pressure, and male impotence.

Causes

Recognized causes of depression include nutritional deficiencies, chemical imbalances, allergies, anxiety, stress, events, and diseases such as AIDS, chronic fatigue syndrome, hypothyroidism, diabetes, and rheumatoid arthritis. Depression can also be caused by environmental toxins and drug abuse, whether prescribed (oral contraceptives, for example), or recreational (alcohol, amphetamines, and cocaine). Nutritional factors that may account for some forms of depression include a deficiency of vitamins, minerals, and amino acids, and an excess of saturated fatty acids and sugar.

Physiological as well as psychological factors can cause depression, and nutritional and lifestyle changes help alleviate depression triggered by both factors.

Diet Suggestions

Diet and nutrition are key factors in achieving a sense of well-being. A good argument for a low-fat, plant protein diet is documented in scientific research that suggests that a diet high in polyunsaturated fatty acids relative to omega-3 unsaturated fatty acids is a risk factor for depression.[1] Limiting or eliminating sugar and caffeine can also help in relieving depression symptoms.[2] Stay clear of processed foods and artificial ingredients such as aspartame, which has been linked to depression because of its methanol content. Use complex carbohydrates, high-fiber foods, raw vegetables and fruits, and their juices to help relieve depression.

Foods That Help

Foods highest in super-unsaturated fatty acids are oily fish such as anchovy, herring, mackerel, salmon, sardine, swordfish, trout, and tuna, as well as cod liver oil. Flaxseed oil is the best source for vegetarians, followed by the oils from hemp, pumpkin seeds, chia, canola, and wheat germ.

Vegetables and grains with high mineral and B-vitamin content (including folic acid, a well-documented "happy" vitamin) can help relieve depression and restore a sense of well-being. For help with depression, eat or juice the following: wheatgrass, wheat germ, alfalfa sprouts, soybeans, legumes, nuts, spinach, kale, brewer's yeast, spirulina, apricot, bananas, cantaloupe, carrots, cabbage, sweet potato, cauliflower, and broccoli. Many of these foods are high in amino acids such as tyrosine, which helps relieve depression.[3] Other foods high in tyrosine include bananas, yogurt, apples, strawberries, beets, watercress, fennel, onion, and garlic. Mango and cashews are high in anacardic acid, which may help relieve depression.

Nutrients and Herbs That Help

Try to avoid the side-effects of antidepressant drugs by substituting natural remedies in the form of food and supplements. Nutrients and herbs can also be helpful for augmenting antidepressant drugs, but check with your doctor before changing your prescribed medications.

Give your system plenty of minerals, including iron, bromine, calcium, lithium, magnesium, potassium, and zinc. Vitamins are equally helpful. Various B-vitamin deficiencies have been linked to depression. Vitamin B6 and B12 have helped many, including women taking oral contraceptives and those experiencing depression related to premenstrual syndrome (PMS). Folic acid especially helps alcoholics and those who are manic-depressive. Vitamin C has been found to be lacking in many victims of depression.[4]

Amino acids are effective for treating depression, especially cases related to women taking oral contraceptives. In addition to tyrosine, L-Phenylalanine and D-Phenylalanine are amino acids with mood-altering properties.

Hormonal imbalances have also been identified as causes of depression, and DHEA may be effective for improving some symptoms, especially for middle-aged and elderly people.[5] Pregnenolone and natural progesterone relieve and help prevent depression in some women.

A promising natural alternative to antidepressant drugs has won favor with both patients and health professionals. S-adenosylmethionine (SAMe) has been used successfully to treat most forms of depression, including major depression, postpartum depression and depression related to drug dependence (though not manic depression). In fact, SAMe has worked better than pharmaceutical antidepressant drugs in relieving some cases of depression. It works quickly and also generates beneficial side-effects in contrast to some of the detrimental side-effects of pharmaceutical antidepressant drugs. SAMe is an antioxidant that can ease the pain associated with conditions other than depression. Taking SAMe supplements is the best way to get quick-acting, noticeable therapeutic benefits.[6]

The star herb for helping treat depression is Saint John's wort. This herb has several qualities that significantly relieve depression. Its link with serotonin is similar to that of Prozac, a leading antidepressant pharmaceutical drug. The flavonol and hypericin in Saint John's wort protects against the toxic enzymes associated with depression.[7]

Ginkgo biloba's ability to improve blood circulation to the brain helps treat depression. Passion flower and valerian are calming to the nervous system. Other herbs that have positive effects on depression are cat's claw, the ginsengs, gotu kola, licorice, and the aromatic oil of lavender rubbed on the forehead.

Helpful Foods, Nutrients & Herbs

For more information, see "Nutrient Sources" & "Glossary"

Foods

Oily Fish	Spirulina	Sweet Potato
Wheatgrass	Apricot	Cauliflower
Wheat Germ	Banana	Broccoli
Alfalfa Sprouts	Yoghurt	Beets
Soybeans	Apples	Watercress
Legumes	Mango	Fennel
Nuts	Cashews	Onion
Spinach	Cantaloupe	Garlic
Kale	Carrots	Barley Grass
Brewer's Yeast	Cabbage	

Nutrients

Iron	Zinc	L-phenylalanine
Bromine	Vitamin B6	D-phenylalanine
Calcium	Vitamin B12	DHEA
Lithium	Folic Acid	Pregnenolone
Magnesium	Vitamin C	Progesterone
Potassium	Tyrosine	SAMe

Herbs

St. John's Wort	Valerian	Ginseng
Ginkgo Biloba	Lavender Oil	Gotu Kola
Passion Flower	Cat's Claw	Licorice

Recipes

I'm So Glad

½	Banana
1 cup	Yoghurt
1 small	Apple, cut and cored
1 tsp	Flax or Wheat Germ Oil
To taste	Pure Water

Yoghurt, bananas, and apples are some of the best sources of the amino acid tyrosine, which according to the *American Journal of Psychiatry*, successfully treats some forms of depression. Flaxseed and wheat germ oils are the highest plant sources of omega-3 super-unsaturated fatty acids, which are needed to counteract depression. Blend all the ingredients together and thin with a small amount of water if too thick.

Heavenly Peace

1 cup	Whole Cashews
2 cups	Cantaloupe or Mango, chopped
2 Tbsp	Wheat Germ
To taste	Pure Water

Cashews, mango, and cantaloupe are high in anacardic acid, an organic acid that has been used as an antidepressive. Wheat germ is the second best dietary source of folic acid (after brewer's yeast) and is one of the best sources of acetylcholine, which is crucial for the health of nerve fibers and the transmission of nerve impulses. It is also high in energy (calories) and the minerals chromium and iron. Blend all the ingredients together and thin with a small amount of water if too thick.

Liquid Pro-Zap

1 cup	Apple Juice
1 Tbsp	Brewer's Yeast
1 Tbsp	Blue-Green, Spirulina, or Chlorella Algae
1 Tbsp	Lecithin Granules
1 tsp	Ginseng Granules or Extract

Pharmaceutical drugs are only an invention of the 20th century. As far back as the ancient Greeks and Chinese, medicines were derived from plants. This liquid plant medicine contains lots of antidepressive compounds in the form of vitamin B12, spirulina, and brewer's yeast. Algaes are superb antioxidants and our best sources of vitamin B12 and nucleic acids, crucial for mental acuity and alertness. Lecithin is the best source of the B vitamin factor choline, which is involved in the manufacture of myelin sheaths for a healthy nervous system. The ginsenosides in ginseng fight fatigue, increase stamina, and feed the nervous system.

While this drink may give you a zap, it is not a drug. Herbs and foods nourish you for the long term in a way that enables higher functioning. Chemicals may spike you up but keep you dependent. Real improvement takes time. Regular consumption of the good nutrients in this drink and others will produce results.

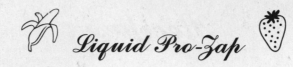

Diabetes

See also Hypoglycemia

A properly functioning body converts food into glucose, a form of sugar that fuels the body's cells. To be effective, however, glucose must be delivered into the cells from the bloodstream. Diabetes is the name for a category of diseases in which the body makes glucose but has trouble getting it into the cells. High blood sugar–the accumulation of too much glucose in the bloodstream–stems from a lack of insulin, the hormone that triggers the cell to accept glucose.

There are two major categories of diabetes. Type 1 diabetes, also called juvenile-onset or insulin-dependent diabetes, results when no insulin is produced. Without regular injections of insulin and proper diet, type 1 diabetics would not survive, because too much glucose would remain in the bloodstream and lead to a diabetic coma. By contrast, the pancreas of type 2 diabetics produces some insulin, but not enough to properly convert food into energy. Also called adult-onset or non-insulin-dependent diabetes, type 2 is much more prevalent than type 1 and can be controlled with diet and exercise.

Hypoglycemia is a blood sugar related condition that arises when blood sugar levels are too low rather than too high.

Causes

Age, heredity, obesity and diet can all lead to diabetes. Sometimes pregnancy can cause temporary diabetes. You cannot change your heredity or your birthday, but you certainly can change your diet. Avoid highly refined and high-fat foods, since they can lead to unhealthy blood sugar levels and obesity.

Unbalanced blood sugar levels can also cause other problems, such as infection, heart disease, circulation problems in the legs, depression, and damage to the kidney, eye, and nervous system. Maintaining proper blood sugar levels can also reduce the risk of these diseases.

Type 1 & 2 diabetics should not consume fish oil supplements because excessive accumulation of it interferes with the ability of the pancreas to produce insulin. The herb ephedra (Chinese ma huang) should also not be used by diabetics, since it can interfere with proper metabolism and further complicate diabetic problems.

Diet Suggestions

Diabetics rely heavily on diet to adjust their blood sugar levels. For most diabetics, type 1, 2, or other types, a high-protein diet is beneficial, but eating protein from animal sources is counter-productive. High fat intake increases the risk of cardiovascular disease and cholesterol, and prevents glucose from getting into the cells where it is most beneficial. Instead, a low-fat, high-protein vegetarian diet is best, including lots of legumes and fresh vegetables, especially those with low natural sugar content.

Foods That Help

Diabetics should look for foods that lower blood sugar levels. These include guava, carob, fenugreek seeds, and bitter melon. Legumes are excellent insulin regulators, and the protein provided by kidney beans and lentils are especially helpful. Flaxseed oil lowers insulin requirements, and evening primrose oil, borage, and black current seed oils, relieve symptoms of diabetic neuropathy and diabetes mellitus because of their high gamma-linolenic acid (GLA) content. Diabetics have difficulty in converting linoleic acid to GLA.[1]

Anecdotal evidence suggests that asparagus juice and celery juice help to restore normal blood sugar levels, as do Jerusalem artichokes, onions, and spinach. Brewer's yeast, a significant source of chromium, helps regulate blood sugar levels, whether too high or too low. Epidemiological evidence suggests that consuming a vegetarian diet may prevent type 2 diabetes.[2] Scientific research indicates that gymnema sylvestre, a tropical herb from India that aids insulin-producing cells in the pancreas, can prevent as well as relieve type 1 and 2 diabetes.[3]

Nutrients and Herbs That Help

Herbs are effective for treating diabetes and other diseases to which diabetics are prone. Agrimony has characteristics that prevent as well as control diabetes. Several herbs–alfalfa, blue cohosh, cat's claw, dandelion, the ginsengs, goldenseal, and stevia–help diabetics by lowering blood sugar levels. Bilberry helps alleviate the eye damage that sometimes occurs with diabetes.

Minerals such as chromium, magnesium, vanadium, copper, manganese, potassium, and zinc are important additions to a diet for controlling diabetes. Biotin and vitamins C and E are known to help diabetics regulate blood sugar levels. And vitamin B12 helps prevent the cardiovascular diseases that sometimes afflict diabetics. Lipoic acid helps counteract neuropathy and cataracts, two conditions that typically affect diabetics. Coenzyme Q10 is known to relieve diabetes as well as other consequences of diabetes.

Helpful Foods, Nutrients & Herbs

For more information, see "Nutrient Sources" & "Glossary"

Foods

Guava
Carob
Fenugreek Seeds
Bitter Melon
Kidney Beans
Jerusalem Artichoke
Flaxseed Oil
Asparagus Juice
Celery Juice
Onions
Spinach
Gymnema Sylvestre
Fish
Brewer's Yeast
Lentils

Nutrients

Chromium
Magnesium
Vanadium
Copper
Manganese
Potassium
Zinc
Coenzyme Q10
Vitamin C
Vitamin E
Biotin

Herbs

Alfalfa Sprouts
Aloe Vera Juice
Agrimony
Blue Cohosh
Evening Primrose Oil
Dandelion
Ginsengs
Goldenseal
Stevia
Cat's Claw
Borage Oil
Black Current Seed Oil

Recipes

Sugar Leveler

4 oz	Tomato Juice
2 oz	Celery Juice
2 oz	Spinach Juice
2 oz	Jerusalem Artichoke Juice
1 oz	Asparagus Juice
1 oz	Alfalfa Sprouts Juice
1 oz	Lemon Juice
2 Tbsp	Tamari
1 Tbsp	Flaxseed Oil

This powerful elixir is strong in taste but loaded with the healing potential to keep your blood sugar balanced. Pick ripe tomatoes since they are the major flavor here and make a better tasting drink. This drink will still be potent medicine, even if you do not have every ingredient.

Insulin Regulator Tea

1 bag or tsp	Cat's Claw *(Una-de-Gato)*
1 bag or tsp	Asiatic Ginseng

Use one teaspoon each of the loose, dried herb or one tea bag each. Asiatic ginseng is the panax variety used in insulin biosynthesis research. Cat's Claw is a high-climbing vine native to the highlands of the Peruvian Amazon. The root contains a higher proportion of the active alkaloids and phytosterols than the inner bark. Between drinks you can supplement with 500mg capsules of cat's claw and 100–200mg capsules of Asiatic ginseng standardized with at least 7% ginsenosides.

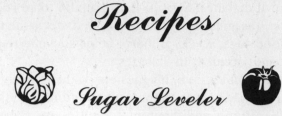

Pancreas Rebuilder

1 cup	Apple Juice
2 Tbsp	Sunflower Seeds
1 Tbsp	Brewer's Yeast
1 ml	Gymnema Sylvestre Extract
½ tsp	Vitamin C Crystals
1 tsp	Flaxseed Oil
To taste	Pure Water

Gymnema sylvestre is a very beneficial herb for diabetics that has the ability to regenerate the islets of Langerhans in the pancreas. These islets are responsible for the production and secretion of Insulin. This blended drink uses 1 milliliter of the liquid extract, but you can also supplement with 200–500mg capsules. Brewer's yeast is our best source of chromium, the primary mineral responsible for regulating blood sugar levels. Sunflower seeds and brewer's yeast are excellent sources of zinc, which is usually deficient in diabetes patients.

Place these ingredients in your blender one at a time in the order listed and blend. Add water only if necessary to thin out your drink.

Energizer for Diabetics

by Dr. Allan Sosin, M.D. and Diane Lara

2 cups	Almond Milk
4 Tbsp	Soy Protein Powder, unsweetened
2 Tbsp	Flaxseed, freshly ground
2 tsp	Vanilla
1 tsp	Cardamom Powder
½ tsp	Cinnamon Powder
¼ tsp	Nutmeg
To taste	Stevia

Blend all ingredients together. Chill and serve. Dr. Allan Sosin is Medical Director of *Whitaker Wellness Institute* in Newport Beach, CA.

Diarrhea

See also Constipation, Colon Problems, Colic, Indigestion, Parasites & Candida, Ulcers, Stress

Our intestinal tract is a roller coaster ride with hundreds of twists and turns, more than any amusement park could hope to build. In some of those dark corners lurks some nasty foreign matter and bothersome organisms that can only cause trouble. Should they become too populous, they will attempt to dominate the intestinal terrain. Our body fights back with a cascading response that like an internal earthquake or a great flood, purges the evil within.

It's a natural response. Diarrhea is one of the body's ways of ridding itself of toxins and foreign materials that cause irritation and inflammation. The intestines secrete extra fluids and the result is cramping and the loose, watery, frequent stools characteristic of diarrhea.

An occasional loose bowel movement is not serious, but frequent loose or watery stools need attention, especially when there is a considerable amount of water passed in the evacuation. Diarrhea affects people of all ages, and is particularly serious for the very young and the elderly. Because this condition often causes dehydration, low blood sugar and chemical imbalances, early treatment can prevent complications.

Causes

Diarrhea is really a side-effect of other conditions. It can be caused by detrimental bacterial and viral infection, parasites, fungi, food poisoning and diseases such as Crohn's disease, ulcerative colitis, irritable bowel syndrome, diverticulitis, cystic fibrosis, and HIV. Bacteria and viruses can be picked up from infected people or through contaminated food and water, which is often the case for travelers. Allergies and food sensitivities can trigger a variety of symptoms, including diarrhea. Lactose (milk) intolerance is one of the most common causes of diarrhea. Other causes include anxiety, mineral imbalances, herbs, and pharmaceuticals. Check with your pharmacist or doctor when experiencing diarrhea after taking a new drug.

Another cause of diarrhea worth mentioning is overly aggressive treatment for constipation. Excess amounts of fiber, vitamin C, magnesium, or herbs taken to relieve constipation can actually work too well and cause diarrhea.

Diet Suggestions

The primary role of nutrition in the treatment of diarrhea is to provide substances that firm up watery stool and to prevent depletions of fluid, sodium, and potassium. Diets consisting of bulk-forming foods and lots of clear liquids to replace lost fluids can help alleviate diarrhea. Coffee, most dairy products, and fats should be avoided, because they can irritate the delicate intestinal lining and provoke rather than cure diarrhea.

When all else fails, fasting is the best way to calm the intestinal tract and stop the discharge. Just skipping a couple of meals and snacks is often enough to quiet the system and reduce the irritation. A longer fast may be needed in more severe cases. Be sure to drink plenty of green (calming) vegetable juices and pure water to insure good hydration.

Foods That Help

Most cases of diarrhea are mitigated by eating foods that add bulk to thicken the stool, such as rice, oatmeal, black beans, bananas, and bran. Yoghurt and other foods that contain active beneficial bacteria, such as lactobacillus, acidophilus, bifidus, and bulgaricus, are essential to ensure a healthy intestinal terrain. They are especially helpful in diarrhea caused by foreign bacteria such as Montezuma's revenge. Fennel, radish, black currants, blackberry juice, and blueberries also help neutralize such "unfriendly" bacteria. While yoghurt and clabbered milk products are traditional sources of friendly bacteria, you can also find them in non-dairy foods such as nut and seed yoghurts, rejuvelac, sauerkraut, and umeboshi (Japanese plum). Fermented soy foods such as miso, tamari, and tempeh, and amazake rice drinks are cultured with friendly bacteria, although they may not be active.

Potassium and zinc are lost during bouts of diarrhea. To restore these essential minerals, eat brewer's yeast, pumpkin and sunflower seeds, ginger, sea vegetables, bananas, soy foods, and almonds, all of which also have bulk-forming properties.

Nutrients and Herbs That Help

Curiously, some remedies for constipation also work for treating diarrhea. Additional fiber with bulk-forming properties can move waste through the intestines to relieve constipation or conversely, to absorb excess fluids and carry away the toxins that cause diarrhea; psyllium and flaxseeds are excellent sources of fiber for either purpose.

Drink herbal and green teas to replenish lost fluids and to add other helpful nutrients to a system disturbed by diarrhea. Blackberry leaf, ginger, and chamomile teas calm the intestinal tract.

Herbs containing tannins, such as blackberry and blueberry leaves, carob, and yellow dock, are helpful, because tannins act as binders. Other helpful herbs include hawthorn berries, bayberry, black walnut, paprika, peppermint, and slippery elm.

Since diarrhea can cause excessive excretion of potassium, sodium, zinc, folic acid, and vitamins A and K, it may be helpful to temporarily increase these supplements.

Healthy intestinal walls are crucial for preventing and curing diarrhea. Colostrum, available in the form of powder, capsules, or tablets, improves the health of the intestinal wall, as does folic acid, which helps repair wall damage caused by acute diarrhea.[1] Supplements of acidophilus or other probiotics (beneficial bacteria) are available in capsules, powder, or fresh liquid acidophilus. They replenish an intestinal tract that has been stripped of beneficial bacteria. Brewer's yeast also helps restore balance in the intestinal tract as well as provide a healthy dose of potassium and zinc.

Charcoal and bentonite clay are highly effective for treating diarrhea. Activated charcoal is very porous and attracts and absorbs gases and toxins as it travels throughout the intestines. It is available in tablets and capsules. Bentonite clay is a colloidal liquid that works similarly to charcoal. Both have a stabilizing and quieting effect on the bowel. Neither is absorbed by the body. However, both can absorb nutrients from your meal as well as toxins so take them on an empty stomach. Take them preferably in the morning or evening, or 2 hours before or 4 hours after meals.

Helpful Foods, Nutrients & Herbs

For more information, see "Nutrient Sources" & "Glossary"

Foods

Almonds	Fennel	Sauerkraut
Amazake Rice	Miso	Sea Vegetables
Bananas	Nut and Seed Yoghurts	Sunflower Seed
Black Beans	Oatmeal	Tempeh
Black Currants	Pumpkin Seed	Tofu
Blackberry Juice	Radish	Umeboshi
Blueberries	Rejuvelac	Yoghurt, active
Clabbered Milk	Rice	

Nutrients

Acidophilus	Flaxseed	Psyllium Seed
Bentonite Clay	Folic Acid	Vitamin A
Brewer's Yeast	Potassium	Vitamin K
Charcoal	Sodium	Zinc
Colostrum	Probiotics	

Herbs

Black Walnut	Chamomile	Bayberry
Paprika	Ginger	Peppermint
Blackberry Leaves	Green Tea	Slippery Elm
Blueberry Leaves	Hawthorn Berries	Yellow Dock
Carob		

Recipes

Smooth-It-Out Smoothie

1–2 cups	Pure Water
1	Banana
½ cup	Blueberries
2 Tbsp	Yoghurt, with active cultures
1 Tbsp	Slippery Elm Powder
1 Tbsp	Carob Powder
2 Tbsp	Oat Bran
1 Tbsp	Brewer's Yeast

Pour 1 cup of pure water into your blender; add the first powders and blend. If you do not have one of the powders, you can make the drink without it. Then add the banana, blueberries, and yoghurt. Last, add enough water to achieve a thick shake consistency.

Parasite Clean Up

2 cups	Pure Water
4 Tbsp	Bentonite Liquid
1 tsp	Honey or pinch of Stevia Powder

This fantastic natural clay absorbs the toxic chemical byproducts, quiets the bowel, and slows down elimination. Put simply, it binds. But, it will also absorb good nutrients, too, so keep those expensive vitamins and health foods away for at least 2 hours after downing. Bentonite is best taken on an empty stomach or upon awakening or retiring. To make your own, follow this recipe. Bentonite powder can be ordered from your pharmacist. Stevia or honey improve its clay-like taste. Ready-made liquid bentonite is also available at your health food store. *(See Resources.)*

Green Calm

3 oz	Spinach Juice
3 oz	Celery Juice
2 oz	Cabbage Juice
2 oz	Cucumber Juice
1 oz	Green Pepper Juice
1 oz	Alfalfa Sprouts Juice

This juice binds and calms the entire digestive tract in addition to replenishing the vital electrolytes that are lost in diarrhea. For ease of juicing, alternate the leafy spinach and cabbage with the stiffer celery, cukes, and peppers. Best to take on an empty stomach.

Quiet Stomach Teas

1 bag or tsp	Chamomile
1 bag or tsp	Green Tea

Steep your tea for 3 minutes following the instructions in the *Power Drinks Basics* chapter. Sip slowly and relax.

Stomach Heater Tea

10	Peppermint Leaves, crushed
¼ inch	Ginger Root, grated

You can use tea bags of powdered ginger and peppermint for convenience. But if you want the best results make this tea fresh. Crush the leaves of peppermint and steep along with the ginger. Grate about ¼ inch of ginger root into 1–1½ cups of water. Steep for 5+ minutes.

Ear Infections

See also Allergies, Cold & Flu, Tinnitus

Pediatricians' offices are often filled with children uncomfortably tugging at their ears. Ear infections affect people of all ages, but children are most prone to this annoyance that causes earache and pain. Because the ears are vital organs responsible for our senses of hearing and balance, any untreated infections can result in hearing loss and dizziness or unsteadiness.

The ear is a delicate, complex organ and has many parts where different types of infection and inflammation can hide and develop. Most infections occur in the middle and inner ear and can recur often. "Glue ear" is a particularly persistent type of ear infection, characterized by chronic accumulation of fluid in the middle ear.

Causes

Ear infection is caused by bacteria from external sources or from bacteria already within the body. A frequent consequence of a cold, flu, or allergy, ear infection indicates that bacteria are growing in the many tiny caverns of the ear.

Recurrent ear infections may be a symptom of allergies. Take steps to eliminate the factors that might cause an allergy. Dairy products are known to be a frequent source of allergies, so avoid them or carefully test small amounts in the diet.

Avoid behaviors such as smoking while pregnant or exposing children to second-hand smoke, both of which increase the risk of childhood ear infections. A common treatment for ear infections is antibiotics. Often, they fail to eliminate the root of the problem or shorten the recovery time. Antibiotics also degrade our immunity by killing probiotic "friendly" bacteria that are essential to a healthy immune system. They eliminate the opportunity for the body to create antibodies resistant to the infecting bacteria, leaving the child more receptive to future infections. Whenever possible, avoid the use of antibiotics and rely on immune boosting herbs and foods.

Diet Suggestions

Bacterial growth indicates a compromised immune system. Sugar is also known to compromise the immune system, so avoid consuming sugar during times of infection and reducing sugar overall in the child's diet. Pesticide-free vegetables, fruits, and whole grains should fill your refrigerator and pantry. Drive away infection by drinking water and nutrient-rich juices that help eliminate toxins from the body while delivering easily absorbed nutrients.

Foods That Help

Foods that are high in vitamins A and C and beta-carotenes help build an immune system that will fight infection. To help the body produce white cells and eliminate bacteria, carrots, squash, and melons, as well as other yellow-orange fruits and vegetables can be combined with legumes, pumpkin seeds, and wheat germ—foods that are high in zinc. Juices blended with these foods, as well as algae and grasses, are a pleasant and efficient way to get the nutrients necessary to strengthen immunity.

Xylitol, a natural sugar found in raspberries and strawberries, has been known to interfere with the growth of some bacteria that may cause ear infections. The berries' bright red color in juices or popsicles is bound to help perk up a cranky, infected child or adult.[1]

Nutrients and Herbs That Help

Anyone who suffers from recurrent infections will benefit by stimulating the immune system with vitamins A and C and by adding enough zinc to the diet in the form of foods and supplements.

Earaches typically accompany ear infections. Treatments in the form of ear drops help reduce the inflammation and pressure caused by infection. Mullein, St. John's wort, and garlic oil dropped into the ear are traditional herbal remedies that reduce the aches and fight bacterial infection. Grapefruit seed extract is a powerful antibiotic and anecdotal evidence suggests that a few drops of diluted GSE can soothe the pain associated with ear infections.[2]

Echinacea may prevent ear infections before they start. By strengthening our immunity, echinacea as tablet or tea, reduces the risk of catching upper respiratory infections. This would include ear infections generated by a cold or flu. Since children are especially prone to ear infection, they may be better prepared to fight off recurrent infections if echinacea is used preventatively.[3]

The Chinese herb osha has been used to reduce middle ear inflammation.

Helpful Foods, Nutrients & Herbs

For more information, see "Nutrient Sources" & "Glossary"

Foods

Algae
Barley & Wheat Grass
Carrots
Garlic
Legumes
Melons
Pumpkin Seeds
Raspberries
Squash
Strawberries
Tofu
Wheat Germ
Yellow-Orange Fruits
Yellow Orange Vegetables

Nutrients

Vitamin A
Vitamin B12
Vitamin C
Vitamin D
Histidine
Quercetin
NAC
Calcium
Grapefruit Seed Extract
Magnesium
Xylitol
Zinc

Herbs

Chickweed
Echinacea
Garlic Oil
Ginkgo
Golden Root
Lavender Oil
St. John's Wort Oil
Osha Extract
Mullein Oil
Ginseng

Recipes

Immunit-Tea

1 bag or tsp	Echinacea
1 bag or tsp	Mullein

Echinacea is the most popular herb for strengthening immunity. Numerous studies have shown its effectiveness for upper respiratory infection. Mullein contains mucilaginous elements that sooth mucous membranes and saponins that help with expectoration. Mullein oil can be dropped directly in the ear. Use loose tea or tea bags. Steep in hot water for 5 minutes.

Immune Smoothie

1	Apple, cut and cored
1 tsp	Spirulina, or other Algae
2 Tbsp	Barley or Wheat Grass Powder
2 Tbsp	Wheat Germ
½ tsp	Vitamin C Powder
1-2 cups	Pure Water
pinch	Stevia, optional

First, cut the apple into quarters and blend them with some of the water. Then, add the remaining ingredients and blend until smooth. Wheat germ needs at least five minutes to soften. Add only enough water to achieve a thick shake consistency. Stevia is a non-sugar herbal sweetener. Use sparingly.

Anti-Bacterial

½ cup	Raspberries
1 cup	Strawberries
1	Grapefruit
To taste	Pure Water

Sort and wash the berries well (See *"Power Drinks Basics–How to Wash Fruits & Vegetables."*) and buy organic berries whenever possible. Fruits and berries are subject to more agricultural sprays than vegetables. Cut the grapefruit in 8 parts and be sure to scrape the white pulp, which contains valuable bioflavonoids. Place the fruit into the blender in stages, adding small amounts of water and pulsing until you achieve a whirlpool and a smooth fruitshake consistency. Grapefruit seeds may be included in this drink although they will make it chewy. This drink is already chewy because of the tiny "stones" in the raspberries. The whole drink can be strained if you prefer a less seedy texture. These fruits contain xylitol, a sugar that can prevent ear infections and does not increase blood sugar.

Eye Problems

Macular Degeneration, Cataracts, Glaucoma, Dry Eye, Conjunctivitis

The eyes are the organs responsible for the sense of sight. Subject to disorders and defects of their own, the eyes are sometimes called windows of the body since they can reflect ill health elsewhere in the body.

Many eye conditions, such as macular degeneration, glaucoma, and cataracts, are primarily the result of aging. Other conditions, such as conjunctivitis and dry eye, are the result of infection and environmental irritants. Common to all eye ailments is increased risk of impaired vision. The central field of vision and/or peripheral vision can be impaired when various parts of the eye are compromised–deprived of oxygen and other nutrients or over-exposed to pollutants, sunlight, and use. Sometimes, eye conditions result in blindness, completely impaired vision.

Macular degeneration affects the light-sensitive cells (rods and cones) in the retina's macula. Particular to the elderly, eyesight is diminished when these cells become damaged and die. As more and more of the vital links to good eyesight die, less and less sight is available.

Glaucoma is damage to the optic nerve caused by increased fluid pressure within the eyeball. This eye disease is most often a result of aging but also indicates other problems in the body, such as diabetes.

Characteristically "cloudy" vision is the result of cataracts, a deterioration of the lenses of the eyes. A relatively simple procedure to remove cataracts has successfully restored clearer vision to people with cataracts.

Conjunctivitis, a common and easily treatable condition, is an inflammation or infection of the membrane lining the eyelids. Some infections are highly contagious, especially among children. Excessive dryness of the cornea and membrane that covers the front of the eyes and lines the eyelids is called dry eye.

Proper treatment of each condition can decrease the threat of total vision loss.

Causes

Infection, vitamin and mineral deficiencies, and foods and environmental factors can lead to damage of the eyes. Changes in the eyes can also be caused by diseases in other parts of the body. Artificial sweeteners, caffeine, alcohol, sugar, lactose, tobacco, steroids, mercury, excessive computer use, and direct sunlight can all cause eye strain and, more threateningly, rob the eyes of perfect vision. Avoiding the entire list of hazards can protect the eyes as well as the rest of our bodies. To reduce the risk of developing macular degeneration and cataracts, avoid smoking in particular.

Conjunctivitis is usually caused by bacteria, viral infection, allergies, and other irritants. Lack of water in the tear ducts is usually the cause of dry eye.

Diet Suggestions

Foods, nutrients, and herbs can strengthen the eyes by improving circulation, fighting infection, and retarding the damage created by natural oxidation. A diet high in antioxidant-rich vegetables, fruits, soy products, and whole grains is the best strategy for getting the basic vitamins and minerals that the body needs for general well-being and good eyesight.

Foods That Help

Foods that are high in antioxidants, such as vegetables, fruits, citrus, soy, and grasses, promote overall eye health because they strengthen the capillaries that prevent lens damage. Grapes, grape seeds, and the berry family, blueberries, raspberries, blackberries, and strawberries, contain plentiful amounts of anthocyanidins and pro-anthocyanidins. These belong to the same family as isoflavonoids and bioflavonoids. These wonderful phyto-medicines protect our eyes against cell degeneration by improving the integrity of the capillaries that supply blood to the retina.[1]

Bilberry, a variety of the blueberry, also known as huckleberry, is one of our best defenses against eye disease. Bilberry improves blood circulation to the eye, retards cataracts, glaucoma, macular degeneration, and relieves eye fatigue caused by reading, driving, and using computers. The list of bilberry's scientifically documented attributes includes relief from both day and night blindness, increased range of vision, improvement of short-sightedness, reduced inflammation, and decreased sensitivity to bright lights.[2]

Fresh wheatgrass juice, strained and dropped into the eyes, is a home remedy used to relax eye muscles and soothe eyestrain. Green, chlorophyll rich vegetables, in general, should be added to the diet for eye health, because they contain vitamins A, B, C, and E. Yellow-orange vegetables, such as carrots, pumpkins, and sweet potatoes, are also rich in pro-vitamin A, beta-carotene, which the body converts to vitamin A. Juices made from carrots, kale, spinach, tomatoes, and melons are a delicious way to get these eye-essential carotenoids. As a source of antioxidants and pro-vitamin A, carrot juice guards against eye infections and prevents cellular deterioration from free radicals. Kale and spinach are especially good protection against macular degeneration. Eating whole grains and nuts adds fiber and minerals to the diet as well as a good supply of vitamin E, which protects cells, including eye cells, from damage.[3]

Oily fish, fish oils, and flaxseed oil can improve our perception of color eyesight because of their docosahexaenoic acid content. DHA is the super unsaturated fatty acid that is vital for the development of the retina. DHA is an animal fat and not available in plants; however, flaxseed oil is a rich source of alpha linolenic acid, which the body converts into DHA.

A tea made from fennel or its seeds clears and refreshes the eyes and is claimed to improve vision. Fenugreek seeds also improve general eye health. And reishi mushrooms have been known to work against inflammation associated with conjunctivitis.

Nutrients and Herbs That Help

Ginkgo biloba is often cited for its powerful antioxidant abilities that neutralize the free radicals that cause eye damage and degeneration. Ginkgo biloba also brings nutrients to the eye by improving circulation, as do gotu kola, hawthorn berry, marjoram, cayenne pepper, ginger, and garlic.

Helpful Foods, Nutrients & Herbs

For more information, see "Nutrient Sources" & "Glossary"

Foods

Bilberry	Grape Seed Extract	Melons
Blueberry	Carrots	Plums
Other Berries	Pumpkin	Garlic
Wheat Grass	Sweet Potatoes	Flaxseed Oil
Tempeh	Tomatoes	Nuts
Kale	Fennel	Reishi Mushrooms
Spinach		

Nutrients

Vitamin A	Vitamin D	Iron
B Vitamins	Vitamin E	Selenium
Lipoic Acid	Zinc	Magnesium
Vitamin C	Chromium	Germanium

Herbs

Calendula	Ginkgo Biloba	Marjoram
Chamomile	Gotu Kola	Cayenne (chili) Pepper
Goldenseal	Hawthorn Berry	Ginger
Eyebright		

Because the eye contains a high percentage of vitamin C, adding this vitamin has marked effects. Most notable are the prevention and cure of cataracts, relief from bloodshot eyes, a cure for conjunctivitis, and easing of inflammation. Vitamin C is also especially helpful for reducing the pressure associated with glaucoma, as is lipoic acid.

Topical treatments for conjunctivitis that are soothing, anti-inflammatory and healing include sterile, cold water, vitamin C solutions, calendula tea, goldenseal ointment, and chamomile compresses. Drinking eyebright tea, as its name implies, helps to relieve conjunctivitis symptoms as well as general eye inflammation and fatigue. Applying eyebright topically is not recommended, because contact of eyebright with the eyes can cause itching and redness.

Eye drops containing vitamin A are effective for relieving dry eye and promoting corneal health. There is some anecdotal evidence that a few drops of mother's milk successfully clears up dry eye. This remedy, however, is limited to those who are fortunate enough to know a generous nursing mother!

Minerals are equally helpful for promoting good eyesight and eye health. Zinc is concentrated in the retina, along with vitamin E, and is therefore necessary for treating macular degeneration. Chromium, iron, and selenium deficiencies can cause poor eyesight. Magnesium and germanium have been especially effective against glaucoma.

Recipes

Eye Blend

1/2 cup	Blueberries
1/4 cup	Raspberries
1/4 cup	Blackberries
1/2 cup	Strawberries
1+ cups	Soy Milk

Blueberries are closely related to the most healing of "eye" herbs—bilberry. All these berries contain plentiful amounts of anthocyanidins and pro-anthocyanidins, powerful antioxidant flavanols that nourish the cells of the retina. They protect against cell degeneration, in general, and therefore also possess anti-cancer and life extension properties. Cranberries and grapes are also rich sources.

Make this drink whenever fresh berries are in season. Buy organic whenever available. Just add soy milk and blend until smooth. If you cannot find all the berries, you can make this recipe with only blueberries and strawberries.

Eye Power Tea

1 bag or tsp	Bilberry
1 bag or tsp	Eyebright

These two herbs are famous for general eye care and for relieving symptoms of inflammation and fatigue. They bring nutrients to the eye by improving circulation. The major natural tea manufacturers package these teas in bags, and they are also available in capsules. Whichever way you consume these beneficial herbs is fine. The loose tea can be found in herb stores and requires a strainer. Steep for 5 minutes, but do not boil. For variety and flavor, add other helpful 'eye' herbs such as fennel, hawthorn berry, and marjoram.

Green Eye Juice

2 oz	Wheatgrass Juice
5 oz	Carrot Juice
2 oz	Kale Juice
2 oz	Spinach Juice
3 oz	Tomato Juice
½ inch	Ginger Root
1 clove	Garlic
pinch	Cayenne Pepper (chili) Powder

This juice is about as green as you can get. Wheatgrass by itself is a powerful eye healer. If any of the ingredients in this juice are unavailable, it will still be powerfully therapeutic.

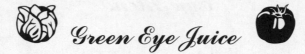

Fatigue

Chronic Fatigue Syndrome

See also Depression, Stress, Mind, Parasites & Candida

Perhaps you are burning the midnight oil or the candle at both ends. Maybe you are just a busy workaholic. Whatever the case, you usually know why you are feeling fatigued. Most often, a good rest will rejuvenate your strength and energies. But what if you rest and are still tired? What if you experience prolonged periods of fatigue? You may be suffering from a health problem that is sapping your energy.

You can experience fatigue in both body and mind. You expect muscle fatigue after exerting yourself physically. And mental fatigue is normal after a hard day's work or after dealing with the typical emotional ups and downs of modern life. Usually, a good night's sleep or a restful weekend will do the trick. But victims of chronic fatigue syndrome (CFS) experience endless, debilitating lethargy. Symptoms of CFS include swollen lymph nodes, low-grade fever, recurring sore throat, muscle pain, poor concentration and memory, headache, and depression. But most debilitating is the relentless, uncompromising exhaustion.

Causes

CFS or general fatigue can be a symptom of any of several underlying conditions. Poor blood circulation, anemia, inability to absorb nutrients, cancer, yeast infections, diabetes, allergies, dehydration, hypoglycemia, hypothyroidism, Lyme disease, and auto-immune diseases can all zap our energy and significantly slow us down. We may not feel like getting out of bed because of factors such as nutritional deficiencies and imbalances, stress, jet lag, PMS, as well as a diet of too much fat, sugar, and food additives.

When the condition is identified, proper treatment can proceed, and you should experience improvement. But when a condition eludes specific diagnosis, CFS becomes the diagnosis of last resort. But what causes CFS? Speculations include suppressed immune system, Epstein-Barr virus, low helper T-cells, impaired or exhausted adrenal glands, and, last but not least, long-term stress.[1]

Diet Suggestions

Whatever the cause, good nutrition can reduce and possibly eliminate the symptoms. A high-energy diet that builds the immune system should include complex carbohydrates that stimulate the metabolism, whole grains and beans that add fiber and protein, soy and some low-fat dairy products for protein and minerals, fish and fish oils for protein, beneficial fatty acids, and lots of water. Use the power of fruits, vegetables, and their juices to provide the vitamins, minerals, and fiber to get you going. Start the day with a high-protein, high-mineral drink that rejuvenates your senses, vitalizes your spirit, and sustains your body.

Foods That Help

Put away the espresso maker and pull out the juicer. Juicing is the best way to get instant energy. Stock your refrigerator with organic fruits and vegetables, which are rich in vitamins, trace minerals, enzymes, electrolytes, and potent phytochemicals. Leave sugary foods and high-fat, processed foods at the bakery and butcher shops. Vegetables rich in potassium, magnesium, iron, calcium, vitamins A and C include alfalfa sprouts, garlic, carrots, spinach, celery, broccoli, cabbage, cauliflower, watercress, and beetroot. Fruits with similar mineral, vitamin and antioxidant power to boost immunity include figs, apricots, apples, bananas, peaches, cantaloupe, avocado, and citrus—lemons, limes, oranges, and grapefruit.

Wheatgrass, barley grass, brewer's yeast, nuts, seeds, soy products, spirulina, and kelp provide readily accessible nutrients that contribute to efficient energy production.

Grains and legumes are high-energy foods that metabolize slowly to regulate your blood sugar gradually, which provides a sustained source of energy. Fiber-rich foods such as oatmeal, brown rice, barley, corn, and legumes are "slow-burning" foods. Mushrooms–maitake, reishi, and shiitake–seem to alleviate fatigue.

Caffeine may give you a boost, but it is only temporary. It merely postpones fatigue, as do the simple sugars in candy bars and donuts.

Helpful Foods, Nutrients & Herbs

For more information, see "Nutrient Sources" & "Glossary"

Foods

Alfalfa Sprouts	Apples	Nuts
Garlic	Bananas	Seeds
Carrots	Peaches	Soy Products
Spinach	Cantaloupe	Spirulina
Celery	Avocado	Kelp
Broccoli	Lemons	Oatmeal
Cabbage	Limes	Brown Rice
Cauliflower	Oranges	Barley
Watercress	Grapefruit	Corn
Beetroot	Wheat Grass	Legumes
Figs	Barley Grass	Mushrooms
Apricots	Brewer's Yeast	

Nutrients

Potassium	Zinc	Vitamin C
Calcium	Iron	Vitamin E
Magnesium	Vitamin A	Coenzyme Q10
Manganese	B Vitamins	Melatonin

Herbs

Ginseng	Gotu Kola	Goldenseal
Astragalus	Guarana	Lavender
Cayenne (Chili)	Kava Kava	Passion Flower
Ginkgo Biloba	Sage	Valerian
Essiac	Echinacea	Reishi Mushroom
Golden Root		

Nutrients and Herbs That Help

Potassium, calcium, magnesium, manganese, zinc, and iron can provide much needed physical and mental energy to those experiencing abnormal fatigue.[2] Because minerals are excreted during exercise, the muscle fatigue brought on by your workout can be alleviated with supplementation.

You should protect yourself with lots of antioxidants, because free radicals may also cause fatigue. B vitamins, especially vitamin B12, provide many benefits for muscle fatigue, general tiredness, and energy production.[3] Coenzyme Q10 is good for boosting the immune system and also helps improve oxygen delivery. Melatonin helps the body absorb and use minerals and is also good for relieving jet lag.

Herbs can also jumpstart sagging energy production. Asiatic, American, and Siberian ginseng help prevent and relieve fatigue. Astragalus, chilies, and ginkgo biloba stimulate the body to produce more energy. Other herbs that prevent and treat fatigue include essiac, golden root, gotu kola, guarana, kava kava, and sage. Echinacea, goldenseal, and oregano are immunity boosting herbs. Calming herbs that help relieve the stress associated with fatigue include lavender, passion flower, and valerian.

Recipes

Glug Zoom!

8 oz	Carrot Juice
2 oz	Alfalfa Sprouts
1 tsp	Blue-Green Algae, Spirulina or Chlorella

Beam me up Scotty! Carrot juice is renown for its abundance of antioxidants. Alfalfa sprouts are rich in phytochemicals and chlorophyll and increase oxygen in the blood and brain. Blue-green algae, in any of its varieties, is a superb brain food for sharpening concentration and alertness. Use organic carrots whenever possible.

Rocket Fuel

1 cup	Apple Juice
2 Tbsp	Tahini
½	Banana
1 Tbsp	Lecithin Granules
1 ml	Gotu Kola, Ginkgo, or Guarana

This drink provides many energizing minerals: potassium, important for the energy conversion of glucose to glycogen; chromium, which helps balance blood sugar and, therefore, energy production; and magnesium, important for the storage and release of glycogen. Tahini is a high-energy food and one of our best sources of coenzyme Q10. Lecithin strengthens the myelin sheaths surrounding the nerve fibers and axons throughout our nervous system.

Blend the banana, juice, and tahini together. Tahini is sesame seed paste. Use raw, untoasted tahini whenever possible. Add 1 milliliter, about 1 dropper full of your favorite energy herbal extract, gotu kola, guarana, or ginkgo. Buy organic ingredients whenever possible.

"C" You Soon!

1	Grapefruit, juiced
2	Oranges, juiced
1 ml	Ginseng Liquid Extract (1 dropperful)
½ tsp	Vitamin C Crystals

"C" You Soon! With the amount of vitamin C in this draft, you will supercharge your immune system and wake up your nervous system. Add to that the many benefits of ginseng for strength, stamina, and energy, and you have a great way to start the day.

Cut the grapefruit and oranges into eighths and remove as many seeds as possible. And don't forget to juice the pulp from inside the rind. Therein rests the miracle flavonoids and their magical curative powers. Buy organic fruits so you can include that rind without the pesticides.

Wheatgrass Cocktail

2 oz	Wheatgrass Juice
3 oz	Celery Juice
2 oz	Kale or Collard Greens Juice
2 oz	Spinach Juice
1 oz	Lemon Juice
1 Tbsp	Tamari
pinch	Cayenne (chili) Pepper

Get ready to rock and roll. Wheatgrass juice is one of the highest energy foods on the planet. You can take it straight, but in this combination it is more delicious and super-charged. These greens are some of our richest sources of magnesium, an important energizing mineral. Take this drink on an empty stomach and sip slowly. Tamari is a kind of natural soy sauce. Choose wheat-free tamari to avoid possible wheat allergies. Add a pinch of cayenne to this drink or just take it in a capsule. This drink will be powerful even if you do not have all the ingredients. Don't drink and drive.

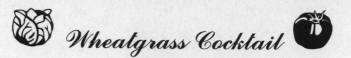

Gingivitis

Periodontal Disease

If you think cavities are bad, listen to this. People over 30 lose more teeth due to periodontal disease than to cavities. Periodontal disease slowly but steadily weakens the connective tissue and bone that hold teeth firmly in place. Early stages of the disease are painless and often go undetected. This lack of detection and corrective treatment can lead to advanced stages that result in tooth loss.

Gingivitis, the simplest and most common type of periodontal disease, is an inflammation of the gums, the connective tissue that covers the underlying section of the teeth. If the sticky film of bacteria called plaque is not removed from the teeth, it irritates the gums, causing inflammation, swelling, and bleeding.

Once the plaque hardens, the gum pulls away from the tooth, leaving pockets that trap even more plaque. Now the disease has progressed from superficial gingivitis to a more deep-seated condition called periodontitis. As the pockets widen and deepen, the tooth loosens. As the remaining tissue and underlying bone are destroyed, the tooth falls out. Surgery, anti-bacterial treatments, dental cleaning and diet can help reverse periodontal disease.

Causes

The cause of periodontal disease is bacteria. Bacteria start the chain of events that leads to tooth loss: bacteria, plaque, gingivitis, periodontitis, and eventual loss of teeth. Prevent bacteria from forming on your teeth by avoiding refined carbohydrates and sugars, both of which cause plaque. Poor dental hygiene and lack of professional dental care further increase the risk of developing periodontal disease, so replace these behaviors with daily brushing and flossing and regular dental appointments.

Excessive phosphorous can also cause periodontal disease by interfering with the absorption of calcium, the bone-fortifying mineral. Soft drinks should be avoided for two reasons: high sugar content and high phosphorous content.

Diet Suggestions

Eating a diet that promotes healthy gums and teeth is as important as brushing and flossing to get rid of plaque before it settles into a cozy pocket. By eating natural, unrefined, and unprocessed foods, many plaque-forming agents never get a chance to adhere to the teeth. A diet high in mineral-rich raw vegetables and fruits is especially helpful.

Foods That Help

Foods high in calcium, magnesium and zinc help prevent and reverse periodontal disease. Calcium helps shrink the pockets of inflammation between the gums and teeth, and strengthens the jawbone to which teeth are anchored. Calcium is found in foods such as dairy products, salmon, sardines with edible bones, nuts, wheat germ, broccoli and leafy green vegetables. Whole grains, nuts, seeds, spinach, kelp, and brewer's yeast, all of which are high in magnesium, also increase bone density.

Zinc is especially helpful for preventing gingivitis because it fortifies gum tissue. A mouthwash containing zinc also helps reduce the amount of plaque near the gums. Oysters contain a substantial amount of zinc. Other sources of zinc include whole grains, bananas, nuts, seeds and brewer's yeast.

Garlic's anti-bacterial properties help in the prevention and care of periodontal disease.

Coenzyme Q10 has a remarkable reputation for curing periodontal disease. Scientific research, including many documented cases of full recoveries, indicates that "coenzyme Q10 dramatically halts the progression of periodontal disease and usually totally heals the damage already done, including the re-growth of previously atrophied tissue."[1]

Salmon and mackerel are good sources of coenzyme Q10 as are rape seed oil, nuts, sesame seeds, whole grains, yellow-orange vegetables, spinach and broccoli. The benefits of coenzyme Q10 can also be acquired in capsule form.

Nutrients and Herbs That Help

Reducing bacteria and inflammation are both desirable for building a defense against periodontal disease. Vitamin C in foods and supplement form is especially helpful as an antioxidant and for fighting bacteria, while vitamins A, C and E help reduce inflammation.

Herbs are also commonly used to treat various stages of periodontal disease effectively. Whether ingested or applied topically as toothpaste and mouthwash, herbs are used primarily to alleviate inflammation and fight infection. Calendula, chamomile, echinacea, and myrrh provide anti-inflammatory and anti-bacterial actions that are necessary for successfully treating gingivitis.

Other natural products that soothe and prevent periodontal disease include toothpaste containing propolis, which alleviates gingivitis by reducing inflammation, and green tea, which prevents bacterial growth, the underlying cause of many cases of gingivitis. Tea tree oil rubbed on the gums also relieves gingivitis.

Helpful Foods, Nutrients & Herbs

For more information, see "Nutrient Sources" & "Glossary"

Foods

Spinach
Leafy Green Vegetables
Yellow-Orange Vegetables
Garlic
Kelp
Wheat Germ
Whole Grains
Broccoli
Brewer's Yeast
Rape Seed Oil
Tea Tree Oil
Sesame Seeds
Bananas
Salmon
Sardines
Nuts

Nutrients

Calcium
Coenzyme Q10
Magnesium
Zinc
Vitamin A
Vitamin C
Vitamin E

Herbs

Calendula
Chamomile
Echinacea
Green Tea
Myrrh

Recipes

Anti-Gingivitis Juice

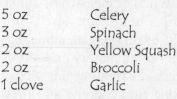

5 oz	Celery
3 oz	Spinach
2 oz	Yellow Squash
2 oz	Broccoli
1 clove	Garlic

This fresh squeezed vegetable juice is one of the best ways to get the live coenzyme Q10, a major antioxidant that has enormous life extension potential. Q10 dramatically halts the progression of gingivitis and relieves the discomfort of gingivitis sufferers within days. If supplementing with Q10, use dosages of 50-75 mg per day.

Green Tea

1 bag or tsp	Green Tea
1 cup	Water, pure

Green Tea helps to prevent gingivitis by inhibiting the growth of the detrimental bacteria streptococcus mutans, which is often the underlying cause. The high quotient of polyphenols in green tea also prevents the formation of plaque on teeth and helps tooth enamel resist dietary acids.[2]

Use tea bags or loose tea to make your own. Steep for 5 minutes. Drink often and keep the hot tea in contact with the gums for as long as possible.

Gum Strengthener

½ cup	Sesame Seeds
½ cup	Apple Juice
1	Banana, sliced
2 Tbsp	Brewer's Yeast
2 Tbsp	Wheat Germ
1+ cup	Water, pure

Brewer's yeast is our finest source of folic acid, and wheat germ is the next best source. Both are better sources than beef liver. People who took 4 mg of folic acid orally per day were able to prevent gingivitis.[3]

First blend blonde sesame seeds in a dry blender. Keep the lid on tight so the little seeds do not fly out. Once they are ground into a meal, add the apple juice, half of the water, the banana and blend. (As an alternative to the sesame seeds, you may use 2-4 Tbsp of sesame tahini.) Next add the brewer's yeast and the wheat germ. Add water to achieve the preferred consistency.

Headache

Migraine

Do you sometimes feel like your head is being squeezed in a vise? Is there a woodpecker searching for breakfast in your skull? You need headache relief! Whether you get the mild and more common tension headaches or the fierce pain of cluster headaches and migraines, you need help. What you eat and drink can make a difference.

A dull ache that affects your whole head is a common tension headache. Migraines, on the other hand, are characterized by a persistent throbbing in the forehead and temple, often accompanied by impaired vision, extreme sensitivity to lights and noise, numbness, and even nausea and vomiting. Similar to migraines, cluster headaches produce pain centralized in the eye. They usually affect only one side of the head, yet differ from migraines in that the pain reoccurs for weeks or months. Exertion headaches are usually short-lived, with pain in the back of the head, while headaches caused by infections, such as sinusitis, flu or the common cold, are characterized by pressurized pain and ache.

Causes

Tension headaches may be caused by anything from screaming people, barking dogs, impending deadlines, and traffic jams, to out-of-town guests. Headaches caused by strenuous exercise or infection are usually temporary and subside once the cause is eliminated. Fasting can also cause headaches as the body begins to rid itself of stored toxins, which reenter the bloodstream temporarily while on their way out.

Allergies are a major cause of headaches, especially migraines. Headaches have been linked to the intake of salt, lactose, caffeine (including chocolate), citrus fruits, onions, birth control pills, artificial sweeteners such as aspartame and monosodium glutamate (MSG), and other food additives.[1] Environmental factors such as the vapors of household chemicals and air pollution can also cause headaches.

Women often complain of migraines while experiencing premenstrual syndrome (PMS). Headaches can also be a side-effect of drugs, which may also cause chronic fatigue syndrome (CFS) and meningitis. Headaches can forewarn of other medical conditions such as stroke, cerebral hemorrhage, and lead or mercury poisoning. And finally, examine your vices. Alcohol and tobacco can cause headaches, especially when overindulged.

Diet Suggestions

A diet high in complex carbohydrates and low in protein is recommended for headache sufferers.[2] Prepare your foods by juicing, steaming, or broiling rather than frying. Fried fats contain aldehydes, which have been linked to migraines. Avoid simple sugars, since unruly blood sugar levels can cause headaches and other problems.

High-protein foods contain tryptophan, an amino acid that is converted to serotonin, which has been known to trigger and worsen some migraines. Beer, wine, milk products, especially cheese, and nuts all contain tyramine, which triggers migraines. Too much protein also leaches our bodies of calcium and magnesium, two important minerals that help prevent and relieve headaches.

Drink lots of water. Dehydration, an unrecognized epidemic in America, is thought to contribute to the onset of migraines. Cut down on alcohol and caffeine and substitute fresh fruit and vegetable juices to rid the body of the toxins that can cause headaches.

Foods That Help

Complex carbohydrates such as whole gains and starchy vegetables help us maintain stability and balance in the face of stress that could easily lead to a headache. Vegetables and fruits are easier to handle because they are low in protein and full of headache-helpful vitamins and phyto-nutrients. Non-dairy foods that are rich in magnesium, calcium, and vitamin D include cauliflower, broccoli, spinach, corn, celery, hot peppers, apples, bananas, kelp, sunflower seed sprouts, brown rice, wheat bran, wheat germ, and soy beans. Carrots and beets help detoxify the liver, which is our front line against headaches caused by toxins.

Although caffeine can sometimes relieve a headache, more often it causes headaches and interferes with the production of melatonin, a hormone that helps relieve headaches. Replace soda and caffeine drinks with fruit and vegetable juices. Juicing with wheat grass adds calcium, magnesium, iron, and vitamins A and C, and it is a good long-term treatment for allergies that may cause headaches.

Helpful Foods, Nutrients & Herbs

For more information, see "Nutrient Sources" & "Glossary"

Foods

Complex Carbohydrates	Corn	Brown Rice
Whole Grains	Celery	Wheat Bran
Whole Grain Pasta	Hot Peppers	Wheat Germ
Kelp	Apples	Soy Beans
Cauliflower	Bananas	Carrots
Broccoli	Sunflower Sprouts	Beets
Spinach		

Nutrients

Magnesium	Vitamin D	Melatonin
Calcium	Iron	Fish Oil

Herbs

Feverfew	Basil	Rosemary
Gingko Biloba	Chamomile	Valerian
Ginger	Marjoram	Willow Bark
Cayenne	Passion Flower	Lavender Oil

Nutrients and Herbs That Help

Magnesium and calcium are the minerals of choice for headache sufferers, because they reduce the spasms that cause head pain and ache. High doses of calcium and vitamin D help relieve migraines, as does vitamin B2 (riboflavin). Some pre-menopausal women find headache relief by taking extra magnesium. Melatonin has been known to help prevent migraines and cluster headaches, and there is some research indicating that omega 3 fatty acids ward off migraines.[3]

Herbs may be your most valuable ally in the fight against headaches. Feverfew has several properties that make it the first herb you should reach for. It prevents the release of serotonin, stops blood from rushing to the head, and reduces inflammation. Feverfew not only shortens the duration of migraines but also reduces both the frequency and intensity of headaches.[4]

Ginkgo biloba also has a good track record for relieving migraine headaches. Ginger helps relieve the nausea associated with migraines, and the wondrous capsaicin (hot red peppers) will take away your cluster headache when applied to the nostril on the same side as the ache.[5]

Remove stress from your life. It couldn't hurt, and your headaches may disappear, too. How about taking some herbs for stress? Try drinking chamomile, passion flower, or valerian tea and start cooking with basil, marjoram, and rosemary. Our great grandmothers massaged lavender oil on their temples for soothing relief.

Recipes

De-Headache Tea

1 bag or ¼ inch	Ginger
1 capsule	Cayenne

Ginger gets the blood circulating, is warming, and reduces inflammation. You can use the convenient tea bags of powdered ginger, but if you want the best results make it fresh. First buy a good-looking piece of ginger root. Grate about ¼ inch of the root into 1–1½ cups of water. Steep for about 15 minutes. If you make more, you can refrigerate it and warm it up quickly later on.

Both ginger and cayenne are proven headache helpers. You can also put a pinch of cayenne powder into your tea, but if this makes it too hot for your taste, simply take a capsule of cayenne powder with your tea. Take cayenne capsules with small amounts of food or drink when you feel a headache coming on. Prevention is easier than cure.

Sea of Tranquility

5 oz	Celery Juice
2 oz	Kale or Collard Greens Juice
2 oz	Alfalfa Sprouts Juice
2 oz	Spinach Juice
1 oz	Wheatgrass Juice
1 oz	Lemon Juice
1 tsp	Spirulina Powder (optional)

This all green cocktail will have a powerfully quieting influence on your nervous system. Make sure you sip it slowly and sit down and relax. Take your time. The object is to get quiet. This drink is an aid, but it can easily be overpowered by your behavior.

These foods are some of the highest dietary sources of calcium and magnesium—minerals that are crucial to maintaining the health and balance of your nerves. In addition, wheatgrass is the highest source of riboflavin, which, in high doses, has been successful in treating migraines. Spirulina, which is optional in this recipe, is our finest food source of vitamin D, another "headache vitamin."

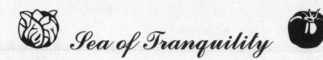

Meyerowitz Water Cleanse

1 Liter Pure Water. Drink in 20 minutes

This is the author's daily constitutional drink. Dehydration is an unrecognized epidemic in America, and is thought to contribute to the onset of migraines. Water helps rid the body of the toxins that often cause headaches.

Always drink the purest water you can find. Get rid of the microwave and put a distiller or water purifying filter in there instead. Timing is everything in this recipe. This much water, a little more than a quart taken within 20 minutes, flushes the intestinal tract from top to bottom. It is an inexpensive self-help tool that keeps the plumbing clear, the body hydrated, and all things running smoothly. Water is one of our top three fundamental healers—along with oxygen and exercise.

Wheatgrass Juice

2 oz Wheatgrass Juice, fresh

Grass juice is very purifying to the blood stream and helps transport oxygen to the cells. In large enough amounts, it serves as a laxative to help clear the bowel. This, along with its potent capacity to detoxify the liver, makes it a superb overall headache prevention system. Wheatgrass is also our finest source of riboflavin, which, in high doses, has been helpful in treating migraines. Grandma would have put a hot cloth on your forehead or soaked it in herbs. Alternate a hot cloth with a wheatgrass dipped cloth. Green is the color of tranquility.

Wheatgrass juice can be purchased at a juice bar. To make your own, grow the grass or buy grown grass and juice it. Be aware that only certain juicer machines will juice its woody fiber. *(See "Juicers, Blenders, & Water Purifiers.")*

Heart Disease

Atherosclerosis, Congestive Heart Failure, Blood Problems, Stroke, High Cholesterol, Hypertension, Heart Attack

See also Stress, & Obesity

A heartfelt greeting to you! Did you know that there are as many heart-related conditions as there are heartbeats in an hour? Heart disease has the ignominious distinction of being the number-one killer in America. It includes a wide range of ailments involving both the heart and circulatory system. Congestive heart failure, heart attack, stroke, atherosclerosis (hardening of the arteries), and hypertension (high blood pressure) are some heart conditions that affect every segment of the population. So, be good to your heart.

With congestive heart failure, the heart cannot pump blood effectively in and out of the heart. Swelling and congestion in the body's tissues are the result. A heart attack occurs when a blood clot forms in the coronary artery. The flow of blood from the heart is stopped, causing some or all of the heart tissue to die. While an interruption of blood flow to the heart results in a heart attack, the successive interruption of blood and oxygen to the brain results in a stroke.

As we age, the inner walls of the arteries become less elastic and more rigid, and they become clogged more easily with accumulated calcium and fat deposits. Cholesterol is a waxy substance that not only clogs arteries but also increases the risk of blood clots and gallstones. Atherosclerosis is the increased narrowing of the our arteries, which eventually interferes with or stops blood flow. Hypertension is abnormally high arterial blood pressure, a major factor in heart health.

Causes

Because the heart has so many important functions and working parts, it is understandable that heart disease has a large number of causes. In addition to heart defects, some of the more common causes of heart disease are aging and lifestyles that include smoking, excessive alcohol consumption, stress, lack of exercise, and–by far the number one cause–poor diet. Poor diet results in a number of suspected causes of heart disease, including nutrient deficiencies, obesity, too much fat and cholesterol accumulation.

Heart disease can be caused by anything that can clog arteries, interfere with regular, strong blood circulation, or damage heart tissue. High cholesterol, high blood pressure, and atherosclerosis can also lead to progressively more serious and debilitating heart ailments as well as ailments in other parts of the body. Other diseases like diabetes and hypothyroidism can also increase the risk of heart disease. Excess cadmium, zinc, cobalt, potassium, and calcium can compromise the heart, and prolonged, strenuous endurance exercise can become not such a good thing for your heart.

Diet Suggestions

Our challenge is to keep blood flowing smoothly in and out of the heart and throughout the body. Here is where diet can make a major difference. Whole grains and high-fiber, low-fat, nutrient-rich fruits and vegetables that are high in plant proteins should make up the major part of our menus. Excess coffee, alcohol, dairy products, sugar, and fat can only complicate the work of the heart, so avoid them to help your heart. Limiting or eliminating sugar, dairy and other saturated fatty acids can help protect you from building up the damaging type of cholesterol (LDL) and other factors that can clog your arteries.

Foods That Help

Juicing with chlorophyll-rich green foods like wheatgrass can help alleviate heart ailments, especially high blood pressure. And don't neglect the yellow-orange vegetables, because they deliver valuable carotenoids and antioxidants for a more healthy heart. Vegetables that lower blood pressure include mushrooms and celery, while carrots and spinach help prevent stroke.

In the fruit category, bilberry, also known as huckleberry, helps keep arteries clear by reducing swelling, increasing capillary strength and blood circulation, and preventing abnormal clotting. Grapefruit and pineapple are also effective artery "scrubbers" that prevent atherosclerosis by breaking down plaque. Bananas are full of potassium and help lower blood pressure, as do kumquats and watermelon.

Peanuts contain resveratrol, a plant fat that prevents and corrects atherosclerosis.[1] Bran, especially oat bran, increases the good cholesterol (HDL) and lowers the bad (LDL) cholesterol.[2]

Garlic, onions, and aged garlic have a wide range of benefits for the heart. Garlic lowers fibrinogen levels, reducing the risk of heart attack and the danger of thrombosis caused by abnormal blood clotting. It contains prostaglandin-like substances that dilate blood vessels, slow the manufacture of cholesterol, and prevent the abnormal blood clotting that causes stroke and heart attack.[3]

Soy lecithin is the best source of the B vitamin factors choline and inositol, and it is a major remedy for preventing and treating atherosclerosis. When patients with elevated cholesterol counts were given lecithin for 30 days, their total cholesterol and triglycerides were reduced (by 33%) as were their LDL (bad) cholesterol (by 38%). Their good HDL cholesterol improved by 46%.[4]

Foods that lower LDL cholesterol directly affect atherosclerosis. Rice bran contains the plant fat gamma oryzanol, which increases good HDL cholesterol and discourages bad LDL cholesterol.[5] Alfalfa, sesame seeds, eggplant, soybeans, and soy products help the body reject rather than absorb dietary cholesterol. Moderate consumption of red wine also prevents bad LDL cholesterol from forming and keeps the arteries clear.[6]

Turn to the sea for more heart helpers. Algae such as chlorella, and sea plants such as kelp and kombu can lower blood pressure. Cod, herring, mackerel, salmon, and tuna also reduce blood pressure due to their high content of super-unsaturated fatty acids. Also rich in super-and poly-unsaturated fatty acids are oils from fish, blackcurrant seed, flaxseed, and olives.

Helpful Foods, Nutrients & Herbs

For more information, see "Nutrient Sources" & "Glossary"

Foods

Wheatgrass
Mushrooms
Leafy Greens
Yellow-Orange Vegetables
Celery
Carrots
Spinach
Bilberry
Grapefruit
Pineapple
Banana
Kumquat
Watermelon
Lentils
Peanuts
Brewer's Yeast
Oat & Rice Bran
Garlic
Onions
Alfalfa Sprouts
Soy Products
Eggplant
Sesame Seeds
Algae
Fish & Fish Oil
Flaxseed Oil
Olive Oil

Nutrients

Calcium
Magnesium
Silicon
Potassium
Chromium
Selenium
Copper
Zinc
Vitamin A
Biotin
Choline
Inositol
Vitamin B1
Vitamin B6
Vitamin C
Vitamin E
Coenzyme Q10
Lecithin

Herbs

Ginseng
Hawthorn
Allspice
Oregon Grape
Bilberry
Black Cohosh
Cat's Claw
Stevia
Chili (Cayenne)
Devil's Claw
Dong Quai
Goldenseal
Gotu Kola
Olive Leaf
Rosemary
Valerian
Green Tea
Forskolin
Ginkgo Biloba
Saffron
Reishi Mushroom
Coltsfoot

Nutrients and Herbs That Help

Minerals keep the heart in good condition and functioning properly. Calcium is good for heart muscle contraction and a steady heartbeat. Magnesium helps energize the heart in general and it dilates the arteries, insuring adequate delivery of oxygen. It also reduces the risk of stroke, protects the heart from the effects of stress, and prevents calcium from building up on artery walls.

People with clear arteries appear to have high levels of silicon. Research shows that just before substances attach to the inner walls of the arteries, silicon levels decrease.[7] The bicarbonate form of potassium regulates blood pressure and people with higher potassium intake have a 50% lower risk of stroke.[8]

Chromium, magnesium, and potassium can help prevent congestive heart failure. Selenium, copper, vanadium, and zinc help break down fatty deposits and protect against atherosclerosis.[9]

Vitamins can reduce and reverse some forms of heart disease. Vitamin A is important to heart health, and the B vitamin factors biotin, inositol, and choline keep the heart beating regularly, lower the risk of heart attack in men, and slow the process that hardens arteries.[10]

Vitamin B1 is effective for treating congestive heart failure patients by helping with normal heart muscle tone and by helping prevent atherosclerosis. Vitamin B6 helps males prevent heart attacks by lowering estrogen levels and breaking up deposits on artery walls.[11]

During a heart attack, vitamin C is called on to help stop damage to the heart muscle. It also helps remove calcium and cholesterol deposits from the artery walls. In tests on humans, vitamin C was proven to reduce the risk of death from stroke.[12] Vitamin E stops blood clots that could cause stroke, lowers elevated estradiol levels in males, and reverses atherosclerosis. Coenzyme Q10 helps the heart maintain its oxygen supply and prevents hardening of the arteries.

Herbs should be a part of any healthy heart regimen. Ginseng provides many benefits to the heart. Asiatic ginseng improves heart energy, Siberian ginseng improves blood circulation, and Asiatic ginseng lowers blood pressure. Ginseng also helped against atherosclerosis.

Hawthorn berries can be used in several ways to help the heart. Sometimes referred to as the "heart herb," hawthorn berries are rich in antioxidants and bioflavonoids. They help to improve blood flow and dilate blood vessels, increase oxygen utilization, promote heart muscle contractions to relieve congestive heart failure, and lower blood pressure.[13]

Other herbs for lowering blood pressure include allspice, oregon grape (barberry), bilberry, black cohosh, cat's claw, chili, devil's claw, dong quai, goldenseal, gotu kola, olive leaf, rosemary, stevia, valerian, and green tea. Herbs that help the artery walls from accumulating plaque include hawthorn, cat's claw, ginkgo biloba, saffron, and reishi mushroom. Chilies and coltsfoot prevent the absorption of dietary cholesterol and chili (cayenne) prevents abnormal blood clotting by stimulating the breakdown of fibrin.

Herbs for preventing stroke include cat's claw and green tea. One study found that people who drank more than five cups of green tea per day reduced their incidence of stroke by 500%.[14]

Recipes

Cardio–Cocktail

2 oz	Wheatgrass Juice
3 oz	Celery Juice
2 oz	Kale or Collard Greens Juice
2 oz	Spinach Juice
1 oz	Lemon Juice
1 Tbsp	Tamari
pinch	Cayenne (chili) Pepper

One of the best things you can do for your cardiovascular system is to drink plenty of juice from chlorophyll-rich, high-energy greens. Taken regularly, this recipe will give you the long range solution to a healthier heart. Wheatgrass juice is one of the highest energy foods on the planet and, together, these greens are our finest sources of the important heart mineral magnesium. Drink on an empty stomach and sip slowly. Tamari is a kind of soy sauce. Choose wheat-free tamari to avoid problems with wheat allergies. Break open a capsule of cayenne pepper and add a pinch to this drink or just swallow the capsule. This drink will still be powerful even if you do not have all the ingredients.

Pressure Cutter

1-2	Grapefruits, juiced
3 oz	Pineapple Juice
½ tsp	Vitamin C Crystals
1 tsp	Flaxseed Oil

You can't expect to reduce blood pressure with one drink or even one exercise session. But the nutrients and phytochemicals in this delicious drink are proven blood pressure reducers. Vitamin C prevents damage to the heart muscle and removes cholesterol deposits from the artery walls. The bromelain in pineapple inhibits the formation of fibrinogen, which is the cause of abnormal blood clotting and a significant factor in cardiovascular disease. The pectin in grapefruit lowers the viscosity of blood, so be sure to include the white pulpy parts of this fruit. The prostaglandin-like compounds in flaxseed oil lower blood pressure and make blood platelets less sticky. Buy organic fruits whenever possible to avoid the risks of pesticides.

Artery Scrubber

1-2 cups	Pure Water
½ cup	Pineapple Juice
2 Tbsp	Oat or Rice Bran
1 Tbsp	Blue-Green Algae, Spirulina, or Chlorella Powder
1 Tbsp	Lecithin Granules
1 Tbsp	Brewer's Yeast
½ tsp	Flaxseed Oil

The algaes are the richest sources of blood-purifying chlorophyll on the planet and reduce blood pressure. Flaxseed also lowers blood pressure, due to its super- and poly-unsaturated fatty acids. Numerous studies have proven the effectiveness of oat and rice bran to increase good cholesterol and lower bad cholesterol. Lecithin has proven in human studies to dramatically reduce total cholesterol, triglycerides, and bad cholesterol. Pineapple is a legendary artery "scrubber." And brewer's yeast is our best source of vitamin B1 thiamine, and vitamin B6 pyridoxine, nutrients that ease congestive heart failure, normalize heart muscle tone, and break up deposits on artery walls.

Blend the ingredients one at a time but begin with only half the water. Add part or all of the rest of the water later as needed to create the consistency you prefer. This drink will be effective even if you are missing one of the ingredients.

Heart Muscle

10 oz	Carrot Juice
2 oz	Alfalfa Sprouts
1 tsp	Spirulina, Chlorella, or Algae Powder
1 clove	Garlic
pinch	Cayenne (chili) Pepper

Pump your chest with these muscle-building ingredients for the heart. Garlic and aged garlic extract have a wide range of benefits for the heart, including reduced risk of atherosclerosis, heart attack, and stroke. Cayenne prevents abnormal blood clotting by stimulating the breakdown of fibrin. Algae and alfalfa are the richest sources of blood-building chlorophyll. Spirulina and alfalfa sprouts are our top sources of magnesium, the most important mineral for the heart muscle. Carrots and cayenne pepper are our best sources of vitamin A. They protect the heart from disease and free radicals. Strive to use organic ingredients, especially carrots, whenever possible.

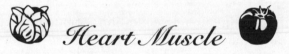

Hemorrhoids

See also Constipation and Colon Problems

Hemorrhoids are probably the most common problem affecting the gastro-intestinal tract. Also referred to as piles, hemorrhoids involve the veins in and around the anus, which is the terminal end of the gastro-intestinal tract. Blood vessels in and around the anus and lower rectum stretch under pressure and become knotted and swollen. Like varicose veins in the legs, hemorrhoids are varicose veins in the anus.

For a fairly non-threatening condition, hemorrhoids get a lot of attention because they can cause such discomfort. They come in different types and sizes: internal and external to the anus, bleeding and non-bleeding, large and small, itchy and non-itchy, painful and not-so-painful.

Causes

Anything that increases pressure on the veins of the anus can cause hemorrhoids. And this can be complicated by weak vein walls. Constipation, diarrhea, pregnancy, heredity, aging, stress, liver problems, and prolonged sitting are common causes.

Diet Suggestions

Drink plenty of water. Eat lots of fiber from plant sources to keep things flowing. And feel good about yourself. Things could be worse!

Foods That Help

Because straining to alleviate constipation is considered a predominant cause of hemorrhoids, preventing constipation eliminates the main cause of hemorrhoids. Good sources of fiber that help relieve constipation are fruits, vegetables, and whole grains, all of which add bulk. Water and carrots are good stool softeners, making passage through the colon easier.

Hemorrhoids can lead to anemia when blood loss is significant. Kelp, a form of algae, helps relieve the iron deficiency associated with anemia. To counteract the effects of blood loss, eat foods that are high in iron and also relieve constipation—wheat and rice bran, the seeds of pumpkin, sesame, and sunflower, wheat germ, soy foods, dried fruits, and lentils. And juice with wheat grass. But beware of a potential vicious cycle: Too much iron can cause constipation.

Vitamin C strengthens blood vessels while it loosens stools, so include black currants, lemons, and lots of yellow-orange fruits and vegetables in your diet.

Helpful Foods, Nutrients & Herbs

For more information, see "Nutrient Sources" & "Glossary"

Foods

Whole Grains	Dried Fruits	Barley Grass
Wheat Germ	Lentils	Black Currants
Carrots	Sesame Seeds	Lemons
Kelp	Pumpkin Seeds	Soy Foods
Rice Bran	Sunflower Seeds	Yellow-Orange Fruits
Wheat Bran	Wheatgrass	and Vegetables

Nutrients

Psyllium Seed	Shark Liver Oil	Vitamin C
Magnesium	Vitamin A	Vitamin E

Herbs

Horse Chestnut	Comfrey	Goldenseal
Butcher's Broom	Calendula	Bilberry
Witch Hazel		

Nutrients and Herbs That Help

Psyllium and flax seeds add bulk to stools, which eases some of the pressure on existing hemorrhoids. Remember to drink lots of water when adding these gelatinous seeds to your diet. Magnesium also keeps things moving through the colon with greater regularity and ease. Supplements of magnesium oxide are especially effective.

Herbs that improve the condition of veins are horse chestnut and butcher's broom. Interestingly, butcher's broom is the sole herbal source of ruscogenin, a steroid that constricts blood vessels. Scientific research verifies that butcher's broom is effective for treating both external and internal hemorrhoids; it improves blood circulation, constricts veins, and calms inflammation.[1] However, be aware that it can also increase blood pressure, and possibly cause mild gastritis and nausea. Butcher's broom is available in the form of capsules, tablets, a tincture, and as a loose, dried herb. Typical dosage is 500mg.

Other herbs that can perceptibly affect the veins involved with hemorrhoids are goldenseal, which constricts veins, and bilberry, which strengthens capillaries.

Hemorrhoids, especially external ones, can become inflamed, itchy, and painful. Topical treatments can be soothing as well as healing. Shark liver oil, known for improving the condition of skin, is a component of a well-known commercial hemorrhoid ointment. Witch hazel, applied as an ointment or in a compress, helps reduce inflammation and swelling. Calendula and comfrey ointments also help ease the discomfort associated with hemorrhoids, while vitamin A and vitamin E creams help relieve the itching that is associated with hemorrhoids.

Recipes

Hemorrhoid Repairman

6 oz	Carrot Juice
3 oz	Celery Juice
1 oz	Wheatgrass Juice
1 tsp	Spirulina or other Algae Powder

Fresh, organic green vegetable juice is one of the fastest ways to sooth irritated and inflamed tissues. Carrots are a good stool softener. Wheatgrass is one of the best ways to stimulate your body's production of iron. Spirulina, blue-green algae, and chlorella add iron and boost chlorophyll. Chlorophyll repairs tissue.[2] This green juice will wash your entire intestinal tract with living enzymes that nourish and heal.

Flax It Through

2 Tbsp	Flaxseeds
1 small	Apple, cut and cored
½ cup	Soy Milk
2 Tbsp	Acidophilus Liquid, or 1 Tbsp Powder
1-2 cups	Pure Water

Put the dry flaxseeds in the blender and blend into a meal. Next add 1 cup of water and blend thoroughly. Then, add the apple, soy milk, and acidophilus. Acidophilus is available as a liquid, a powder, or in capsules. It adds friendly bacteria to your intestinal tract and solves a wide variety of problems. Let this drink sit in the blender for 10 minutes prior to drinking. This allows the flax to absorb water. After this, if it becomes too viscous, add more water or soy milk to achieve a desirable thick shake consistency.

Iron Vessel

1–2 cups	Pure Water
2 Tbsp	Rice or Wheat Bran
½	Banana
½	Papaya, ripe
2 Tbsp	Tahini
2 Tbsp	Wheat Germ
½ tsp	Vitamin C Crystals

Rice or wheat bran, wheat germ, and sesame seeds are some of our richest foods in iron. Tahini is sesame seeds ground to a paste. Try to buy raw tahini. Iron-rich foods are helpful in cases of significant blood loss and constipation. Vitamin C crystals work to strengthen blood vessels and loosen stools. Papayas contain the valuable digestive enzyme papain, and bananas ease constipation.

Start with half the water and add the ingredients slowly in the order listed, blending between each. Add additional water at the end to achieve your desired thick consistency. If you do not have all ingredients, try it anyway. These recipes are versatile.

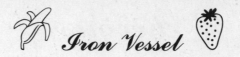

Hypoglycemia

See also Diabetes, Anemia, Fatigue

How many times have you eaten a candy bar or sweet snack hoping to get some quick energy? Yes, it does the trick ... for a short while. But soon you feel more tired than you did before. If this sounds like you, than you may be suffering from hypoglycemia–insufficient blood sugar in the bloodstream. While high blood sugar (diabetes) is menacing, hypoglycemia, or low blood sugar, is also troublesome.

A sugary snack is quickly converted into glucose, a source of energy. However, the body needs to move the excess accumulation of glucose in the bloodstream into the cells. The brain receives a message telling it to produce insulin, the hormone responsible for the moving process. Too much glucose in the bloodstream, however, triggers too much insulin production. Consequently, too much glucose exits the bloodstream and leaves the body fatigued because of lower blood sugar levels. This in turn triggers a craving for more sugar, which perpetuates an unstable cycle of fluctuating insulin and blood sugar levels.

Causes

Hypoglycemia is generally caused by poor diet, especially one high in refined sugar. Avoid simple sugars, such as fructose, glucose, and sucrose, which convert too quickly in the bloodstream. Sucrose can do double damage, because it increases the excretion of chromium, a mineral that is vital for stabilizing blood sugar levels. Abstain from alcohol because of its high sugar content and other complicating effects. Avoid caffeine and nicotine, both of which are known to interfere with the adrenals, which are often associated with hypoglycemia.

Diet Suggestions

Diet is the keystone for controlling hypoglycemia. Because carbohydrates convert food into usable energy more quickly than protein, you should eat several small meals that are high in complex carbohydrates in order to maintain higher blood sugar levels. Also, increase your intake of fiber in the form of grains and bran to help slow the release of insulin, which will prevent lower levels of blood sugar.

Foods That Help

Foods that tackle hypoglycemia by safely increasing blood sugar levels include nuts, whole grains, and spirulina, a type of blue-green algae. Brewer's yeast, a significant source of chromium and vitamin B3, helps regulate blood sugar levels, whether the levels are too high or too low. The chromium content in wheat bran, wheat germ, apples, navy beans, spinach, potato, and especially parsnip makes these valuable foods for a person with hypoglycemia; each helps improve the body's metabolism of glucose. Fennel is a tasty way to treat hypoglycemia, since it reduces the craving for simple sugar carbohydrates.

Foods high in vitamin C, which complements chromium, include citrus fruits, guava, strawberries, broccoli, and sweet peppers, especially red sweet peppers. Fenugreek, flax, and guar seeds are also good blood sugar stabilizers.

Nutrients and Herbs That Help

Chromium, magnesium, and potassium are important minerals in a diet intended to prevent hypoglycemia. Vitamin C has a dual role in treating hypoglycemia: it is a vital nutrient concentrated in the adrenal glands and it enhances the effects of chromium. Chili (cayenne) pepper and parsley are good herbal sources of vitamin C. Vitamin B3, also known as niacin, is helpful in controlling blood sugar levels.[1]

Ginseng is the most important herb for treating low blood sugar. Because of its influence on the adrenal glands and in improving the body's metabolism, ginseng increases blood sugar levels for hypoglycemics. Other herbs that help normalize blood sugar include dandelion, goldenseal, and licorice.[2]

Helpful Foods, Nutrients & Herbs

For more information, see "Nutrient Sources" & "Glossary"

Foods

Apples
Brewer's Yeast
Broccoli
Citrus Fruits
Fennel
Fenugreek Seed
Flaxseed
Guar Seed
Guava
Navy Beans
Nuts
Parsnips
Potatoes
Spinach
Spirulina
Strawberries
Sweet Peppers
Wheat Bran
Wheat Germ
Whole Grains

Nutrients

Chromium
Magnesium
Potassium
Vitamin B3
Vitamin C

Herbs

Chili (Cayenne)
Dandelion
Ginseng
Goldenseal
Licorice Root
Parsley

Recipes

Glucose Tolerance Tea

1 bag or tsp	Licorice Root
1 bag or tsp	Asiatic Ginseng

Use one teaspoon or one tea bag each. Asiatic ginseng is the panax variety of ginseng used for insulin biosynthesis research. Licorice is a source of chromium. In between drinks you can chew on a licorice stick or take a supplement along with 100–200mg capsules of Asiatic ginseng standardized with at least 7% ginsenosides. *(See "Power Drinks Basics—How to Brew Tea."*)

Sugar Stabilizer

1–2 cups	Pure Water
1 small	Apple, cut and cored
1 Tbsp	Spirulina or other Algae Powder
1 Tbsp	Brewer's Yeast
2 Tbsp	Bran, Oat or Wheat
2 Tbsp	Wheat Germ
2 Tbsp	Sunflower or Pumpkin Seeds
½ tsp	Vitamin C Crystals
pinch	Stevia Powder

This smoothie is loaded with fiber from the apple and bran, chromium support from the yeast, vitamin C and wheat germ. Sunflower seeds provide long term energy enhancing the blood's ability to maintain its sugar. Stevia is a naturally sweet herb that is unrelated to sugar and does not affect blood glucose levels.

First, blend the small apple (or half of a big one) in the water. Then add the remaining ingredients one or two at a time.

Sugar Leveler

4 oz	Tomato Juice
2 oz	Celery Juice
2 oz	Spinach Juice
2 oz	Jerusalem Artichoke Juice
1 oz	Asparagus Juice
1 oz	Alfalfa Sprouts Juice
1 oz	Lemon Juice
2 Tbsp	Tamari
1 tsp	Flaxseed Oil

This powerful elixir is loaded with the healing potential to keep your blood sugar balanced. Pick ripe tomatoes since they will make for a better tasting drink. Tamari is a natural soy sauce available in health food stores. Its saltiness helps counter cravings for sugar.

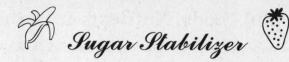

Indigestion

Heartburn, Flatulence, Stomach Problems

See also Nausea, Colon Problems, Constipation, Diarrhea

Digestion is the process of breaking down the food we eat into smaller and simpler bits, which then penetrate the gastrointestinal wall and fuel our bodies. Indigestion is anything that interferes with that process–any number of bothersome conditions that keeps the food in the gastrointestinal tract from entering our bloodstream where it can nourish our cells.

Symptoms of indigestion are flatulence, heartburn, acid imbalance, nausea, stomachache, and stomach upset. Flatulence is excessive digestive track gas, which escapes through belching or passing wind. Eating a spicy pizza with the works may cause heartburn—that burning pain in your delicate esophagus caused by acid escaping from what you thought was your cast iron stomach. Too little or too much acid causes problems. If you are nauseous or have a tummy ache, chances are your stomach is rebelling and asking for some form of relief.

Causes

Can you hear your parents' warnings? "Chew your food. Eat more slowly." Let's face it, eating and running just doesn't fit with a healthy lifestyle, and eating on the run often leads to indigestion. What happens to the undigested food? It sits in your stomach, causing discomfort and slowing you down rather than providing energy and increased productivity. Over-eating also burdens the digestion process. Our bodies were designed for enough stomach acid to facilitate digestion of a reasonable amount of food. It seems that God never anticipated the modern American diet. What happens to that remaining undigested food?—Problems!

Bacteria, viruses, food allergies and sensitivities, and gastrointestinal disease typically cause most types of indigestion ranging, from short-lived annoyances to chronic discomfort. Some foods are tougher than others. Legumes and foods with high sulfur content–eggs, broccoli, cabbage and cauliflower–are more prone to cause gas and indigestion.

Age and stress can rob the digestive tract of gastric juices and enzymes needed for complete digestion. Also, a high-fat diet and undigested protein and carbohydrates often cause flatulence, acid indigestion, and heartburn. Gallstones, ulcers and hiatus hernia can also lead to heartburn.

Antacids, a common over-the-counter remedy for indigestion, can actually cause more indigestion. Antacid, as its name implies, neutralizes acid, which is not okay when the problem is too little acid to begin with. The result can be further depletion of necessary stomach acid, possibly prolonging indigestion.[1]

Diet Suggestions

Prevention is the best cure for indigestion. Eat unprocessed foods, raw fruits and vegetables, and foods that develop beneficial bacteria in the gastrointestinal tract. Additionally, by limiting high-fat proteins and carbohydrates, you will improve digestion. Slowly eat or drink small meals, chewing carefully and completely.

Alcohol, dietary fats, and caffeine cause indigestion, so if you're bothered by indigestion steer clear of your morning ritual of donuts and coffee and your evening chili dog and beer.

Foods That Help

Beneficial bacteria–bifidus, bulgaricus and acidophilus–are necessary for a healthy digestive tract, especially for the prevention of flatulence. Yoghurt that contains active cultures is a good source of beneficial bacteria. If you do not take dairy foods, try seed yoghurt and rejuvelac. *(See recipe below, also "Power Drinks Basics" and "Sproutman's Kitchen Garden Cookbook" by this author.)* Raw sauerkraut, and fermented soy foods such as miso, tempeh, and tamari are also beneficial. Umeboshi, a very sour Japanese plum, creates the perfect environment for beneficial bacteria to flourish. Garlic kills unhealthy bacteria, but don't overdo it because too much garlic causes flatulence.

Decreasing the time it takes for food to pass through your digestive tract can eliminate many potential causes of indigestion. Barley, rice, oats, and similar grains add bulk to the digestive contents and help speed digestion. Bran from oats, rice, and wheat keep things moving along, as does flaxseed and psyllium seed.

Celery and fennel are good vegetables for alleviating flatulence, as are fennel, caraway, and dill seeds. Potato juice is especially helpful for relieving heartburn. Kiwi fruit has a cooling effect on heartburn, because it contains protein digesting enzymes. Bananas protect the stomach and stimulate the production of stomach lining cells that secrete gastric juices. Although most legumes cause flatulence, adding kombu, a type of kelp (seaweed) to your beans helps as does changing the cooking water.

Nutrients and Herbs That Help

Based on the number of indigestion remedies that dominate shelf and counter space in drug stores, hotel shops, highway rest stops and airports, indigestion is a common complaint. Avoid indigestion aids that contain aluminum. Instead, to relieve heartburn try zinc, vitamin A, and vitamin E supplements or chew magnesium tablets. To protect the stomach from irritation, take coenzyme Q10 and vitamin B1.

That sprig of parsley served with your dinner does a lot more than look pretty on the plate; it aids digestion by increasing blood circulation to the stomach and helps relieve gas. Find time and a quiet corner to drink a cup of tea made with chamomile, ginger, or peppermint, each a key digestive herb and helpful for its calming, anti-inflammatory properties.[2]

Other herbs that aid and relieve indigestion include allspice, aniseed, lemon balm, feverfew, goldenseal, oregano, cinnamon, spearmint, ginger, and aloe vera juice. Licorice helps produce mucin, a substance that protects against stomach acid and other harmful substances.[3]

Bitter herbs have long been known to stimulate digestion. Wormwood, gentian, barberry, oregon grape, blessed thistle, and devil's claw all stimulate the flow of gastric juices.[4]

Another category of digestive aids is absorbent substances such as charcoal and bentonite clay, which have sponge-like properties that absorb gas and toxins in the digestive tract. Do not take these with food and nutrients or they will absorb them as well.

Helpful Foods, Nutrients & Herbs

For more information, see "Nutrient Sources" & "Glossary"

Foods

Banana
Barley
Caraway Seed
Celery
Dill Seed
Fennel
Garlic
Kiwi
Kombu
Potato
Yoghurt

Nutrients

Bentonite Clay
Charcoal
Coenzyme Q10
Licorice
Magnesium
Vitamin E
Vitamin B1
Vitamin A
Zinc

Herbs

Allspice
Aloe Vera Juice
Aniseed
Blessed Thistle
Devil's Claw
Chamomile
Ginger
Peppermint
Feverfew
Gentian
Goldenseal
Oregano
Cinnamon
Spearmint
Lemon Balm
Oregon Grape
Parsley
Wormwood
Barberry

Recipes

3 Stomach Settlers

1 bag or tsp	Ginger
1 bag or tsp	Peppermint
1 bag or tsp	Licorice
1 bag or tsp	Cinnamon
1 bag or tsp	Chamomile

These are 3 separate teas. Any of them can be taken as an after meal tea. If a hot tea feels good to you, then be sure to drink it hot. Heat can be beneficial to digestion because it increases circulation to the stomach. Somtimes these teas work best after the stomach has had time to settle, 1-3 hours after eating. No one can determine "when" is best, better than you.

Gas Eater

3-6 Tbsp	Bentonite Clay liquid

Okay, so you overate! It wasn't your fault, right? These things happen. Thank God, there's bentonite. This fantastic natural clay absorbs toxic chemicals and fumes. It will also absorb nutrients. So, keep those expensive bottles of vitamins and health foods out of reach for at least 2 hours before or after taking this liquid clay. Bentonite is best taken upon awakening or retiring. Liquid bentonite is available at your health food store or see *Resources.*

Rapid Transit

1-1½ cups	Pure Water
2 Tbsp	Oat Bran
½	Apple, cut and cored
2 Tbsp	Wheat Grass Powder
2 Tbsp	Acidophilus Liquid, or 1 Tbsp Powder
2 Tbsp	Sunflower Seeds

Gotta keep things moving! Let's face it, everything has a schedule, even your insides. If you've ever had to call your plumber because of a clogged pipe, then you know just how much trouble this kind of thing can be. Nobody likes a cesspool. So, let's get with the program and have one of these drinks every morning. After all, the best way to get up and go, is to get up and GO!

Soothe Me Up, Scotty!

7 oz	Celery Juice
3 oz	Cabbage Juice
1 oz	Potato Juice
1 oz	Parsley Juice
1 oz	Aloe Vera Juice
½ oz	Fennel Juice
½ inch	Ginger Root
1-2 Tbsp	Tamari

This juice calms the stomach. For ease of juicing, alternate the delicate leafy vegetables with the stiffer celery and cabbage. Tamari is a naturally aged soy sauce that prepares the intestinal tract for good bacteria to flourish.

Rejuvelac-Nondairy Acidopilus

½ cup	Soft Wheat Berries
6–7 cups	Pure Water
	Makes approximately 2 quarts

This is a homemade acidophilus drink. You may feel like you are brewing something here. You are—good health! First, obtain a half gallon jar, and a sprout bag or sprouting jar. *(The author invented the Flax Sprout Bag; see "Resources.")* Although rejuvelac can be made with unsprouted grain, sprouting the wheat delivers a wealth of vitamins and enzymes to the water. You may use common hard wheat, but soft wheat is preferred because it is sweeter.

Start by sprouting ½ cup of soft wheat berries for 3 days in a sprout bag. First soak the berries for 10–12 hours, then rinse twice daily. Mix or chop the 3-day-old sprouts in a blender filled with about 3 cups of water. Chop or break open the sprouts by blending for about 5-10 seconds. Next, pour the water and the sprouts into the half gallon jar. Fill the jar to the top with additional water and let it sit for three days in a shady spot at 65°–75°F. Cover the top with your sprout bag, cheesecloth or a screen. Your rejuvelac must breathe. A mason jar is very convenient for this since it has a removable inner lid and allows for easy placement of a cheesecloth or screen. Stir the mixture twice daily. Yes, twice; this is very important. It mixes up the enzymes and develops live organisms. A chopstick or other long utensil is useful. Smell your mixture each day to monitor its maturation. Making rejuvelac is like baby-sitting. Although these baby organisms are too small to see, they still need your tender care. So, don't walk out on your rejuvelac or, like a baby, it will develop a bad smell! *(For more about rejuvelac, read "Sproutman's Kitchen Garden Cookbook" by this author.)*

Liver Problems

Lupus, Hepatitis, Jaundice, Halitosis

See also Skin Problems, Fatigue

As the largest internal organ of the body, a healthy liver is related directly to overall health and vitality. The liver performs several important tasks within the body. It stores blood and constantly filters it to remove harmful toxins; it rids the body of dead blood cells, secretes hormones and enzymes, supports digestion, converting what we eat into life-sustaining nutrition, and even regenerates its own damaged tissue.

When the liver is malfunctioning, the consequences range from sluggishness to life-threatening illness. Skin conditions, jaundice (yellowing of skin and eyes), fatigue, and digestive disorders such as halitosis (bad breath), can all result from liver malfunction. Hepatitis, cirrhosis, and lupus are more serious liver conditions, which can be fatal if not treated. Hepatitis is an inflammation of the liver, cirrhosis is a chronic, progressive inflammation of the liver, and lupus is an auto-immune disease that affects primarily women and causes the body to attack its own connective tissues, including connective tissue in the liver.

Liver spots (also known as age spots because they occur in older people) are deposits of extra pigment on areas of the skin that have been exposed to light. Liver spots indicate an aging liver that has accumulated an excess of the pigment lipofuscin, which remains as a side effect of free radical damage.

Causes

Because the functions of the liver are many, the causes are equally diverse. If we have overtaxed our liver with too much fat and alcohol, it may not be able to keep up with its job of removing toxins. The result is a toxic buildup that manifests as skin disorders such as psoriasis and acne, as well as digestive disorders, jaundice, fatigue, and halitosis.

Viruses are usually the cause of hepatitis, but some medications and conditions like lupus can also cause hepatitis. Liver problems may also be caused by mineral and metal toxicity, especially from arsenic, sodium, nickel, mercury, and aluminum. Overworked or damaged adrenal glands can result in reduced liver function.

The cause of lupus is unclear, but genetic predisposition, supplemental estrogen, and environmental factors are considered likely initiators. Systemic lupus erythematosus (SLE) can lead to hair loss, muscle weakness, numbness, inflammation of the kidneys, water retention, and increased risk of miscarriage.

Halitosis can be caused by many factors, including liver ailments and digestive blockages related to liver functions. The causes of liver spots are age and exposure to sunlight and ultra-violet radiation.

Diet Suggestions

Since toxic substances can harm the liver, it is important to periodically cleanse the liver with a detoxification diet. Fresh organic vegetables, fruits, and grasses are the best way to cleanse the liver–and the rest of you–of toxins. Avoid alcohol, caffeine, processed foods, and sugar, especially if you have liver problems. These substances can further damage the liver. Steer clear of excess animal fats and fats that are adulterated, saturated, or hydrogenated. They are hard to digest and pose special problems for a compromised liver.

Foods That Help

Start juicing regularly with beets and greens rich in magnesium, chlorophyll, and vitamins A, C, and E, such as wheat and barley grass, kale, collards, Swiss chard, parsley, alfalfa, spinach, and cabbage. Fruits rich in minerals, B vitamins, and vitamins A and C, such as melons and citrus, are especially cleansing. The heat of hot lemon tea helps arouse a sluggish liver. Add a teaspoon of olive oil to stimulate the release of excess bile that congests the liver. A diet rich in plant foods is generally easier on the liver than fatty animal foods. Sunflower seeds, soybeans, wheat germ, and their oils, are great sources of vitamin E.

Other chlorophyll-rich foods include spirulina, chlorella, and blue-green algae. Algaes are the highest sources of chlorophyll and are high in protein. Too much protein, however, slows detoxification, so consider low protein alternatives such as alfalfa sprouts and wheatgrass. Chlorophyll also assists in the production of red blood cells.

Nutrients and Herbs That Help

Vitamin C protects the liver and effectively treats liver disease. Choline, a B-vitamin factor, works to ease symptoms of hepatitis. Lupus patients benefit from vitamins E, A, and B. In one study, large doses of vitamin B5 (pantothenic acid) and vitamin E generated improvement in 100% of the patients.[1] Vitamin B12 helps heal lesions, and vitamin A rebuilds a healthier immune system in lupus patients.[2] The hormones DHEA, pregnenolone, and testosterone help treat and prevent further development of lupus. Fish oils help prevent kidney complications for people affected by lupus, and the minerals germanium, potassium, and magnesium are needed for general liver health.

Herbs can be good detoxifying agents and help restore good health to a damaged liver. Silymarin, a bioflavonoid with protective, antioxidant properties found in milk thistle, helps a variety of liver ailments, both mild and chronic, by preventing toxins from entering liver cells.[3]

Dandelion, tumeric, and gentian help maintain normal bile flow and can alleviate hepatitis. The red berries of the Chinese vine schisandra contain lignans with strong antioxidant qualities, which have generated complete recovery for 76% of hepatitis patients tested.[4] Lignans are a group of phytochemicals that behave like plant estrogens. They are not dietary fiber.

Cat's claw and the Chinese herbs gotu kola and codonopsis have been used to mitigate lupus symptoms. Reishi mushroom may provide some relief for people suffering from chronic hepatitis, while karawatake and maitake mushrooms have been used to treat some forms of hepatitis.

Drinking herbal tea helps flush toxins from the liver, and chamomile tea can help eliminate halitosis. Cinnamon and parsley are also effective remedies for bad breath. Chewing cloves or the seeds of coriander, dill, or fennel leaves a pleasant taste in your mouth while removing offensive odors. Gargling with sage tea, salt water, or tea tree oil is another remedy for halitosis.

Helpful Foods, Nutrients & Herbs

For more information, see "Nutrient Sources" & "Glossary"

Foods

Alfalfa Sprouts	Cantaloupes	Soybeans
Algae	Collard Greens	Spinach
Apricots	Kale	Strawberries
Barley Grass	Kelp	Swiss Chard
Black Currants	Lemons	Tofu
Brewer's Yeast	Nuts	Wheat Germ
Broccoli	Oranges	Wheatgrass
Cabbage	Rhubarb Juice	

Nutrients

Choline	Pregnenolone	Vitamin B12
DHEA	Testosterone	Vitamin C
Germanium	Vitamin B6	Vitamin A
Magnesium	Vitamin B5	Vitamin E
Potassium		

Herbs

Cat's Claw	Dill Seeds	Milk Thistle
Chamomile	Fennel Seeds	Parsley
Cinnamon	Gentian	Sage
Cloves	Gotu Kola	Schisandra
Codonopsis	Karawatake Mushroom	Tea Tree Oil
Coriander Seeds	Maitake Mushroom	Tumeric
Dandelion	Reishi Mushroom	

Recipes

Hot Detox Tea

½	Lemon, squeezed
1 tsp	Fennel or Dill Seeds
1 ml	Silymarin Liquid Extract (1 dropperful)

Drinking hot tea stimulates a sluggish liver and flushes toxins. Of all the citric fruits, lemon is the most potent detoxifier for the liver and gall bladder. Fennel and dill seeds are both highly aromatic herbs used for treating halitosis. Add silymarin, an extract of milk thistle, and you have a full liver treatment program. *(For more about lemon, see "Citrus Fruits.")*

Liver Rejuvenator

8 oz	Carrot Juice
2 oz	Wheatgrass Juice

Vitamin A heals lesions and rebuilds the immune system of lupus patients. Carrots are our most famous source of beta-carotene, the precursor animals need to manufacture vitamin A. Use organic carrots to avoid adding more pesticides for the liver to break down. Wheatgrass is renown as a liver detoxifier and stimulant. It is so potent that many people cannot tolerate more than 2-3 ounces at a time. Carrots make wheatgrass more palatable. Higher doses of wheatgrass juice can be taken in rectal implants, which deliver wheatgrass from the colon directly to the liver. *(For more, see "Wheat Grass and Barley Grass.")*

Citrus Liver Purge

1	Grapefruit, juiced
1	Lemon, juiced
1 tsp	Olive Oil
½ tsp	Vitamin C Crystals

Vitamin C both treats and prevents liver disease. This juice is supercharged with vitamin C. The small amount of olive oil serves to stimulate the flow of bile. Limit it to a teaspoon, since larger amounts will burden the liver. This is a great way to start your day.

And don't forget to juice the pulp from inside the citrus rinds. Therein rests the miracle flavonoids and their magical curative powers. Buy organic fruits so you can include that rind without the pesticides.

Master Cleanser

by Elson M. Haas, M.D.

2 Tbsp	Fresh Lemon or Lime Juice
1 Tbsp	Pure Maple Syrup
pinch	Cayenne Pepper
8 oz	Pure Water

This "lemonade diet" or fast eliminates toxins and fats. The lemon acts as a cleanser and astringent; it squeezes toxins from the tissues and stimulates the liver to detoxify. The pure maple syrup provides a steady energy source with its simple sugar. The cayenne pepper gives heat to the body, aids the circulation, and acts as a diuretic, helping excess fluids to be cleared through the kidneys. Drink 8-12 glasses a day. Eat or drink nothing else except water and herb tea.

Dr. Elson M. Haas is the author of several books including *Staying Healthy with the Seasons, The Detox Diet,* and *The False Fat Diet.* He is founder–director of the *Preventive Medical Center of Marin,* an integrated health care facility in San Rafael, California.

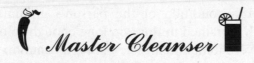

Lyme Disease

See also Chronic Fatigue Syndrome, Arthritis, Parasites & Candida, Skin Problems

Lyme is a lovely coastal town in Connecticut. However, its beauty masked an unpleasant secret. Scientists discovered that the bites from certain infected ticks, carried mostly by deer and mice in the northeastern United States, transmit a species of detrimental bacteria that causes a potentially distressing inflammatory disease.

A bull's-eye rash often indicates the spot where the tick bit and the presence of Lyme disease. The consequences of a tick bite vary depending on the condition of the person's immune system and whether the tick remained in the skin long enough to transmit infection. Mild to severe joint and muscle pain is a common symptom, but there can be intermittent discomfort, ranging from flu-like symptoms to fatigue, backache, stiff neck, and headaches. In the worst cases, more serious complications develop, causing chronic arthritis and affecting the heart and nervous system.

Causes

The cause of Lyme disease is clear: a bite from an infected tick. Gardening, walking the dog, and almost any outdoor activity increase the chances of being bitten. You can minimize exposure by wearing protective clothing and, whenever possible, avoiding the grassy and wooded areas favored by white-tailed deer.

Once bitten, people with Lyme disease need to seek treatment as quickly as possible to minimize the possibility of complications. Take steps to rebuild your immune system and stop the detrimental bacteria from multiplying.

Diet Suggestions

Consume foods and nutrients that help build immunity, reduce inflammation, and counteract the imbalances caused by antibiotic treatment. Whole, unrefined foods, organic vegetables and fruits, yoghurt, and brewer's yeast are especially curative. Avoid counterproductive foods such as sugar, alcohol, caffeine, hydrogenated fats, and refined foods, especially those containing chemical additives.

Foods That Help

Once properly diagnosed, Lyme disease is treated with antibiotics, which kill the detrimental bacteria. Antibiotics also kill good bacteria in the body, however, so you have to reintroduce good bacteria into your system with foods that contain them. The most common is unsweetened yoghurt containing active acidophilus cultures. But there are nondairy sources, too. Other good sources of friendly bacteria include nut and seed yoghurts, rejuvelac, sauerkraut, sourdough breads, amazake rice drinks, umeboshi, and soy miso, tamari, and tempeh. You can also buy liquid acidophilus concentrate in dairy or nondairy form or as capsules or powder. Not only do they repopulate your gut, they also beat the bad bacteria down. They are called "probiotics" because they promote a natural intestinal ecology that inhibits the growth of harmful organisms, unlike antibiotics which kill the organisms.[1]

Garlic, onions, and chives, all members of the allium family, contain the sulfur compound allicin, which kills many kinds of bacteria.[2] Other foods that inhibit bacteria include grapes and the Japanese seaweed nori.

The bee products propolis and royal jelly contain potent antibacterial proteins that are effective against everything from the common cold to candida albicans, e-coli, salmonella, and AIDS. Even honey can inhibit bacteria.[3] *(See "Bee Pollen.")*

Foods such as papaya, celery, parsley, spinach, cabbage, dandelion greens, brussels sprouts, lettuce, and carrots are high in glutamine, an amino acid that enhances our immunity and fights bacteria.[4] Although glutamine can also be taken in supplement form, it is more easily absorbed when you drink juices high in this valuable nutrient. Certain types of bacteria cannot tolerate chili or hot pepper dishes.

Helpful Foods, Nutrients & Herbs

For more information, see "Nutrient Sources" & "Glossary"

Foods

Grapes	Celery	Papaya
Barley Grass	Chives	Parsley
Brewer's Yeast	Dandelion Greens	Seaweed (Nori)
Brussels Sprouts	Garlic	Spinach
Cabbage	Lettuce	Yoghurt
Carrots	Onions	

Nutrients

Acidophilus	Vitamin B6	Vitamin C
Copper	Vitamin E	Vitamin D
FOS	Vitamin B1	Zinc
Glutamine	Vitamin A	

Herbs

Aloe Vera	Echinacea	Lavender
Barberry	Fenugreek	Marjoram
Burdock	Rosemary	Tea Tree Oil
Cinnamon	Horseradish	Thyme
Cloves	Hot Peppers	

Nutrients & Herbs That Help

Certain anti-inflammatory vitamins and trace minerals help build immunity and can be used to fight Lyme disease. Vitamins A, B1, and D stimulate the immune system, while Vitamins C and E strengthen the immune system. A deficiency of vitamin B6 can interfere with the immune system's effectiveness.

Copper works to reduce sensitivity to pain and inflammation, which are prevalent symptoms of Lyme disease. Copper and silver both have strong antibiotic and antiviral properties.[5] Zinc is another mineral that promotes a healthy immune system.

Aloe vera cream or lotion and tea tree oil applied topically can soothe the skin rash caused by a tick bite, and it can also prevent bacterial skin infections. Olive leaf and echinacea are both immune-enhancing herbs that also fight bacteria and viruses.[6] Barberry, burdock, rosemary, thyme, and fenugreek are bacteriostatic, meaning they create an inhospitable environment for bacteria. Hot pepper (also called capsicum or cayenne) can overpower certain bacteria, as can cinnamon, cloves, horseradish, lavender, and marjoram.[7]

Recipes

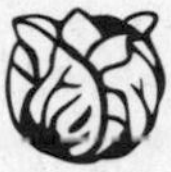

Anti-Biotic V-8

5 oz	Tomato Juice
3 oz	Celery Juice
1 oz	Lemon Juice
1 clove	Garlic, juiced
1–2 Tbsp	Tamari (Soy Sauce)
1–2 tsp	Acidophilus Powder
½ tsp	Vitamin C Crystals
1 ml	Echinacea Liquid Extract (1 dropperful)
pinch	Cayenne (hot) Pepper

This is a yummy antibiotic juice. Tomatoes are a good source of FOS (fructo-oligosaccharides), which nourish friendly intestinal bacteria. Garlic is an antimicrobial herb, and lemon and vitamin C create an acid environment that is beneficial to good bacteria but inhibits the bad kind. Tamari is a natural soy sauce aged with friendly bacteria. Boost this formula with acidophilus, bifidus, bulgaricus, or any probiotic powder you choose. Probiotics (beneficial bacteria) are also available as liquids or capsules, or you can make your own homemade acidophilus drink called rejuvelac *(see "Rejuvelac," p. 203)*. Last but not least, cayenne pepper and echinacea are both natural antibiotic herbs.

2 Anti-Lyme Teas

1 bag	Cinnamon (or 1 inch Stick)
1 bag or tsp	Cloves
To taste	Royal Jelly

1 bag or tsp	Echinacea
1 pinch	Cayenne Pepper
To taste	Honey

In the first tea, cinnamon and cloves inhibit the growth of bacteria, fungi, and molds. If you use cinnamon sticks, steep for 10+ minutes to get the full infusion. Royal jelly is a proven bactericide and is also delicious, since it is related to honey.

In the second tea, echinacea, cayenne, and honey all fight bacteria. Cayenne is super hot, so start with a tiny pinch; you can always add more. If you do not have cayenne powder, break open a cayenne capsule. Cayenne is also known as capsicum or chili pepper. If you find cayenne too spicy, enjoy the tea with just echinacea and honey.

Basic Nut And Seed Yoghurt

1 cup	Cashews
1 cup	Pure Water

Blend the cashews with water until smooth. If you achieve the consistency of heavy cream, you have added the proper water-to-nuts ratio. Pour into a pint jar and cover with a cheese cloth, towel, napkin, or other loose fitting cover, allowing for air transfer. Set your jar in a warm place that will maintain a yoghurt temperature of about 90°-100° F. It is done when the taste is tart or sour, approximately 6 to 8 hours later. *(For more about nut and seed yoghurts, read "Sproutman's Kitchen Garden Cookbook" by this author.)*

Nausea

Motion Sickness & Morning Sickness

See also Indigestion, Ulcers, and Diarrhea

Ugh! Just discussing this subject can upset your stomach! You know the feeling: Your stomach is unsettled, jittery, aching. It even threatens to defy gravity. Food is the last thing you want near you. Nausea is feeling sick in the stomach and trying to resist the involuntary impulse to vomit. Nausea and vomiting are natural reactions to irritations in the stomach.

Causes

Since the stomach is the hub of lots of activity, there are many things that can disturb its delicate balance. Common causes of nausea are overeating, drinking too much, food poisoning, food allergies, food additives such as monosodium glutamate (MSG) and aspartame, pharmaceutical drugs and the stomach "bug," or flu. Alcohol, caffeine, and over consumption of rich or unhealthy foods can also wreak gastrointestinal havoc. Of course, there are physiological sources of nausea, such as disease and obstruction of the gastrointestinal tract.

Common stomach disturbances that cause nausea and vomiting are morning sickness during pregnancy and pre-menstrual syndrome and motion sickness while traveling. People with ear ailments and imbalances are also susceptible.

Diet Suggestions

Food is often the last thing you want when you are nauseous or vomiting, yet once you can bear the thought of putting something in your mouth, try juicing. Juicing is the easiest way to add nutrition without upsetting a sensitive tummy. If you can't get to the juicer, eat small, frequent meals prepared with calming, bland foods or go on a mono diet (one food), such as apples. If this is still too much, give it a rest. Fast for a couple of meals or the whole day! You won't die and it will give your system a chance to catch up and restore its equilibrium.

Pregnant women who eat a lot of saturated fat from meat and poultry may experience more morning sickness than those who eat a vegetarian diet.[1] Of course, anyone, not only pregnant women, can benefit from the reduced demands of a vegetarian diet on the digestive system.

Foods That Help

To calm a jittery stomach, try drinking juice made with ginger, non-acidic fruits or green vegetables. Often mineral and vitamin deficiencies are the result of purging an unsettled stomach. Drinking vegetable juices made from organic vegetables is an ideal way to add essential minerals and vitamins while boosting energy.

When you are ready to tackle solid food, try brown rice, wheat germ, hot soups, barley, or dry, whole-grain breads. Foods high in magnesium and potassium are good; these include apples, bananas, carrots, spinach, celery, brown rice, and tofu. If food does not appeal to you at all, be sure to drink pure water or take soup broth, which will keep you hydrated and provide minerals.

Helpful Foods, Nutrients & Herbs

For more information, see "Nutrient Sources" & "Glossary"

Foods

Apples
Bananas
Carrots
Spinach
Celery
Wheat Grass
Tofu
Brown Rice
Wheat Germ
Sunflower Seeds
Soy, Rice, and Oat Milk
Barley Grass

Nutrients

Vitamin B1
Vitamin B6
Vitamin C
Vitamin K

Herbs

Ginger
Cinnamon
Lavender
Licorice Root
Pennyroyal
Peppermint
Spearmint
Raspberry Leaf

Nutrients and Herbs That Help

Taking vitamin C in conjunction with vitamin K relieves morning sickness, and in human studies, 150mg/day of vitamin B6 remedied morning sickness for most participants.[2] Travelers can take vitamin B1 to help prevent motion sickness.

Herbs are effective as anti-emetics—substances that counteract nausea and relieve vomiting. While ginger is the most effective anti-nausea herb, a tea made with cinnamon, lavender, licorice root, pennyroyal, peppermint, or spearmint will also do the trick. Try ginger, peppermint, spearmint, or raspberry leaf tea for nausea related to either morning or motion sickness. In fact, research confirms that ginger is more effective than prescription drugs for treating motion sickness.[3] Lavender oil dabbed on the temples is another old time remedy for travel sickness.

Be aware that over consumption of some herbs and vitamins can sometimes cause nausea. This list includes, in part, black cohosh, which can also be an abortive herb, blessed thistle, goldenseal, and very large doses of nutmeg, and vitamins A and D.

Recipes

Stomach Smoother

½	Banana, yellow
1 small	Apple, cut and cored
2 Tbsp	Wheat Germ
1+ cup	Soy, Rice, or Oat Milk

Let's face it, bananas smooth things out. Apples are soothing, too, because of their pectin content. Both are rich in magnesium and potassium. Soy, rice, and oat milks are easier to digest than dairy milk and thus preferred for an upset stomach. They also eliminate any questions of lactose intolerance for milk sensitive people. Blend all the ingredients together and sip slowly.

Grandma's Tummy Teas

1 bag or Tbsp	Ginger
1 bag or Tbsp	Cinnamon
1 bag or Tbsp	Licorice Root
1 bag or Tbsp	Peppermint
1 bag or Tbsp	Raspberry Leaf Tea

These are 3 separate teas. Any of them can settle an upset stomach. Use fresh ginger whenever possible. Just grate a ¼ inch piece into 1–1½ cups of water. Use cinnamon and licorice root sticks, instead of powders, if available. Steep all of these roots for 15-30 minutes. Make enough so that you can refrigerate the leftover teas and warm them up quickly later. Peppermint and raspberry are leaf teas and are finished steeping in just a few minutes. Drink these teas hot. Heat can be beneficial to digestion because it increases circulation to the stomach.

Un-Chicken Soup

5-7 cubes	Tofu, cut in ½ inch cubes
1 cup	Brown Rice and Barley Broth
1 tsp	Miso Paste
½ tsp	Ume Plum Paste or Vegetable Powder

Hot drinks and soup broths are often just what the doctor ordered. You've heard of chicken soup? Well, here is a similar but, perhaps, more ethical remedy.

Cook the rice and barley together using 2/3 cup of rice and 1/3 cup of barley grains in a pot of approximately 3-4 cups of pure water. Simmer over a low flame until the grains are soft. Use the broth for this recipe. Miso paste and ume plum paste are both excellent for digestion. They are found in health food and Asian grocery stores. If ume is unavailable, substitute with a vegetable broth powder.

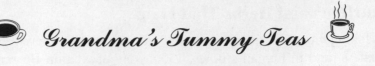

Parasites & Candida

See also Fatigue, Colon Problems, Indigestion

Fungi, bacteria, viruses, protozoa, and worms. This list of human parasites scares up a frightening vision. Once properly diagnosed, however, prevention and treatment are readily available through diet and natural remedies.

Parasites cause a wide range of serious problems with far-reaching consequences. Malaria, for example, is a type of parasitic protozoa. But more often, it is intestinal parasites we hear about.

Candida is the term for a group of toxic yeast-like microorganisms that are responsible for the presence of parasites in the human mouth, throat, intestine, and genital/urinary tract. As yeast reproduces, toxins build up in the body. After a long-term presence in the intestines, yeast can develop into fungi that root themselves into the intestinal walls, creating *leaky-gut syndrome* and weakening the immune system. Vaginal infections (vaginitis) in women are also the result of overabundant yeast production.

Causes

Unsanitary conditions, improperly cooked food, polluted drinking water, allergies, and antibiotics all contribute to the risk of contracting a parasite. While antibiotics are typically taken to kill the harmful bacteria in the body, they often destroy much of the good bacteria, too. Once both the good and bad bacteria are gone, the yeast that normally live harmlessly in the body have more room to grow and spread, causing an imbalance that leads to an infection. Avoid oral antibiotics if at all possible.

Diet Suggestions

Animal fats can be another vehicle through which parasites can enter your body. By eliminating foods such as pork and sausage you can reduce your risk of contracting parasites. Eat more vegetables than fruit, since fruit contains sugar, the primary food of parasites and yeast. But make sure that any raw fruits and vegetables you eat are properly washed to avoid introducing a parasite into your system. *(See "Power Drinks Basics–How to Wash Fruits & Vegetables.")*

Because yeast feeds on sugar, also avoid refined sugars and refined carbohydrates. This includes all kinds of sweets including those made with "healthy" sugars such as organic cane crystals, molasses, honey, maple syrup, rice syrup, and barley malt. Naturally sweet foods such as fruits and fruit juices also feed yeast. Anything that contains fructose, sucrose, maltose, glucose, or any "-ose" is sugar.

If you keep feeding your yeast, they will remain hearty enough to resist the most powerful antifungal agents. Consider non-sugar sweeteners. Stevia is a good substitute for artificial sweeteners such as saccharin and aspartame, which should be avoided. This naturally sweet herb comes in its original form–green leafy flakes–or as a purified, white powder.

Also, consider reducing your intake of caffeine, alcohol, bread, and vinegar, all of which contribute to yeast production. Because yeast grows best in an alkaline environment, a diet high in acidic foods helps prevent and cure yeast infections.

Foods That Help

The good news is that most parasitic conditions can be eliminated through dietary changes. Foods can be our friends or our foes. If you have parasite problems, call on your best friend: garlic—*raw* garlic. You've heard it wards off vampires, right? For garlic, parasites are, well, small game. Garlic exerts antibacterial, antiviral, antifungal, and anti-yeast action that eliminates tape worms, round worms, and candida.[1] Onions, pumpkin seeds, and pineapple are also formidable parasite fighters.

It is essential to increase the consumption of foods containing active lactobacillus acidophilus. Also known as probiotics, lactobacillus, acidophilus, bifidus, bulgaricus, as well as others are friendly bacteria that fight unfriendly bacteria for dominance in the intestinal terrain. Put plainly, you need ground troops to fight this war, and probiotics are your army. Dairy yoghurt and clabbered milk products are the traditional probiotic foods, but so are these nondairy foods: nut and seed yoghurts, rejuvelac, sauerkraut, sourdough breads, amazake rice drinks, umeboshi, miso, tamari, and tempeh. Acidophilus, can be taken for curative or preventative treatment of yeast and parasites and may be taken vaginally or orally in the form of liquid, capsules, or powder.

Acidic foods, like cranberries, create a hostile environment for candida. Carrots and spirulina also discourage the unruly reproduction of parasites. Kelp, wakame, herring, apricots, and lemon extract are enemies of intestinal parasites, too.

Nutrients and Herbs That Help

Fructo-oligosaccharides (FOS) nourishes lactobacillus and other friendly bacteria. It is found in tomatoes, onions, garlic, and bananas. Grapefruit seed extract (GSE), a highly concentrated citric acid, kills a broad range of bacteria, including those that cause flatulence and body odor, and it is used by campers instead of iodine to purify water of giardia and e-coli.[2] For parasites, take 25-75 drops in pure water throughout the day. Bentonite liquid, made from a clay, absorbs the toxic byproducts of parasites, thus unburdening your immune system. Take 3-4 tablespoons on an empty stomach in the morning, or if you wish more, again before bedtime. Trace minerals zinc and copper help the body resist infection, while lemon grass oil, goldenseal, and biotin enhanced with folic acid help prevent and suppress the proliferation of yeast and other detrimental fungi. Tea tree oil applied topically has been known to inhibit yeast production, and boric acid capsules inserted vaginally have been successful in treating vaginitis.

The antifungal properties of agrimony and black walnut inhibit the growth of parasites, as does germanium and cinnamon. Echinacea has compounds that are famous for their ability to support the immune system. Skullcap and propolis are effective against detrimental fungi, as are lemon balm, lavender, and rosemary. Tea made with bayberry, chamomile, wormwood, or nettle helps expel intestinal parasites, while feverfew, horseradish, gentian, and olive leaf work similarly. Wormwood is also effective against malaria.[3]

Due to the unfortunate popularity of parasites, which has become a silent epidemic, there are many wonderful anti-parasitic and anti-candida herbal formulas for sale at natural vitamin stores and pharmacies. These formulas are more potent than any homemade teas.

Helpful Foods, Nutrients & Herbs

For more information, see "Nutrient Sources" & "Glossary"

Foods

Blue-Green Algae
Chlorella
Yoghurt, Unsweetened
Nut and Seed Yoghurts
Rejuvelac
Sauerkraut
Amazake Rice Drink
Umeboshi
Miso
Tamari
Tempeh
Cranberries, Unsweetened
Carrots
Onions
Pumpkin Seeds
Pineapple
Spirulina
Wakame
Kelp
Herring
Apricots
Lemon

Nutrients

Acidophilus
Probiotics
FOS
Vitamin C
Vitamin E
Boric Acid
Zinc
Copper
Biotin
Folic Acid
Bentonite

Herbs

Garlic
Stevia
Agrimony
Black Walnut
Germanium
Cinnamon
Echinacea
Bayberry
Tea Tree Oil
Lemon Grass Oil
Goldenseal
Skullcap
Propolis
Lemon Balm
Lavender
Rosemary
Chamomile
Wormwood
Nettle
Feverfew
Horseradish
Gentian
Olive Leaf

Recipes

Parasite Clean Up

3-4 Tbsp Bentonite Liquid Clay, daily

Are you having a bad-air day? Is your stomach complaining that it is running a hotel for unwanted guests? And what a mess they make! Parasites leave toxic residues, especially when they are being killed off. So if you are using antimicrobial herbs, grapefruit seed extract, or other anti-candida supplements, you need to protect yourself from the overload of toxins. Thank God, there's bentonite.

This fantastic natural clay absorbs toxic chemicals and gases. It also absorbs nutrients, however, so keep those expensive vitamins and health foods out of reach for at least 2 hours. Bentonite should be taken on an empty stomach or upon awaking or retiring. Liquid bentonite is available at your health food store. *(See "Resources.")*

Grapefruit Seed Extract

25-75 Drops Grapefruit Seed Extract (GSE), daily

The seeds of grapefruits contain flavonones and polyphenols that act as powerful solvents. You have undoubtedly seen citrus solvents in the cleaning section of your housewares store. Well, it can clean your insides, too. GSE is available in liquid or capsules. For parasites or candida, take 25-75 drops in pure water over the course of the day. Ten drops in 8 ounces of water is an easy-to-take dilution. It tastes like acid, so it's best to just take your medicine and get it over with. However, you may prefer to mask the taste with some apple, orange, or grapefruit juice.

Because GSE kills unfriendly bacteria and fungi, it is used to treat flatulence, foot and body odor, and candida. It also eliminates e-coli, giardia, and salmonella. Use it as a wash to sanitize your raw fruits and vegetables before you put them through your juicer. *(See "Power Drinks Basics–How to Wash Fruits & Vegetables.")* GSE is also available in capsules at your health food, vitamin, and pharmacy stores. *(See also "Citrus Fruits.")*

Good Riddance Potion

7 oz	Tomato Juice
3 oz	Celery Juice
1	Lemon, juiced
1-2 cloves	Garlic, juiced
1-2 Tbsp	Tamari, Wheat-Free
1 ml	Black Walnut Extract (1 dropperful)
2 tsp	Acidophilus Powder
½ tsp	Vitamin C

Tomatoes are a good source of FOS (fructo-oligosaccharides), which nourish the friendly bacteria in the gut. Garlic is an antimicrobial herb, and lemon and vitamin C create an acid environment that is good for beneficial bacteria but inhospitable for the other kind. Black walnut is a powerful antimicrobial herb. Last but not least, implant friendly bacteria with acidophilus, bifidus, bulgaricus, or any other probiotic powder you choose. Probiotics (beneficial bacteria) are available as liquid acidophilus, in capsules, or as a homemade drink. *(See "Rejuvelac" page 203.)*

PMS & Menopause

Hot Flashes, Premenstrual Syndrome

See also Urinary Tract Infections, Depression, Pregnancy, Power Drinks for Physical Performance

The joys of being a woman come with a badge of courage: enduring premenstrual syndrome, menopause, and hot flashes. Centered around the female reproductive process, menstruation, or the lack of it, creates changes in the female body that often require physical, mental, and spiritual care.

As cyclical menstruation nears, many women experience premenstrual syndrome (PMS), a range of symptoms that can occur a few days before menstruation starts and can last a few days beyond the onset. (Some women experience some of these symptoms during ovulation, too.) The list includes varying degrees of anxiety, mood swings, irritability, insomnia, carbohydrate cravings, depression, and memory loss, as well as fainting, fatigue, headaches, vertigo, water retention, abdominal bloating, weight gain, breast tenderness, aggravated varicose veins, constipation, diarrhea, acne, oily skin and hair, cramps, nausea, and vomiting.

Many of these same symptoms are present during menopause, when the aging female body adjusts to lower hormone levels and the end of reproductive capabilities, usually between the ages of 45 and 55. This list of possible symptoms also includes a few more inconveniences, like night sweats, hot flashes, vaginal dryness, and reduced sexual drive.

Causes

Fluctuating hormonal levels account for many cases of PMS, and declining levels of melatonin, estrogens, progesterone, and testosterone cause the symptoms of menopause, when the ovaries end the production of eggs.

More specifically, water retention, which is thought to trigger PMS, is caused by low levels of the hormones progesterone and adreno-corticosteroid. Menopausal symptoms and the end of egg production are primarily tied to decreased estrogen levels, which can also make post-menopausal women more susceptible to bone loss, male-pattern baldness, and osteoporosis. In an effort to regulate the body's temperature, hot flashes are nature's response to erratic hormonal levels.

Diet Suggestions

A low-fat, high-fiber diet that includes abundant vegetables, fruits, whole grains, and soy products will increase the body's ability to circumvent and minimize the symptoms of PMS and menopause.[1] If you crave carbohydrates, try to eat complex carbohydrates and foods high in magnesium. To help reduce irritability, ease digestion, control weight, and promote restful sleep, limit your consumption of dairy fat and meat.

Because decreased estrogen levels increase the risk of heart disease and osteoporosis, eat foods and take supplements that foster a healthy heart and strong bones—namely a low-fat diet that is rich in calcium. Regular exercise and a positive attitude reduce the symptoms of PMS and menopause and promote a general sense of well-being.

Sugar, alcohol, and caffeine interfere with the body's ability to deal with symptoms related to the female reproductive system. Also, reduce salt consumption, since sodium fosters water retention.

Foods That Help

Whether you are menopausal or premenopausal, reach for soy foods often. Soybeans contain phytoestrogens, substances that imitate estrogen and provide high-quality protein. Soybeans can be eaten in a variety of forms—as tofu, soy milk, tempeh, and roasted soy nuts.

Alfalfa and red clover sprouts and alfalfa powder contain high levels of phytoestrogens and isoflavones, which can bind to estrogen receptors but lack the side effects of the real hormone.[2] Flaxseeds and evening primrose oil contain high amounts of GLA and LNA, two omega oils purported to mitigate the symptoms of PMS. Oats, cashews, almonds, and apples provide a secondary source of foods that enhance estrogen.

Foods rich in calcium and magnesium include soy foods, wheat germ and bran, alfalfa sprouts, algae, flaxseeds, legumes, nuts like almonds and cashews, sunflower and sesame seeds, green leafy vegetables, sea vegetables and algae, wheat and barley grass, and brewer's yeast.

To help relieve swelling and bloating, start juicing with natural diuretics such as grape, watermelon, parsley, cucumber, celery, grapefruit, lemon, lime, asparagus, and watercress.

Nutrients and Herbs That Help

Vitamin B6 helps restore normal hormonal levels and is effective for calming anxiety-related symptoms and edema caused by PMS. Supplements of vitamin A work similarly by increasing the low progesterone levels that cause PMS symptoms.[3]

Vitamin E relieves PMS discomfort centered in the breasts and can also relieve hot flashes and vaginal discomfort related to menopause.[4]

Magnesium may be a woman's best friend, since it relieves several PMS symptoms—irritability, fatigue, depression, carbohydrate cravings, and edema.[5] Calcium is another favorite for relieving PMS symptoms and for fortifying the menopausal body against osteoporosis.

Herbs have many beneficial qualities for dealing with changes that affect the female body, for the monthly cycle of premenopausal women and throughout the menopause process. Chaste berry (also known as vitex) has been used since the days of Hippocrates to relieve many female ailments. Due to its ability to stimulate and regulate female hormonal levels, it aids in childbirth, can relieve hot flashes during menopause, and works to relieve PMS symptoms—headaches, breast tenderness, bloating, fatigue, carbohydrate craving, nervousness, anxiety, irritability, and depression.[6]

Like soy, some herbs, because of their phytoestrogen content, "fool" the menopausal body into thinking that estrogen levels are still high. These herbs include black cohosh, aniseed, Mexican wild yam, and licorice. Black cohosh is especially preferred by menopausal women, because it relieves hot flashes, depression, and vaginal problems. Dong quai is often chosen by women, since it helps restore hormonal balance and relieve pain during PMS and menopause.[7] Supplements of isoflavones extracted from soy are also helpful because of their phytoestrogen content.

Wild yam is recommended by many herbalists for PMS and morning sickness. Mexican wild yam is not progesterone, however, nor can your body turn wild yam into progesterone. It may help in some way with menopausal problems, but it may not be the cure-all some have claimed.

Need hot flash relief? Try vitamin E, topical creams containing natural progesterone, vitex, dong quai, black cohosh, and the bioflavonoid, hesperidin contained in the pith of unripened citrus fruits. Also try the herbs mullein, buchu, and olive leaf.[8] To calm nerves, try valerian, skullcap, chamomile, and passion flower.

Helpful Foods, Nutrients & Herbs

For more information, see "Nutrient Sources" & "Glossary"

Foods

Tofu
Soy Milk & Cheese
Tempeh
Oats
Almonds
Alfalfa & Red Clover Sprouts
Apples
Figs
Apricots
Lemons
Wheat Grass
Wheat Germ
Bran
Legumes
Kelp
Sesame Seeds
Sunflower Seeds
Flaxseeds & Oil
Spinach
Broccoli
Sea Vegetables
Oranges
Brewer's Yeast
Grapes
Watermelon
Barley Grass

Nutrients

Vitamin A
Vitamin B6
Vitamin E
Magnesium
Calcium
Evening Primrose Oil
Isoflavones
Hesperidin
Flaxseed Oil

Herbs

Chaste Berry
Black Cohosh
Dong Quai
Aniseed
Mexican Wild Yam
Licorice
Mullein
Buchu
Olive Leaf
Valerian
Skullcap
Chamomile
Passion Flower
Juniper Berries
Green Tea

Recipes

PMS Cocktail

5 oz	Celery Juice
2 oz	Kale or Collard Greens Juice
2 oz	Alfalfa Sprouts Juice
2 oz	Spinach Juice
1 oz	Wheat Grass Juice
1 oz	Lemon Juice
1 tsp	Spirulina Powder (optional)

These foods are our highest dietary sources of calcium and magnesium—minerals that are crucial to maintaining the health and balance of your nerves and alleviating irritability, fatigue, depression, carbohydrate cravings, and edema. Celery and lemon are diuretics, and alfalfa sprouts are one of our best sources of dietary phytoestrogens. This all-green PMS cocktail will have a powerfully quieting influence on your nervous system. Sip it slowly and sit down and relax

Watermelon Diuretic

6 oz	Watermelon Juice

While adding many ingredients is tasty and very nutritious, simplicity is a virtue. Watermelon is a terrific diuretic and makes as delicious a drink as any. Be sure to juice the rind as well as the red part. But be careful not to drink too much. Only six ounces is recommended, because this drink is very high in natural sugars and water, and too much will increase bloating rather than cure it. Buy organic melon whenever possible.

Estrogen Elixir

2 Tbsp	Oat or Wheat Bran
1 cup	Soy Milk, Vanilla flavor
1 tsp	Brewer's Yeast
1 tsp	Bee Pollen
To taste	Pure Water

Soy foods are a fantastic source of phytoestrogens and isoflavones. Bran is one of our best sources of magnesium, while bee pollen is very rich in calcium. Brewer's yeast contains lots of both minerals. Brewer's yeast is also our finest source of pyridoxine, vitamin B6, which normalizes hormonal levels.

Purchase a soy milk brand that you like, since its flavor will dominate this drink. If you wish additional sweetness, replace the bee pollen with a teaspoon of liquid royal jelly, another honey-like bee product. Add the ingredients in the order listed, blending after each one. Add only enough water to achieve the thickness you desire.

Calcium Calm

1 + cup	Oat Milk, Vanilla flavored
½	Banana, green
1–2 Tbsp	Tahini, raw
1 Tbsp	Bee Pollen

Oats play a role in supporting estrogen regulation, while tahini (ground sesame seeds) is our best source of calcium. Green bananas are rich in flavonoids and fiber. Bee pollen is an excellent source of calcium.

Add the ingredients in the order listed, blending after each one. Oat milk is available in health food stores and makes a delicious substitute for dairy or soy milk. To make your own oak milk, see *"Power Drink Basics."* Add the tahini one spoonful at a time. Raw tahini has an entirely different flavor than the common toasted variety and is healthier. Add a little water if necessary to achieve the thickness you desire.

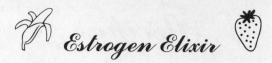

Pregnancy

and Diet for Nursing Mother

See also Nausea

Oh boy! Oh girl! Having a baby is an amazing process that places tremendous demands on your body and requires special attention. During pregnancy and nursing, women are indeed eating for two (or more) and need to nourish everyone involved. Additionally, pregnant women are susceptible to morning sickness, heartburn, varicose veins, leg cramps, back pain, constipation, hemorrhoids, anemia, high blood pressure, and swelling due to water retention. After delivery, these increased nutritional requirements remain, especially for lactating mothers and those experiencing postpartum depression.

Diet Suggestions

Digestion will be easier if you eat frequent, small meals rather than a few large ones. Each meal should be a positive contribution to the health of the mother and baby to reduce the risk of birth defects, to guarantee sufficient vitamins and minerals, and to fortify the mother for the demands of pregnancy, delivery, and breast-feeding. Eat the freshest organic vegetables and fruits, whole grains, legumes, and sufficient protein from low-fat sources such as fish and soy products. Also be sure to increase your intake of water.

Sugar and foods that deplete calcium (chocolate, coffee, and salt) should be avoided. Problems are known to arise for the mother and baby when pregnant women use caffeine, alcohol, tobacco, recreational drugs, and certain pharmaceutical drugs.[1] Avoid them at all costs.

Foods That Help

Kelp, parsley, alfalfa, and leafy green vegetables such as kale, spinach, and watercress work extra hard to deliver vitamin K and iron and prevent fatigue and anemia. Green algae, kelp, brewer's yeast, wheat and barley grass, wheat germ, flaxseeds, bananas, berries, figs, dates, most legumes, lentils, nuts, oysters, salmon, cucumber, cabbage, asparagus, avocado, alfalfa sprouts, green beans, mushrooms, cauliflower, pumpkin, and corn are all rich in folic acid as well as vitamin K and calcium. Build up your protein intake (depending on your dietary persuasion) by eating more fish or soy products and natural protein sources such as spirulina, chlorella, blue green algae, wheat and barley grass, bee pollen, and brewer's yeast.

Nutrients and Herbs That Help

Because women need twice the normal amount of folic acid during pregnancy, it is important to take in enough of this water-soluble B vitamin.[2] Without this vitamin, the risk for birth defects and low birth weight is increased. Niacin, a form of vitamin B3, and choline are also important for healthy, well-developed babies.

Requirements for calcium also double during pregnancy.[3] To reduce the risk of preeclampsia (a form of toxemia), premature delivery, leg cramps, and high blood pressure you should increase your calcium intake from food sources and supplements (1,500 mg per day).

Vitamin K and vitamin C, taken together, help alleviate morning sickness. Vitamin B6 also helps with morning sickness, and it can also relieve postpartum depression.[4] Flaxseed oil, because of its alpha-linolenic acid, and DHA (docosahexaenoic acid) are crucial for the development of intelligence, memory, and sight of the fetus and infant.[5]

Herbs are often a good alternative to pharmaceutical drugs, since they affect not only the pregnant woman but the unborn baby as well. A tea made with ginger, peppermint, spearmint, and raspberry leaf helps relieve morning sickness. Red raspberry leaf, nettles, and dandelion leaf are rich in vitamins and minerals and help ease digestive problems.[6] Red raspberry leaf and nettle also increase the flow of milk and continue to work after delivery by boosting Mom's energy. Another herb that is especially helpful after delivery is calendula, which accelerates healing.[7] During and after pregnancy, calendula can be applied topically as a good remedy for hemorrhoids and varicose veins. Nettle leaf is good for relieving swollen tissue, while basil improves blood circulation. Heartburn, often experienced during pregnancy, can be relieved by slippery elm lozenges or by placing a drop of peppermint oil on the back of the tongue.

Helpful Foods, Nutrients & Herbs

For more information, see "Nutrient Sources" & "Glossary"

Foods

Alfalfa Sprouts	Cauliflower	Parsley
Almonds	Chlorella	Pumpkin
Avocado	Collard Greens	Seeds
Bananas	Corn	Soy Products
Barley Grass	Cucumber	Spinach
Bee Pollen	Figs & Dates	Spirulina
Blue-Green Algae	Kale	Watercress
Bran	Kelp	Wheat Germ
Brewer's Yeast	Legumes	Wheat Grass
Cabbage	Mushrooms	

Nutrients

Calcium	Folic Acid	Vitamin B6
Choline	Iron	Vitamin C
Evening Primrose Oil	Niacin	Vitamin K
Flaxseed Oil	Vitamin B3	

Herbs

Basil	Green Tea	Raspberry Leaf
Calendula	Nettle Leaf	Slippery Elm
Dandelion Leaf	Peppermint Oil	Spearmint
Ginger	Peppermint	

Substances that pregnant women should avoid are arginine, yohimbe, barberry, blue cohosh, chaste berry, ephedra, goldenseal, juniper, passion flower, schisandra, arbutin, pennyroyal, melatonin, and some pharmaceutical drugs. Check with your doctor. Scientific research indicates that pregnant women should avoid excessive consumption of linoleic acid in the form of oils from safflower, evening primrose, soybean, corn or sunflower seed, since it may interfere with the growth of the fetus.[8] Midwives, however, may use these oils to induce late pregnancies, and they are safe and healthful for the new and nursing mother.

Recipes

Morning Sickness

1 bag or tsp	Peppermint or Spearmint
1 bag or tsp	Raspberry leaf
1 bag or tsp	Nettle
1/4	Lemon, juiced

These herbs help relieve morning sickness. They are also rich in vitamins and minerals that help ease digestive problems. Red raspberry leaf and nettle also increase milk flow and work to boost energy after delivery. Steep your tea bags or loose tea for a minimum of 5 minutes. Add a squeeze of lemon last.

Calcium Caravan

1-2 cups	Pure Water
1 small	Apple, cut and cored
2 Tbsp	Wheat or Barley Grass Powder
1 tsp	Spirulina
2 Tbsp	Brewer's Yeast
2 Tbsp	Pumpkin Seeds
pinch	Stevia Powder

Spirulina, wheat grass, and brewer's yeast are three top calcium foods. Use whole leaf grass powder rather than grass juice powder to add fiber to this drink. This, along with the apple, will keep things moving. Wheat grass, brewer's yeast, and pumpkin seeds are also tops in iron. Stevia is an alternative sweetener that replaces the use of sugar during pregnancy. By restricting the use of sugar, mother's-to-be can avoid the potential for gestational diabetes.

Begin with 1 cup of water in your blender and slowly add the remaining ingredients in the order listed. You may need additional water to achieve a whirlpool in the blender and a smoothie consistency.

Iron Mobile

1–2 cups	Pure Water
2 Tbsp	Bran, Rice, Oat, or Wheat
½	Banana
1 small	Apple, cut and cored
3 Tbsp	Tahini
1 Tbsp	Bee Pollen
½ tsp	Vitamin C Crystals

This drink adds fiber to your diet and keeps things moving when the thoroughfare gets a little cramped during pregnancy. Sesame seeds are the highest dietary source of calcium. Tahini is sesame seed paste. Try to obtain raw, organic tahini from your health food store. Rice bran is one of our finest sources of iron, followed closely by bee pollen and sesame seeds.

Begin with 1 cup of water in your blender and slowly add the remaining ingredients in the order listed. Since some of the ingredients are thickeners, you may need to add additional water to achieve a whirlpool in the blender as well as a smoothie consistency.

Prostate Problems

Benign Prostatic Hyperplasia, Cancer

See also Cancer, Urinary Tract Infections

Talk about the prostate gland and men get squeamish. Attention to prostate health, however, is critical, since a large percentage of men over 50 experience prostate abnormalities. When abnormalities are detected and treated early, there is much less reason to worry.

Enlarged prostate and prostate cancer are the two most common conditions involving the prostate. As the name suggests, enlarged prostate, also known as benign prostatic hyperplasia (BPH), is a swelling and inflammation of the prostate gland. It is not usually life-threatening in itself, but can cause discomfort and urinary obstruction. And it can mask the more serious condition of prostate cancer. Because of its proximity to the bladder, an enlarged prostate increases the risk of bladder and urinary tract infections. It can cause frequent or painful urination, urine retention and, if left untreated, can lead to kidney damage and incontinence.

The most common cancer in men is prostate cancer, and the odds of malignancy increase as men age. An enlarged prostate and/or frequent, painful urination may be symptoms of prostate cancer. PSA (prostate-specific antigen) is a dangerous foreign protein that stimulates the growth of cancer cells. Screening for elevated levels of PSA is one way to diagnose prostate cancer.

Causes

You work hard, eat well, and exercise regularly. Unfortunately, however, just growing older increases the risk of developing an enlarged prostate and prostate cancer. Enlarged prostate glands are caused by certain enzymes such as 5-alpha reductase, aromatase, the protein kinase C, zinc deficiencies, and the hormones prolactin and dihydro-testosterone (DHT).

Prostate cancer has been linked to excessive consumption of saturated fatty acids. In fact, excessive consumption of red meat increases the risk of developing prostate cancer by 200%! Obesity also increases the risk of prostate cancer.[1]

Diet Suggestions

To reduce your risk of developing prostate problems, eat a low-fat, high fiber diet. Limit your intake of red meats, animal fats, and dairy, all of which increase the risk of prostate cancer according to epidemiological studies. Oysters, pumpkin and sunflower seeds, brewer's yeast, pecans, nuts, and whole grains are the best sources of zinc. Beans, lentils, peas, and brans provide the much needed fiber.

Foods That Help

Eat nuts and seeds, especially pumpkin seeds, which are great sources of zinc. Rice and soy foods also protect against prostate cancer. Soybeans contain isoflavonoids, which reduce swelling and provide protective hormonal support. Miso contains genistein, another isoflavonoid that counteracts the damaging activity of the protein kinase C.

Tomatoes, especially cooked tomatoes and tomato sauce, contain the powerful antioxidant lycopene, which stops cancer cell growth by interfering with "growth factor-1," an insulin-like compound that stimulates the growth of prostate cancer cells.[2] Beets provide a rich source of minerals for bladder and kidney health and have been used in Europe to treat prostate cancer. Garlic interferes with the production of PSA and 5-lipoxygenase to help stop the growth of prostate cancer cells.[3] Kiwi, honeydew, peaches, and oranges are good sources of the powerful antioxidant lutein, which reduces the risk of several cancers including prostate cancer.

Nutrients and Herbs That Help

Minerals are most important for prostate health. Zinc is especially critical for a healthy prostate, because it counteracts the conversion of testosterone into dihydro-testosterone (DHT) by obstructing the enzyme 5-alpha reductase. In one study, zinc reduced the size of the prostate in 75% of the men.[4] Magnesium, copper, and selenium are also essential for prostate cancer prevention and proper mineral balance.

Vitamins A, C, D, and E are good prostate cancer preventatives, and vitamin C helps reduce prostate cancer cell multiplication. Vitamin D may benefit the prostate by helping turn cancer cells into normal cells and preventing excess production of PSA.[5] One study showed that beta-carotene (provitamin A) reduced prostate cancer by 36% compared with men taking a placebo.[6]

Citrus pectin helps prevent cancer cells from spreading to other places in the body and is known to specifically prevent the spread of prostate cancer cells.[7] And coenzyme Q10 may extend the life expectancy of men afflicted with prostate cancer. Since human prostate epithelial cells contain melatonin receptors, supplementation with the hormone melatonin may help shrink an enlarged prostate gland.[8]

Many herbs prevent and treat prostate problems. These include nettle, pygeum, goldenseal, parsley, epilobium, and green tea. But the real prostate superstar in the herbal kingdom is saw palmetto. Studies have repeatedly proven that saw palmetto works as well as any drug to reduce the inflammation and pain of an enlarged prostate. Its valuable phytosterols prevent the conversion of testosterone into DHT, the acknowledged cause of BPH. It also tones the bladder muscles, reducing the urgency and frequency of urination.[9]

Nettle works alone or with saw palmetto to increase urinary flow. In addition to its ability to prevent an enlarged prostate in the first place, nettle is effective for preventing benign enlarged prostate cells from becoming malignant.[10]

The evergreen pygeum offers multiple benefits: it prevents the enzymes that raise PSA levels; helps increase the flow of urine; and has a great success rate for reducing the pain and inflammation of an enlarged prostate.[11] Goldenseal's anti-inflammatory properties help shrink an enlarged prostate, and green tea reduces the size of existing tumors.[12]

Bovine and shark cartilage can prevent the formation of the blood vessels that support tumors. The bee products propolis and bee pollen contain the compound galangin, which provides relief for even chronic cases of prostate enlargement. Look in your health food stores and natural pharmacies for herbal formulas that include the combined power of several of these western and Chinese herbs to reduce PSA levels and kill cancer cells.

Helpful Foods, Nutrients & Herbs

For more information, see "Nutrient Sources" & "Glossary"

Foods

Beans, Peas
Bee Pollen
Bee Propolis
Beets
Brewer's Yeast
Carrots
Honeydew Melon
Miso
Nuts & Seeds
Oranges
Oysters
Parsley
Peaches
Kiwi
Pecans
Pumpkin Seeds
Sunflower Seeds
Rice
Soybeans
Tomato
Tomato Sauce

Nutrients

Beta-Carotene
Bovine Cartilage
Citrus Pectin
Coenzyme Q10
Copper
Vitamins C + E
Vitamin A
Vitamin D
Zinc

Herbs

Garlic
Goldenseal
Green Tea
Nettle
Pygeum
Saw Palmetto

Recipes

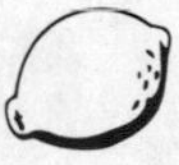

Prostate Purge

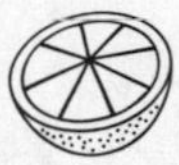

1	Grapefruit, juiced
1	Lemon, juiced
1 ml	Saw Palmetto Liquid Extract (1 dropperful)
½ tsp	Vitamin C Crystals

Vitamin C slows the rate at which prostate cancer cells multiply. Citrus pectin obstructs the spreading of prostate cancer cells. Don't forget to juice the pulp from inside the rind to get the miracle of the pectin and flavonoids. Buy organic fruits so you do not have to worry about the pesticides. Saw palmetto contains fatty acids, sterols, and esters to reduce DHT and ultimately the size of the prostate.

Miso Soup

12 oz	Pure Water, hot
1-2 Tbsp	Miso, blonde
6 cubes	Tofu
1/4 inch	Ginger, grated
1/2 clove	Garlic, grated

Soy foods are a wonderful addition to the diet for prevention of prostate problems. They contain powerful isoflavonoids that reduce inflammation and provide protective hormonal support. Miso contains the isoflavonoid genistein, which counteracts one of the causes of prostate troubles, the damaging protein kinase C. Ginger is an excellent source of the valuable mineral zinc. Garlic stops prostate cancer cell growth.

First obtain a good tasting miso. Miso comes in many flavors. Blonde, or yellow, miso is mild tasting. The darker the miso, the stronger the taste. If you like the miso, you'll like the soup. Using your blender, blend the miso, water, grated ginger, and garlic until smooth. Pour into a pot, add small cubes of tofu, and simmer until hot, approximately 3-5 minutes.

Carotenoid Cocktail

5 oz	Tomato Juice
3 oz	Spinach Juice
3 oz	Carrot Juice
1/2 inch	Ginger Root

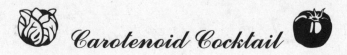

Tomatoes have gotten red-hot press lately because of their high lycopene content and the discovery that the powerful antioxidant carotenoid interferes with the growth of prostate cancer cells. Cooked tomatoes have more lycopene than fresh, but there is also an abundance of living enzymes and phytonutrients in the fresh that more than compensate. Another famous carotenoid is beta-carotene from carrots. This pre-cursor to vitamin A significantly reduces the likelihood of contracting prostate cancer. Spinach is a great source of coenzyme Q10, which extends the life expectancy of prostate cancer victims. Ginger is a major source of zinc and gives a kick to this juice.

Zinc Drink

1–2 cups	Pure Water
2 Tbsp	Sunflower Seeds
2 Tbsp	Pumpkin Seeds
2 Tbsp	Oat, Rice, or Wheat Bran
1 small	Apple, cut and cored
1 Tbsp	Brewer's Yeast
1 Tbsp	Bee Pollen
Pinch	Stevia

Sunflower, pumpkin seeds, and brewer's yeast are our top sources of the most important mineral for prostate health, zinc. Sunflower and bee pollen are both excellent sources of vitamin D, which prevents excess production of PSA. Bee pollen also reduces BPH. Fiber is an important part of any prostate health program, and bran and apple pectin provide our best fiber.

Start by blending the sunflower and pumpkin seeds to a meal in a dry blender. Then add 1 cup of water and blend until smooth. Then slowly add the bran and apple, adding only enough water as needed to maintain a whirlpool in the blender and achieve your desired consistency. Stevia is a natural, non-sugar sweetener to be added last and sparingly.

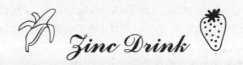

Skin Cancer

Skin is the largest organ in the body. This expansive organ is both tough and delicate—tough in its role as protector of our whole body, and delicate in its vulnerability. One disease to which this organ is vulnerable is skin cancer, a group of cancers that takes the form of malignant tumors on the skin.

There are three types of skin cancer: basal cell carcinoma, squamous cell carcinoma, and malignant melanoma. Basal cell carcinoma is a benign, slow-growing type of cancer that invades areas under the skin but does not spread to other areas in the body. Squamous cell carcinoma, however, occurs on the external surface of the skin and is regarded as more dangerous, because it can metastasize to other places in the body. Both of these types of skin cancer, which occur primarily on sun-exposed skin, are easily treated and seldom fatal.

The third, less common, and most dangerous type of skin cancer is malignant melanoma. Melanomas can spread across the skin or they can grow inward, which is more dangerous, because the cells invade other organs. Early detection and treatment are critical for survival.

Causes

Excessive exposure to the sun is a known cause of skin cancer. If possible, avoid direct, prolonged exposure to the sun and wear protective clothing and sunscreen. People with a fair complexion, blue or green eyes, and blond or red hair are especially vulnerable. Environmental radiation, such as unshielded fluorescent lighting, microwaves, damage to the earth's ozone layer, and medical radiation (X-rays) have damaging effects on the skin, one of which can be basal cell carcinoma. Awareness and avoidance of these perils can reduce the risk of developing skin cancer.

The list of causes and increased risk of skin cancer is diverse. Continued use of the oral contraceptive pill for more than five years increases the risk of skin cancer, while increased risk of malignant melanoma has been linked to excessive consumption of alcohol. Ironically, titanium dioxide, a common ingredient in sunscreens, may actually cause skin cancer.

Of special note is the link between the number of childhood sunburns and the risk of developing malignant melanoma later. The greater the number of childhood sunburns, the greater the risk of developing skin cancer as an adult.[1] Curiously, obese people have a greater risk of developing malignant melanoma than non-obese people.

Foods That Help

Garlic and onions are good for preventing many types of cancer, including skin cancer. Cumin and poppy seeds help prevent squamous cell carcinoma, while scientific research in mice indicates that flaxseeds help stop the metastasis of melanoma.[2]

Another preventative measure against skin cancer is drinking red wine and/or juicing grapes and raspberries. The beneficial acid resveratrol, found in these fruits, stops the conversion of healthy skin cells into cancerous cells.[3] Juicing also aids the process of cleansing and detoxifying, which has produced positive results in the treatment of all skin cancers.

Tea, especially green tea, stops the initiation, promotion and progression of skin cancer. Green tea extract is especially effective for preventing the development of melanoma.[4]

Nutrients and Herbs That Help

Squalene from shark liver oil capsules (also some in wheat germ, rice bran, and olive oils) is effective for treating both squamous cell carcinoma and malignant melanoma. The oil stops the formation of new blood vessels that help a tumor to grow. Because it deactivates skin carcinogens, topically-applied squalene shows promise in preventing skin cancer.[5]

Beta-carotene and selenium have properties that both prevent and cure squamous cell carcinoma. Vitamins A, B6, and E work similarly for melanomas. Vitamins C and E, and para aminobenzoic acid (PABA), a water-soluble B vitamin found in many sunscreens, also help prevent skin cancer. PABA is a super skin nutrient that helps with everything from scleroderma to wrinkles. Nobel prize winner Linus Pauling proved that cancer patients can increase their life-expectancy dramatically by simply supplementing with vitamin C.[6]

Herbs can also be very helpful. Cat's claw decreases the visible size of some skin cancers, while hops restrains the development of cancer-causing agents. Ginseng can prevent the growth of melanoma cells and convert melanoma cells back to normal pigment cells in the skin.[7]

Helpful Foods, Nutrients & Herbs

For more information, see "Nutrient Sources" & "Glossary"

Foods

Shark Cartilage
Garlic
Onion
Seeds
Rhubarb
Black Currants
Grapes
Raspberries
Red Wine

Nutrients

Selenium
PABA-Para Amino-benzoic Acid
Vitamin A
Vitamin B6
Vitamin C
Vitamin E
Squalene

Herbs

Cat's Claw
Chaparral
Hops
Ginseng
Green Tea
Black Tea
Flaxseeds

Recipes

Flaxseed Tea

2 Tbsp	Flaxseeds, Brown or Blonde
½	Lemon, Juiced, or 2 Tbsp of Apple Juice)

Flaxseeds, due to their high lignan content, have demonstrated the potential to stop the metastasis of melanoma and the proliferation of breast cancer cells. *(For more information, see Fluxseeds page 323.)* Heat the seeds in 1-1½ cups of water and let boil for 3 minutes. The seed will foam up with a viscous ooze. Pour the brew, foam and all, into your cup, using a strainer to filter out the seeds. You can flavor this drink by adding a squeeze of lemon or 2 tablespoons of apple juice.

A Berry Anti-Mutagen Juice

6 oz	Grape Juice
1 oz	Raspberry Juice (or other berry juice)
½ tsp	Vitamin C Crystals

Resveratrol is the name of the healthful compound in grapes, berries, and red wine. Technically speaking, it is a sterol produced by the plant as a protective mechanism against insects, pathogens, and weather, similar to the adrenalin response in people. Resveratrol behaves like an anti-mutagen when ingested. It stimulates the production of enzymes that protect our cells against cancerous invaders. It is found in the skin of grapes, raisins, and most berries. Vitamin C increases cancer survival. Juice your grapes and add a touch of vitamin C.

Skin Rejuvenator Juice

6 oz	Carrot Juice
2 oz	Aloe Vera Juice
1 Tbsp	Wheat or Barley Grass Powder
1 Tbsp	Brewer's Yeast

This simple recipe is a bonafide beta-carotene and PABA booster. Make your carrot juice and add bottled aloe vera juice. Although aloe vera can be juiced at home directly from the fresh plant, it is difficult and good quality aloe juice is widely available in health food stores. Yeast is our finest source of PABA, a B vitamin that is in every sunscreen. It is a super skin nutrient that helps with everything from scleroderma to wrinkles. Wheatgrass contains high amounts of PABA as well as beta-carotene. Make your juice and stir in the powders.

Green Tea

1 bag or tsp	Green Tea

Green tea is a powerful antioxidant and immune system enhancing herb with known benefits for cancer. It is particularly effective in counteracting the degeneration of body tissues. *(For more, see "Green Tea.")* If using loose tea, steep for 3 minutes before drinking. *(See "Power Drinks Basics—How to Brew Tea.")*

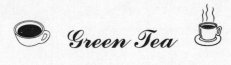

Skin Problems

Dermatitis, Eczema, Psoriasis

We've all heard the adage "beauty is skin deep." Well, sometimes things can affect the skin from the outside to detract from its beauty, but more often, what goes on inside the body is responsible for the skin's beauty or lack of it.

Dermatitis is a general term applied to any superficial inflammation of the skin caused by an outside factor. Several sources of irritants can cause itchy, red, scaly patches on the skin. Contact dermatitis that appears just by touching some irritants can cause great discomfort, as anyone who has suffered from poison ivy will tell you. Eczema is a type of dermatitis usually found in patches on the elbows, knees, wrists and neck of (primarily) infants and children whose bodies may have trouble using fatty acids.

Psoriasis is a similar skin disease that appears on the scalp in addition to elbows, knees and wrists. Psoriasis also differs from dermatitis in other ways: it is classified as an auto-immune, chronic skin disease; it more often affects adults; and is the result of the production of excess skin cells, so the disorder produces thickened areas of silvery, scaly patches that can bleed when scratched. Psoriasis can also cause hair loss, and people with psoriasis may be at an increased risk for larynx and lung cancer.

Causes

Surface contact with an irritant can cause contact dermatitis. Determining the cause of eczema and psoriasis, however, is less apparent. Allergies, especially gluten and milk, are thought to cause eczema and psoriasis, and drinking coffee–not caffeine–has been implicated as a cause of eczema.[1] Excess copper and keratin are possible causes of psoriasis and aspirin, alcohol and tobacco, can make it worse. Thin walls of blood vessels can compound the problem by allowing toxins to be absorbed into the blood stream. These toxins try to exit the body through the skin, causing disruptions like psoriasis.

Since toxins try to escape through the skin, poor liver and kidney function interfere with adequate toxin removal and cause skin problems. Some skin problems are thought to be caused or made worse by excessive stress.

In addition to allergies, deficiencies of minerals and vitamins can cause eczema and other forms of dermatitis. Calcium, potassium, zinc, nickel, selenium, silicon, sulfur, biotin, and inositol deficiencies may be part of the cause. You may inherit a predisposition to skin problems and some medications can also cause them.

Diet Suggestions

As stated, skin ailments often indicate that the body is not getting rid of toxins. A diet that cleans the body of toxins is helpful for "cleaning" the skin. A high fiber, high mineral diet with lots of vegetable protein helps clear up skin problems and prevent further flare-ups. Drinking lots of water can help wash away toxins that cause skin problems. More importantly, fasting and juicing with vitamin and mineral-rich vegetables and fruits can flush toxins out of the body, leaving clear, clean skin. Eliminating gluten and dairy can improve skin problems caused by allergies. And taking an ocean swim (salt water) or adding cider vinegar to your bath water can also soothe irritated skin.

Foods That Help

Eating lots of fresh fruit can reduce the incidence of psoriasis. Rice, especially if it replaces gluten, can greatly help allergic people afflicted with psoriasis. If you have psoriasis or eczema, try drinking rhubarb juice to relieve itching and pain.[2]

Green drinks made with barley or wheat grass help rid the body of toxins while providing minerals, vitamins, and chlorophyll. Eating lots of carrots, tomatoes, garlic and onions translates into improved psoriasis. Carrots are especially helpful for detoxifying the liver and kidneys while providing beta-carotene. Beet greens and other leafy green vegetables and yellow-orange vegetables provide necessary vitamins A and C, beta-carotene and minerals. And grandma used to rub a slice of potato on the skin to soothe eczema.

Make sure to include fiber-rich foods to maintain a clean colon. Colon health is directly related to skin health. Include bentonite clay to absorb colonic toxins and add flaxseed or psyllium colon cleansing drinks to your diet. One of the best cleansers is pure water, so drink lots of it to flush out your system. Acidophilus, as yoghurt, powder, liquid, or capsules helps maintain a healthy intestinal terrain. Healthy skin inside means healthy skin outside. If a milk allergy is the source of your skin disorder, buy non-dairy probiotic powder, or try some homemade rejuvelac *(see page 203.)*

Nutrients and Herbs That Help

Minerals and vitamins are very beneficial for preventing and healing psoriasis and eczema. Potassium sulfate helps reduce scaling associated with psoriasis. People afflicted with psoriasis have low levels of zinc and nickel, so extra doses of each can help return the skin to more normal condition.[3]

Vitamin A, both in the diet and applied topically, reduces skin cell thickening and attacks the root problems of some causes of psoriasis. It is also used to treat dermatitis and eczema in children.[4] Vitamin D also provides benefits internally and topically. Scientific research using topical applications of vitamin D produced improvement of psoriasis lesions in 100% of the trial participants.[5] Vitamin B12 relieves dermatitis and eczema and also has a track record of totally reversing many psoriasis cases.[6] Other B vitamins that help eczema and dermatitis include biotin, inositol, B2 and para aminobenzoic acid (PABA). Vitamin E helps relieve dermatitis and psoriasis symptoms, and vitamin C is good for respiration and general health. Coenzyme Q10 may help psoriasis because it improves the immunity of the skin.

Herbs are often-used remedies for treating and preventing psoriasis, eczema and dermatitis. Effective topical relief comes in the form of soothing gels, creams and shampoos that contain herbs such as aloe vera, calendula, chamomile, comfrey, chickweed, and gotu kola. Creams containing capsaicin (red pepper) provide a different type of relief that works by acting on sensory nerves. When first applied, capsaicin produces a burning sensation but eventually desensitizes nerves that generate pain and itching. But do not use capsaicin on broken skin and avoid contact with sensitive areas such as eyes.

To relieve flaking, itching and irritation, helpful oils that are applied topically include apricot kernel, jojoba, lavender, neem, sesame seed, tea tree, emu, wheat germ, and fish oils.

Herbs that work from the inside out include Oregon grape (barberry), goldenseal, burdock, milk thistle, sarsaparilla, yellow dock and wild oat. Burdock and milk thistle help purify the blood and promote good liver function. Oregon grape and goldenseal have both been known to help prevent the thickening of skin cells implicated in psoriasis because of their high bernamine and berberine content.[7] Sarsaparilla contains a saponin that may bind the endotoxins that can cause psoriasis. In one study, 62% of psoriasis sufferers taking sarsparilla improved and 18% achieved complete recovery.[8] To reduce inflammation, try boswellia or sarsaparilla. Red clover, bitter melon, and reishi mushroom also relieve skin discomfort.

Oregon grape, also known as barberry, deserves special note. This herb has anti-inflammatory and antibacterial qualities. More importantly, since chronic skin disease has been linked to compromised liver function, Oregon grape supports the immune system and liver to eliminate the source of psoriasis and eczema. Tea made from the root of Oregon grape increases the liver's ability to filter toxins. Oregon grape also inhibits the production of lipoxygenase, an enzyme that has been implicated in causing psoriasis. Oregon grape tops the list of helpful herbs, but it may take some time and patience for it to work its magic.[9]

Fatty acid deficiencies of alpha linolenic acid and linoleic acid are implicated in psoriasis and eczema outbreaks. Flaxseed, borage seed, olive, and evening primrose oils are good sources of these essential fats. Fish oils are rich sources of DHA and EPA *(see "Glossary" and "Power Drinks for the Mind"),* which successfully reduced the redness, itching, and scaling of psoriasis sufferers in trials. Add fish oils to your diet or apply them topically.[10]

Helpful Foods, Nutrients & Herbs

For more information, see "Nutrient Sources" & "Glossary"

Foods

Barley Grass
Beet Greens
Carrots
Flaxseed
Fresh Fruits
Garlic
Leafy Green Vegetables
Onions
Potatoes
Psyllium
Rhubarb Juice
Rice
Tomatoes
Wheat Grass
Yellow-Orange Vegetables
Yoghurt

Nutrients

Biotin
Coenzyme Q10
DHA
EPA
Inositol
Nickel
PABA
Potassium Sulfate
Vitamin A
Vitamin B2
Vitamin B12
Vitamin C
Vitamin D
Vitamin E
Zinc

Herbs

Aloe Vera
Apricot Kernel Oil
Barberry
Bitter Melon
Borage Oil
Boswellia
Burdock
Calendula
Capsaicin
Cayenne
Chamomile
Chickweed
Comfrey
Emu Oil
Evening Primrose Oil
Fish Oils
Flaxseed Oil
Goldenseal
Gotu Kola
Jojoba Oil
Lavender Oil
Milk Thistle
Neem Oil
Olive Oil
Oregon Grape
Red Clover
Red Pepper
Reishi Mushroom
Sarsaparilla
Sesame Seed Oil
Tea Tree Oil
Wheat Germ Oil
Wild Oat
Yellow Dock

Recipes

Liver Lover

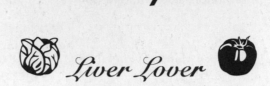

10 oz	Carrot Juice
2 oz	Beet Juice
2 Tbsp	Wheat or Barley Grass Powder
1 tsp	Spirulina Powder
1 clove	Garlic

Your skin will thank you every time you down these liver-loving ingredients. Liver function and skin health are closely related. Grass powders from barley or wheat, help rid the body of toxins while providing minerals, vitamins, and chlorophyll. Carrots are especially helpful for detoxifying the liver, as are beets and garlic. These vegetables are also a rich source of the important healthy-skin vitamins A, C, D (from spirulina), beta-carotene, and minerals. Try to use organic ingredients, especially carrots, whenever possible.

Skin Healer Tea

1 bag or tsp	Oregon Grape
1 bag or tsp	Sarsaparilla

These two herbs are powerful medicines to reduce inflammation, prevent thickening of skin, and control bacteria, all necessary in the fight against skin disease. Tea made from the root of Oregon grape improves liver function and counteracts an enzyme that causes psoriasis. These teas are available in tea bags, and Oregon grape is also available in capsules. *(See "Power Drinks Basics—How to Brew Tea.")*

Colon Clear

2-3 Tbsp	Flaxseed or Psyllium Seed
½-1	Apple or Banana
2-3 Tbsp	Bentonite Liquid
2 Tbsp	Green Foods Powder
2 Tbsp	Probiotic Powder
1-2 cups	Pure Water

Flax and psyllium both develop a mucilage that enhances regularity. Psyllium is available as a powder and flax is available as seeds and powder. You can grind the flaxseed into a meal with your blender. Flax is gentler than psyllium seed, which can be too strong for some. Put the dry flaxseeds in the blender and blend into a meal. Next add the bentonite and one cup of water, and blend thoroughly. Add the apple or banana, and your favorite green powder. Green powders usually include wheat and barley grass and algaes such as spirulina. Probiotic powders include acidophilus and other friendly bacteria. You should also consider a non-dairy acidophilus *(see rejuvelac, p. 203).* All these products are available at your health food store. Let this drink sit for ten minutes to allow the mucilage to expand. Then add more water as necessary to achieve a milk-shake consistency. Also try drinking hot flaxseed tea *(see "Skin Cancer")*.

Sleep Disorders

Insomnia

See also Stress, Fatigue

Do you count sheep endlessly as you struggle to fall asleep, even when you're exhausted? Do you race against the clock as you try to get back to sleep in the middle of the night? You are not the only one. Many people of all ages experience insomnia, the state of being awake when you want to be asleep.

Most people have occasional sleepless nights or awake before they intend to wake up. Occasional insomnia is very common and inconvenient but nothing to worry about. However, some people experience more frequent or even chronic insomnia, which deprives the mind and body of needed rest.

Causes

The causes of insomnia are as numerous as the nights you have probably stayed awake. Common causes include stress, jet lag, restlessness, overwork, pre-menstrual syndrome, stimulants and pharmaceutical or recreational drugs. Shun all sources of caffeine–coffee, tea, caffeinated soft drinks, chocolate, and some pharmaceuticals–especially close to bedtime. Also avoid nicotine and alcohol. Insomnia may also be caused by adrenaline, often a product of stress, and ephedrine, which mimics the actions of adrenaline.

Longer-term insomnia can be caused by major depression, anxiety, grief, changes in medications, menopause, certain foods and herbs, chronic constipation, and diseases such as hyperthyroidism and Lyme disease. Take steps to identify the cause(s) and find ways to eliminate or reduce the source of insomnia. Avoid the ginseng family of herbs, since they are stimulants that could keep you awake. Stay away from the herb feverfew, since it interferes with the production of serotonin, a helpful hormone for sleep. Also, watch out for excessive copper in your diet, because it may over-excite your nerves.

Diet Suggestions

Because so much insomnia is related to stress, a diet high in the B vitamins is desirable for more peaceful, uninterrupted sleep. Eating carbohydrates is known to increase serotonin, a hormone that reduces anxiety and promotes sleep. If you love coffee and chocolate but can't sleep, perhaps this is the time to start thinking about reducing the caffeine in your diet. Eat a larger lunch instead of stuffing yourself with a seven-course dinner late in the evening.[1]

Foods That Help

Carbohydrates and foods high in Vitamin B1 and B6 can help. Apricots, bananas, wheat germ, whole grains, brown rice, legumes, brewer's yeast, and nuts improve the quantity and quality of sleep by increasing serotonin, the hormone that calms the nervous system. Honey aids in the production of serotonin. Some of these foods are also high in calcium, lithium, and magnesium, all of which help serotonin production.

Mushroom lovers claim that eating reishi mushrooms eases mild insomnia, and juice fans say that drinking apple or grapefruit juice at night helps. Lettuce and dill seeds also have a sedating effect on the central nervous system.

If you want to increase the likelihood of a good night's sleep, your evening meal should not consist of a cola, burger, and chocolate cake. Rather choose a glass of apple juice or a cup of chamomile tea, a mushroom sandwich on whole grain bread, and some nuts. You may think a night cap of a banana-based drink with brewer's yeast will attract the monkeys, but it might also keep the sheep at bay.

Nutrients and Herbs That Help

Nutrients that affect the nerves can be used to treat insomnia. Calcium, lithium, and magnesium are minerals that help serotonin do its job of calming the central nervous system. Another natural hormone, melatonin, can help to regulate the body's clock and is especially helpful for insomnia that affects the elderly, since the body's production of melatonin decreases with age. It is also known to help young and middle-aged adults.[2]

Aromatic oils can help induce restful sleep. Lavender oil and neroli oil, an easily vaporized oil from the blossom of bitter orange, are especially pleasant. They are known to lessen anxiety and depression and sedate the central nervous system.[3]

Other herbs that quiet the central nervous system, promote the onset of sleep, or improve the quality of sleep are marjoram, passion flower, black cohosh, chamomile, valerian, St. John's wort, gotu kola, hops, kava kava, and wild oats.[4]

Helpful Foods, Nutrients & Herbs

For more information, see "Nutrient Sources" & "Glossary"

Foods

Apple Juice	Brown Rice	Legumes
Apricots	Dill Seeds	Lettuce
Bananas	Grapefruit Juice	Nuts
Brewer's Yeast	Honey	Wheat Germ

Nutrients

Calcium	Melatonin	Vitamin B1
Lithium	Serotonin	Vitamin B6
Magnesium		

Herbs

Black Cohosh	Kava Kava	Reishi Mushrooms
Chamomile	Lavender Oil	Valerian
Gotu Kola	Neroli Oil	St. John's Wort
Hops	Passion Flower	Wild Oats

Recipes

Sleep Tight Smoothie

1 cup	Apple Juice
8-12	Almonds
1	Banana, small and ripe
2 Tbsp	Wheat Germ
1 Tbsp	Brewer's Yeast
1 Tbsp	Honey
To taste	Pure Water

First blend the juice with the nuts and honey. Then blend the banana and add the remaining ingredients. The preferred consistency should be that of a milk shake. You can add any amount of water at the end to achieve the consistency you desire.

Good Night Tea

1 bag or tsp	Valerian
1 bag or tsp	Passion Flower
1 bag or tsp	Chamomile
1 bag or tsp	Hops

Drink hot approximately one hour before bedtime.

De-Stress Tea

1 bag or tsp	St. John's Wort
1 bag or tsp	Kava Kava

Steep for a few minutes and drink hot. These herbs will have a quieting influence on your nervous system over the long term. They have sedative properties but are safe to enjoy any time of day.

Stress

See also Ulcers, Hypertension, Depression, Fatigue

Climb the corporate ladder. Lose your job. Overspend on your credit card. Break up with your significant other. Present the annual budget. Meet a deadline. Run a marathon. Give birth. Get stuck in traffic. Prepare for the holidays. Live with sickness or pain. Stress is any factor that threatens the body's natural balance.

An ailment of the nervous system, stress overworks the adrenals, the body's stress-regulating center. When the body is under stress, adrenaline is released, which helps us meet the challenge before us. Too much adrenaline, however, is toxic and leads to a variety of symptoms and conditions.

Causes

The causes of stress are as varied as the symptoms it produces. Physical, chemical, mental, emotional, psychological, or traumatic stress manifests through symptoms such as nail biting, headaches, indigestion, allergies, muscle aches, high blood pressure, anger, fear, sadness, anxiety, and depression.

Sure you can take herbs and supplements, but unless you discontinue the lifestyle routines that cause the stress, you will be fighting a losing battle. For many, this directive is virtually impossible. Nevertheless, you should work toward eliminating the major sources of stress. Small changes can have large positive effects. For example: avoid a sedentary lifestyle, exposure to environmental toxins, and foods containing caffeine, chemicals, and additives.

Diet Suggestions

Diet is a practical and gratifying approach to stress reduction and management. Eating more of a vegetarian diet would be a good foundation for dealing with most conditions relating to stress. Juicing with vitamin-rich vegetables, nut milks, and algae is fortifying and can bring noticeable relief.

Foods That Help

Mineral deficiencies have been known to fuel stress symptoms. Eat foods high in iron, magnesium, and phosphorus: algae, wheat germ, wheat and rice bran, brown rice, yoghurt, raisins, wheat grass, lentils, soybeans, nuts, watercress, beet root, celery, spinach, cauliflower, broccoli, bananas, liver, clams, shrimp, and kelp. These help to calm the system and build resistance. A hot cup of herbal tea is great because, in addition to the therapeutic effect of the herbs, tea drinking itself is a calming activity.

Pumpkin, sesame, and especially sunflower seeds are good mineral sources, while nuts, such as almonds, hazelnuts, brazil nuts, cashews, peanuts, pistachios, and walnuts provide protein as well as important stress-reducing minerals.

Foods rich in the B vitamins help counter the effects of stress. Of special note is brewer's yeast. This dietary wonder should be added to foods and drinks since it is an extraordinary source of minerals and B vitamins, as well as being an immune system booster.

Nutrients and Herbs That Help

Vitamins A, B5, C, and E revive and improve the adrenal glands, one of the stress centers of the body. In fact, the adrenal glands contain the highest concentration of vitamin C in the body. Vitamin B3 helps control stress-induced anxiety, nervousness, and irritability. Para Aminobenzoic Acid (PABA), a water-soluble B vitamin, helps reduce stress and depression.

Herbs are important for controlling and eliminating stress. Chaparral supports vitamin C as a protector against stress. Chamomile helps prevent excess production of adrenaline, while hops sedates the central nervous system. Including parsley and alfalfa in juices enhances the flavor while delivering important nutrients.

Ginseng helps the body deal with the effects of stress and prepare the body for the next onslaught of stress. As aids to the adrenal system, ginseng helps ease several conditions, including sleep disorders, anxiety, and hypertension.

Is there a new road being built outside your office window? Or perhaps a fussy baby crying nearby? Or music blasting on the neighbor's stereo? Scientific research indicates that holy basil lowers corticosterone levels of subjects stressed because of loud noise.[1] Saint John's wort is a major anti-depressive herb. So, if your anxiety is leading to depression, don't forget to drink this tea or supplement with this herbal remedy.

A massage with lavender oil is the perfect soothing activity for rebounding from stressful situations.

Helpful Foods, Nutrients & Herbs

For more information, see "Nutrient Sources" & "Glossary"

Foods

Algae	Lentils	Cauliflower
Wheat Germ	Soybeans	Broccoli
Wheat & Rice Bran	Nuts	Bananas
Brown Rice	Watercress	Clams & Shrimp
Yoghurt	Beet Root	Liver
Raisins	Celery	Kelp
Wheat Grass	Spinach	Brewer's Yeast

Nutrients

Iron	Vitamin B5	Vitamin C
Magnesium	Para Aminobenzoic Acid (PABA)	Vitamin E
Phosphorous		
Vitamin A		
Vitamin B3		

Herbs

Alfalfa	Siberian Ginseng	Hops
Parsley	Chamomile	Lavender Tea
American Ginseng	Holy Basil	St. John's Wort
Asiatic Ginseng		

Recipes

Calm Down Juice

3 oz	Celery Juice
2 oz	Spinach Juice
1 oz	Broccoli Juice
1 oz	Watercress Juice
1 oz	Wheatgrass Juice
1 oz	Alfalfa Sprouts or Parsley Juice

Green is the healing color of nature. Green juices have a soothing effect on the nervous system. This is dramatically opposed to orange colored juices such as carrot and orange, which are bright and sweet and provide instant energy. Drink green juices slowly and rest and they will reward you with long term energy and deep cellular nourishment.

De-Stress Teas

1 bag or tsp	Asiatic Ginseng
1 bag or tsp	Chamomile
1 bag ortsp	Holy Basil
1 bag or tsp	St. John's Wort
1 bag or tsp	Hops
1 bag or tsp	Catnip

You can't go wrong with any of these herbs, whether drunk separately or together. Choose 1 tea bag or 1 tsp each and make enough for the whole day. The ginsenosides in Asiatic ginseng counteract the toxic effects of excessive stress and reduce the "alarm stage" of stress—the stimulation of the adrenal cortex.[2] Chamomile reduces the excessive secretion of adrenocorticotropic hormone (ACTH) in response to stress. Hops sedates the central nervous system. Holy basil protects against loud noise stress.

Anti-Stress Smoothie

(Dairy and Non-Dairy)

1+ cups	Yoghurt or Soy Milk
2 Tbsp	Raisins
1	Banana
1 Tbsp	Brewer's Yeast
½ tsp	Vitamin C Crystals
½ cup	Pure Water

This smoothie is a rich source of B vitamins. The B-vitamin family is crucial to any anti-stress diet because these vitamins, along with vitamin C, are exhausted by stress. PABA (para aminobenzoic acid), niacinamide (vitamin B3), inositol, and pantothenic acid (vitamin B5) all protect the body against the effects of stress. This drink is also a good source of iron and phosphorus, two minerals whose deficiency can cause stress and magnesium, which reduces stress by improving the functions of the adrenal glands.

Start with ½ cup of water and blend the raisins. Raisins may also be pre-soaked. Choose yoghurt or soy milk, depending on your dairy preference. Then add the banana and remaining ingredients one at a time. Vitamin C crystals are available in any health food store. Add more or less water to achieve your desired consistency.

Tinnitus

See also Ear Infections

When a tree falls in the woods, what do you hear? Hopefully, just a falling tree. But if you also hear an ocean, you probably have tinnitus. An estimated 30 million Americans live with a 'white' noise that always exists for them in the background. It could be a ringing, humming, buzzing, roaring, or clicking; in any case, it is a most frustrating ailment. Frustrating, too, for those around the tinnitus sufferer who are constantly responding to pleas for repetition.

Causes

While the etiology of tinnitus is unknown, there are several contributing factors. The most common are: loud noises, loud music, infection, inflammation, head trauma, and drugs such as aspirin, quinine, and antibiotics. Tinnitus has also been linked to allergies, anemia, and heavy metal toxicity. Because the jawbone is intricately connected with the ear, a misaligned temporomandibular joint (TMJ) may cause it. To this end, stress is also likely to be a factor.

Nutrients and Herbs That Help

Anything that improves blood circulation to the head will help, such as aerobic exercise, inversion boards, and inverted yoga postures. The nutraceuticals vincamine and vinpocetine, derived from the seeds of the periwinkle plant, improve blood circulation and oxygen to the brain.[1] Forty-seven percent of tinnitus sufferers exhibit a vitamin B12 deficiency. B12 enhances the ear's ability to conduct nerve impulses.[2] Since toxic overload from heavy metals may be a contributing factor, chelation therapy may help, using the synthetic but safe amino acid EDTA. Eardrops of the popular sulfur compound MSM, according to some users, may also help.

Black cohosh, in tincture or by capsule, is a medically accepted treatment for tinnitus in many Latin American countries.[3] Ginkgo improves tinnitus by stimulating blood circulation to the brain. Seventy-four percent (74%) of people taking ginkgo in a three month experiment had their symptoms alleviated.[4] Zinc sulfate (a form of zinc) relieved tinnitus in test subjects taking doses of 600mg daily.[5]

The berries of the Chinese herb ligustrum are used for tinnitus in Asia. Fenugreek seeds and kava kava help tinnitus because of their calming effect on the nervous system.

Helpful Foods, Nutrients & Herbs

For more information, see "Nutrient Sources" & "Glossary"

Foods

Algae
Barley Grass
Beets
Brewer's Yeast
Cabbage
Carrot
Celery
Ginger
Parsley
Pecans
Spinach
Sunflower Seeds
Wheat Germ
Wheat Grass

Nutrients

Choline
Manganese
Vitamin B12
Zinc
EDTA
MSM

Herbs

Black Cohosh
Fenugreek Seeds
Kava Kava
Ginkgo
Ligustrum
Vincamine
Vinpocetine

Recipes

4 Ear Teas

1 bag or tsp	Fenugreek Seeds
1 bag or tsp	Kava Kava
1 bag or tsp	Black Tea
1 bag or tsp	Hops

These are 4 separate teas. Fenugreek seeds and kava kava help tinnitus by quieting the nervous system. Kava kava also helps improve blood circulation. If you wish to supplement your diet with this South Pacific shrub, 200-300mg per day is recommended. Hops and black tea are both excellent sources of manganese, a valuable mineral for the ear.

Wheatgrass Juice

2 oz	Wheatgrass Juice, fresh

Grass juice is very purifying to the blood stream and helps transport oxygen to the cells. It soothes the tissues of the intestinal wall and, in larger amounts, purges the bowel. This, along with its potent capacity to detoxify the liver, make it a superb overall system cleanser and nourisher. Many users strain wheatgrass through a cloth and put drops in their nose, eyes, and ears. *(For more information, see "Wheat Grass and Barley Grass.")*

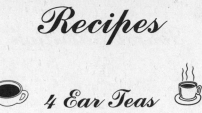

Sound Nutrition

½ cup	Apple Juice
½	Banana, ripe
1 Tbsp	Spirulina or Blue-Green Algae
1 Tbsp	Brewer's Yeast
2 Tbsp	Pumpkin or Sunflower Seeds
4	Pecans
1 Tbsp	Lecithin Granules
1 cup	Pure Water

A great source of tinnitus fighting nutrients. Pumpkin and sunflower seeds are rich sources of zinc. Pecans are an excellent source of manganese. Algae, spirulina, and yeast are our best sources of vitamin B12 (more than any animal food). Lecithin is our finest food source of choline.

First blend the apple juice and banana, then add the powders and the seeds. Add water last and as much as necessary to achieve the thickness you prefer. The consistency should be that of a milk shake. A ripe banana is one that is just beginning to show spots and has lost all of its green complexion. If you have the time to first soak your sunflower seeds in the water, it softens them and starts an enzyme release process–as in germination–that assists digestion. If you like to chew your drinks, which is always a good idea, just blend the seeds for a few seconds.

Toothache & Cavities

See also Gingivitis

Ugh! When it aches, it aches! Put in clinical terms, when the pulp of the tooth–the part of the tooth that contains blood vessels and nerve fibers–becomes irritated, it hurts! Depending on the cause, a toothache can be merely annoying or unmercifully agonizing.

Let's get to the *root* of this problem. The most frequent source of a toothache is bacteria. When food and drink pass over the teeth, bacteria come along with it. If the teeth are not rinsed, brushed, and flossed, bacteria will interact with sugars and starches to form a sticky film of bacteria on the teeth—the dreaded plaque. This interaction also produces acids that weaken the hard surface of teeth and penetrate the pulp. The result is tooth decay–caries or cavities–and eventually a toothache. Once the nerves are exposed to air, heat, and cold, you'll feel it.

Causes

The major cause of toothache is tooth decay, but a cracked tooth or advanced gum disease (see *Gingivitis*) can also cause it. For strong, healthy, pain-free teeth, do not allow food, especially sugars and starches, to remain on the teeth. Special care should be taken for babies who drink bottles of milk as they fall asleep. By rinsing, brushing, and flossing the teeth, the risk of tooth decay is greatly reduced. While fruits are very valuable foods, some such as apples, grapes, and dried fruits such as raisins contain lots of sugar and are known to create cavities. Be sure to brush soon after eating.

Probably the greatest cause of caries is lack of maintenance. Most of us brush because we have to and we are creatures of habit. Children have not yet embraced the concept. But the sound of a roaring drill closing in on your face is an educational experience. It is a visceral example of prevention being better than cure. Canceling dental appointments, albeit an instinctive reflex, will eventually be more painful than keeping them.

Diet Suggestions

Stop the sugar! One of the most effective means of reducing toothaches and the cavities that accompany them, is a change of diet. Reduce your intake of sugary cakes, cookies, and candies and emphasize more whole, unprocessed foods, especially those that are high in calcium and other minerals, which fortify the teeth and bones. Start juicing with mineral-rich vegetables to ensure the health of your teeth and mouth.

Foods That Help

Because one percent of the body's calcium is stored in the teeth, calcium-rich foods such as sesame seeds, sea vegetables, algaes, dark, leafy greens, and dairy products are needed to maintain strong teeth. Carrots are also high in calcium and can be juiced together with cucumbers, which are high in silicone, for a drink that strengthens both bones and teeth.

Iodine, which improves the health of teeth, is found in milk products, pineapple, fish, peanuts, kelp, iodized table salt, and vegetables, such as onions, spinach, tomatoes, carrots, and watercress. Dairy products, nuts, spinach, fish, and wheat germ are rich in magnesium and phosphorous, minerals that concentrate in the teeth.

The caffeine in coffee, tea, and cocoa can prevent tooth decay in a way similar to fluoride by strengthening tooth enamel.[1] Of course, the sugar that usually comes with chocolate and coffee would outweigh any potential benefit. The tannins and polyphenols in tea, especially green tea, are proven fighters of the bacteria that cause tooth decay.[2] Cherry juice blocks an enzyme necessary for the formation of plaque, and herbalists often recommend rhubarb juice for strengthening tooth enamel.

Tea tree oil can be massaged onto the gums for temporary relief of a toothache, and bee propolis can be used either as food or in a mouthwash to reduce plaque.[3]

Nutrients and Herbs That Help

Vitamin D, magnesium, and calcium are critical for the formation of healthy bones and teeth. Besides building strong teeth, calcium and vitamin B5 help soothe the discomfort caused by grinding teeth (bruxism).

Fluoride is the infamous mineral that protects against cavities. While it has proven effective in strengthening tooth enamel, controversy surrounds the political and commercial implications of government laws that force everyone to use it via their drinking water. Sodium fluoride is poisonous in high doses. Since there are so many ways to apply fluoride topically to the teeth, it is unnecessary to universally legislate its ingestion. Molybdenum, another mineral, found in peas and lentils, can also reduce cavities, since people with higher amounts in their diet have fewer cavities.[4]

Like tea tree oil, clove oil can be massaged onto the gums for temporary relief from the discomfort of a toothache. A clove tucked between the cheek and aching tooth will also lend some relief, as will chewing on fresh ginger root. Hops, paprika, and rosemary also provide some temporary relief for pain of a toothache.

Helpful Foods, Nutrients & Herbs

For more information, see "Nutrient Sources" & "Glossary"

Foods

Broccoli	Flaxseeds	Rhubarb
Carrots	Kelp	Sardines
Cherry Juice	Nuts	Spinach
Cucumbers	Onions	Tomato
Dairy Products	Peanuts	Watercress
Fish	Pineapple	

Nutrients

Bee Propolis	Iodine	Phosphorous
Calcium	Magnesium	Vitamin B5
Fluoride	Molybdenum	Vitamin D

Herbs

Cloves	Hops	Rosemary
Ginger	Paprika	Tea Tree Oil
Green Tea		

Recipes

Green Tea

1 bag or tsp	Green Tea

As a dental aide, green tea helps prevent gingivitis by deterring the formation of plaque on teeth, and it strengthens tooth enamel against the invasion of acids. *(For more, see "Green Tea.")* Steep for 3 minutes.

Strong Teeth

5 oz	Celery Juice
2 oz	Kale or Collard Greens Juice
2 oz	Spinach Juice
1 oz	Wheatgrass Juice
1 tsp	Spirulina Powder

These foods are some of the highest dietary sources of calcium and magnesium. Spirulina is also the richest plant source of vitamin D. These three nutrients are vital for the formation of strong enamel and the prevention of caries. Calcium and magnesium are also fundamental to healthy nerves, which you may need in case of a toothache.

Black Cherry Juice

Cherries block the enzyme that leads to plaque formation. They are also capable of lowering uric acid levels in bones and joints. Black cherry juice is rich in the bioflavonoids needed for healthy gums.

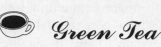

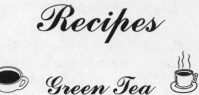

Ulcers

See also Colon Problems, Indigestion

Peptic ulcers are infections of the digestive tract's membranes. Like other infections, the area becomes irritated and inflamed and sores develop causing pain, discomfort and sometimes bleeding. Heartburn is also a symptom of peptic ulcers.

How do ulcers develop? The same gastric juices that digested last night's dinner found weak spots in the stomach's protective mucous lining. Like salt in an open wound, these stomach enzymes (pepsin) and acids irritate the weak spots and create sores or actual holes.

The most common types of peptic ulcers occur in the first part of the intestines (duodenal ulcers) and in the stomach (gastric ulcers). If pain is felt on an empty stomach, chances are the ulcer is duodenal; if pain is felt after a meal, it is likely in the stomach.

Causes

Let's get it straight, once and for all: Chili peppers do not cause ulcers, and neither does stress. Although factors such as spicy foods, stress, alcohol, and smoking can exacerbate an existing ulcer, none are thought to be the original cause. Detrimental bacteria–specifically, helicobacter pylori–are the primary cause of ulcers. When the bacteria are stronger than the stomach's acids, they work through the protective mucous lining, exposing the stomach or intestines to corrosive gastric juices. This same strain of detrimental bacteria can also cause gastritis, a precursor of gastric ulcers, and can possibly cause some types of stomach cancer.[1]

Diet Suggestions

The best foods for an ulcerated digestive tract are those that minimize acid production and have anti-inflammatory properties. To avoid overworking your digestive tract, eat small meals and limit protein from animal sources. Instead, eat organic vegetables, fruits and cultured dairy products to add fortifying nutrients and good bacteria to fight the bad bacteria. Extra fiber should help duodenal ulcers because it slows the movement of food and acidic fluid from the stomach to the intestines.[2]

To speed healing, avoid anything that weakens the mucous membrane or increases stomach acidity, namely, aspirin, citrus fruits, caffeine, smoking, and alcohol. Research has shown that sugar also increases stomach acid, and salt increases the risk of gastric ulcers. Limit your intake of both to prevent or heal ulcers.[3]

Foods That Help

Wherever ulcers form in the digestive tract, two foods are especially helpful: cabbage and unripe bananas or plantain. Long-standing scientific studies confirm that cabbage juice heals peptic ulcers quickly and effectively. Juice cabbage for a calming drink known to reduce healing time by over 70%.[4] Raw potato juice also has healing properties for the stomach.

Unripe bananas and plantains soothe most types of existing peptic ulcers and can prevent new ulcers from forming. For a tasty remedy, sauté unripe bananas and plantains like vegetables. Increase the potential of healing by drizzling the sautéed fruits with honey, an effective agent for stopping the growth of the detrimental bacteria associated with peptic ulcers.

Cow's milk, which has often been prescribed for ulcers, neutralizes stomach acid, while the calcium and protein in milk stimulate production of more acid. Substitute almond milk or soy milk for cow's milk. Cultured dairy products such as yoghurt, kefir, and buttermilk provide protein as well as the beneficial bacteria needed to counteract detrimental bacteria.

Foods rich in zinc and vitamins A and C help heal ulcers. Eat broccoli and yellow-orange fruits as well as vegetables like cantaloupe, yams, carrots, and winter squash. Avoid citrus fruits, which can irritate and further damage the stomach lining.

Helpful Foods, Nutrients & Herbs

For more information, see "Nutrient Sources" & "Glossary"

Foods

Cabbage	Almond Milk	Broccoli
Green Bananas	Soy Milk	Yams
Plantains	Yoghurt	Carrots
Potato Juice	Kefir	Winter Squash
Honey	Buttermilk	

Nutrients

Vitamin A	Silicon	Glutamine
Vitamin C	Calcium	Irish Moss
Zinc	Coenzyme Q10	Bioflavonoids
Lithium	Melatonin	

Herbs

Chilies	Chamomile	Slippery Elm
Licorice	Bilberry	Marshmallow

Nutrients and Herbs That Help

Vitamin A and zinc are the nutritional champions for healing all types of ulcers. Take extra supplements to help shorten healing time, and add extra vitamin C and garlic to your diet for protection against helicobacter pylori, the bacteria that can cause ulcers and stomach cancer.[5]

Lithium, silicon, calcium, and coenzyme Q10 should all be on your supplement list for the prevention of gastric ulcers. Melatonin is known to help ulcerative conditions provoked by stress. Glutamine, an amino acid, supports and helps heal the cells that line the small intestine and stomach.

Not only do chilies not cause peptic ulcers, they have been used to treat and prevent ulcers. Capsaicin, the substance that makes chilies red, helps inhibit detrimental bacteria and protects the mucous lining of the digestive tract.[6]

Raw licorice root provides two major benefits for preventing and healing ulcers: It can increase the production of mucin, a protective substance for the stomach and intestinal lining. Additionally, licorice appears to discourage the production of helicobacter pylori.[7]

Other helpful healing aids include bilberry, which works to strengthen blood vessels in the digestive tract, chamomile, and bioflavonoids, known for their anti-inflammatory properties. Slippery elm and marshmallow also soothe some of the discomfort associated with gastric ulcers. Irish moss, a type of red algae, can be taken in powdered form to help calm irritated mucous membrane in the digestive tract.

Recipes

Ulcer Repair

6 oz	Carrot Juice
1 oz	Potato Juice
1 oz	Cabbage Juice
1 oz	Spinach Juice
1 oz	Broccoli Juice
pinch	Cayenne (chili) Pepper

There is a great deal of research demonstrating the ability of raw cabbage juice to heal stomach ulcers. Potatoes are also healing for the stomach. Spinach and broccoli together are the highest vegetable sources of coenzyme Q10, which can prevent gastric ulcers. Vitamin A is necessary for healing ulcers, and carrots are one of our best sources of pro-vitamin A. Cayenne actually kills helicobacter pylori, the bacteria known to cause certain kinds of ulcers. This fresh juice provides these nutrients in a highly concentrated, not to mention delicious, form.

Tummy Tamer

1 bag or tsp	Chamomile
1 bag or tsp	Licorice Root

Chamomile is known for its anti-inflammatory properties. Licorice increases the production of protective substances in the intestinal lining and discourages the growth of ulcerative bacteria. These teas can be taken separately or in combination. If using cut licorice roots, steep for 15 minutes.

Gastric Healer

1+ cup	Soy or Almond Milk
2 Tbsp	Oat or Wheat Bran
1	Banana, green
1 Tbsp	Slippery Elm, powder
1 tsp	Honey (optional)

Soy or almond milk can be used to replace cow's milk to neutralize stomach acid without stimulating acid secretion or aggravating milk allergies. Bananas and slippery elm soothe peptic ulcers and oat bran provides fiber, which is an ulcer preventative. Honey inhibits the growth of detrimental bacteria associated with peptic ulcers. Non-dairy milks are widely available at health food stores. Blend all ingredients together and add more 'milk' or water to achieve desired consistency.

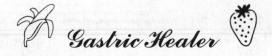

Urinary Tract

Cystitis, Bladder, & Urinary Infections

See also Parasites, Female Problems, Prostate Problems

The urinary tract consists of the kidneys, the ureters (the tubes between the kidney and bladder), and the bladder and the urethra (the final exit tube). These are the organs of the body that produce, store, and eliminate urine. Urinary tract infections (UTI) occur in any of these organs.

Women suffer from UTI more frequently than men and children, but anyone is susceptible. Symptoms of UTI include painful or burning urination, urinating in small amounts, frequent or urgent need to urinate, cloudy urine, blood in the urine, and strong urine odor.

Although some people are prone to recurrent infections, treatment for most UTI is simple and effective, especially if started immediately.

Causes

UTI is usually triggered by bacteria that enters the kidneys from the bloodstream and travels downward or by bacteria that enters the urethra and travels upward. The most common infections, urethritis (infections in the urethra) and cystitis (infections in the bladder or lower urinary tract), often occur together and are caused by bacteria traveling upward.

Cystitis results when bacteria multiply faster than the urine can remove them. Women are more prone to this infection than men, because the female urethra is much shorter and more exposed than the male urethra; the bacteria do not have to travel as far to enter the bladder. Sexual activity is a common avenue for introducing this bacteria into the female bladder through the urethra. One preventive measure for avoiding this annoying infection is to drink adequate water before sexual intercourse and empty the bladder immediately after.

Diet Suggestions

If you are experiencing pain, irritation, and inflammation, you must avoid food and drink that will further irritate the bladder. Eliminate spicy foods, fats, caffeine, sugar, and alcohol. Sugar impairs the ability of white blood cells to destroy bacteria, and alcohol suppresses the immune system. These foods increase irritation and make it harder for your immune system to rebound. You should also limit dairy products, red meats, and shellfish, which increase the acidity of the bloodstream, thus helping to promote bacterial infection.

Foods and Liquids That Help

Your best therapy is water! Since frequent urination flushes bacteria from the bladder, it is essential to drink eight to ten 8-ounce glasses of water per day. But don't quench your thirst just yet. Pour a big glassful of unsweetened cranberry juice. This tart member of the bilberry family is an age-old remedy for treating and preventing kidney stones and recurrent UTI. Cranberry juice restrains e-coli, the most common UTI bacteria, from anchoring itself to the bladder walls.[1]

Any foods that enhance your immunity should be devoured. This is war. There are millions of bacteria and only one of you. You must reduce their numbers while you increase your resources. Foods high in vitamin A will build your immune system and fight infection. These include spirulina, blue-green algae, chlorella, wheat and barley grass, carrots, kale, collards, sweet potatoes, spinach, hot red peppers, beef liver, and cod liver oil. Beta-carotene is the plant version (precursor) of vitamin A. It is converted into vitamin A by our bodies when we need it. So eat your carrots, squash, melons, and lots of other yellow-orange fruits and vegetables.

It is essential to eat more foods containing active lactobacillus acidophilus. Also known as probiotics (as opposed to antibiotics), lactobacillus, acidophilus, bifidus, bulgaricus, and so on are the friendly bacteria that fight unfriendly bacteria for dominance in our system. Dairy yoghurts and clabbered milk products are traditional probiotic foods but so are these nondairy foods: nut and seed yoghurts, rejuvelac, sauerkraut, sourdough breads, amazake rice drinks, umeboshi, and soy miso, tamari, and tempeh. Acidophilus can be used for both curative or preventative purposes and can be taken vaginally or orally in liquid, capsules, or powder.

Natural apple cider vinegar has long been used to fight infections. The early Greeks and Romans kept vinegar vessels handy, and even Christopher Columbus brought barrels of vinegar on his voyage to America to prevent scurvy and fight germs. Vinegar is a major source of acetic acid. The friendly bacteria and natural acidity of this healthy drink act as a powerful intestinal cleanser in addition to helping maintain the body's crucial acid/alkaline balance. While lemon juice also helps balance pH, it does not contain the friendly bacteria to fight germs and line the intestines.

Foods high in zinc help us produce white blood cells and eliminate bacteria. Some of the best sources (in order) are oysters, brewer's yeast, ginger, beef liver, flaxseeds, sunflower seeds, wheat and barley grass, brazil nuts, bee pollen, egg yolks, peanuts, oats, almonds, spirulina, buckwheat, oats, peas, and tofu.

Nutrients and Herbs That Help

Nutrients and herbs can help inhibit the growth of bacteria that causes UTI and can also alleviate symptoms when an infection occurs. Healing as well as preventative measures against UTI rely on maintaining the proper acidity in the urinary tract. Increased consumption of acidic foods and liquids, such as cranberries, vitamin C, lemon juice, and the herb goldenseal inhibit the growth of bacteria and prevent bacteria from sticking to the walls of the bladder. These acid tasting foods should not be confused with "acid-forming" foods, which instead create acidity in the bloodstream and promote bacterial growth.

Vitamin C is a well decorated (and documented) hero when it comes to UTI. It not only stimulates the production of interferon in our immune systems, but also significantly acidifies the urine. High doses of at least 5,000 milligrams per day are widely recommended by urologists.[2]

Other herbs also fight bacteria. Uva ursi (bearberry) contains the active ingredient arbutin, which is converted into the bactericide hydroquinone. Diuretic herbs such as goldenseal, parsley, and juniper berries encourage the production of urine, which increases the opportunities to eliminate bacteria.

UTI sufferers who drink pineapple juice can count on relief. Not only will the pineapple slightly acidify the urine, but in a double-blind study its protein-digesting enzyme bromelain successfully eliminated inflammation and pain.[3] Goldenseal also soothes inflamed mucous membranes in the urinary tract.

Helpful Foods, Nutrients & Herbs

For more information, see "Nutrient Sources" & "Glossary"

Foods

Water 80oz/day
Oysters
Brewer's Yeast
Spirulina
Blue-Green Algae
Chlorella
Wheat Grass
Barley Grass
Carrot Juice
Kale and Collards
Sweet Potatoes
Spinach
Hot Red Peppers
Bee Pollen
Sunflower Seeds
Flaxseeds
Beef Livers
Yoghurt
Rejuvelac
Sauerkraut
Fish Livers
Cod Liver Oil
Cranberry Juice
Pineapple Juice
Apple Cider Vinegar
Black-Eyed Peas
Tofu
Wheat Germ
Lemon Juice

Nutrients

Vitamin C
Vitamin A
Bromelain
Zinc

Herbs

Goldenseal
Uva Ursi
Juniper Berries
Parsley
Ginger

Recipes

Meyerowitz Water Cleanse

1 Liter	Pure Water. Drink in 40 minutes, 3 times daily

Flushing your urinary tract is one of the simplest and effective treatments for UTI. It effectively lowers the bacterial count giving your immune system a better chance to fight back. Drink it on an empty stomach three times per day.

Always drink the purest water you can find. Get rid of the espresso machine and put a water distiller or purifier in its place. Timing is everything in this recipe. This much water (a little more than a quart) flushes the urinary tract from top to bottom. It is an inexpensive self-help tool that keeps the plumbing clear, the body hydrated, and all things running smoothly. Water is one of our top three fundamental healers (along with oxygen and exercise). (*For more on water, see "Juicers, Blenders, & Water Purifiers."*)

Apple Cider Vinegar

2 Tbsp	Apple Cider Vinegar, raw
1+ cup	Pure Water

Use only raw, unfiltered, cloudy vinegar made from organic apples. It should be golden in color and have visible "cobwebs" of the bacterial cultures that result from the natural fermentation process. Shake your vinegar bottle well. You may adjust the ratio of vinegar to water to suit your taste. Drink it on an empty stomach in the morning and evening, or every few hours.

Bacteria Chaser

6 oz	Cranberry Juice
6 oz	Pineapple Juice
1/2 tsp	Vitamin C Crystals

These proven performers for urinary tract infections combine to give you the best ammunition against invading bacteria. But you must drink, drink, drink. This is one disease where volume of liquid is part of the cure.

Pineapple is easy to juice and very delicious. Cranberries can be juiced, but it may be more economical to buy bottled cranberry juice. Vitamin C crystals are also tart, so this is a fairly sour-tasting drink, which is one of the reasons it is effective. Vitamin C can also be taken in tablet form throughout the day.

Spicy Lemon Tea

1 cup	Pure Water, hot
1	Lemon, squeezed
1 pinch	Cayenne Pepper

Of all the citric fruits, lemon is the most potent detoxifier. It kills some types of intestinal parasites such as roundworms, and it contains limonene, a volatile oil that has been used to dissolve kidney and gall-stones.[4] *(For more, see "Lemon.")* Cayenne, a hot red pepper, is the second highest source of provitamin A, which is a major vitamin for fighting infections. Open a capsule and sprinkle a pinch into your tea. If it is too spicy, just take 2 capsules 3 times daily with food. Feel the heat!

Weight Loss

Overweight/Obesity

See also Power Drinks for Longevity and Physical Performance

If our bathroom scales could talk, what stories they would tell! While official definitions of overweight and obesity may help in clinical settings, the term "excess body fat" is a more easily understood and universal definition. We all know when we have gained weight and that extra weight prevents us from feeling our best.

Dieting has been the standard remedy for losing unwanted weight, yet it is not always effective. Instead, lifestyle changes that permanently alter eating and exercising habits have proven more effective for long-term weight control. Maintaining a fit weight reduces our risk for many ailments, such as diabetes, certain cancers, high blood pressure, and cardiovascular disease.

Plain and simple: find a combination of good eating habits and adequate exercise that allows you to burn more calories than you eat.

Causes

Perhaps the increasing numbers on the scale are the result of aging, a night on the town, or several nights on the sofa instead of the treadmill. Or perhaps, it is just the lower rate of metabolism that occurs naturally as we age. Both reduce our body's ability to burn calories efficiently and increase our accumulation of weight.

Pharmaceutical drugs and medical conditions such as hypothyroidism prevent efficient metabolic functions, and the result is obesity.[1] Women often experience a gain in weight during pre-menstrual syndrome (PMS) and menopause. Insulin resistance, the process of converting excess blood sugar into body fat instead of energy, is another common cause of obesity. Another cause is the presence of excessive triglycerides that get stored as body fat rather than being burned. Alcohol not only increases the risk of obesity but also interferes with weight loss.[2]

Diet Suggestions

Increase your consumption of protein and fiber, and reduce your consumption of fats, sugar, and carbohydrates. Replace the sugary, over-processed snack that you crave with low-fat protein, preferably from plant sources such as soy.[3] Check labels and choose products with fewer calories from fat. Remember, losing weight requires a stable diet of foods that easily convert to energy rather than fat. Quickly converting foods include fresh fruits and vegetables, whole grains, legumes, soy products, fish, and shellfish.

Fiber and water are necessary components for losing and controlling weight. In addition to keeping the digestive system moving, both fiber and water fill our stomach, leaving both less room and less desire for eating that doughnut or fried chicken.

Helpful Foods, Nutrients & Herbs

For more information, see "Nutrient Sources" & "Glossary"

Foods

Fruits & Vegetables
Clams
Crabs
Oysters
Salmon
Papaya
Artichoke
Garlic
Onions
Oat Bran
Wheat Bran
Soy Beans
Tofu
Kelp
Grapefruit
Kiwi
Spirulina
Flaxseed Oil
Mustard Seeds

Nutrients

Chromium
Brewer's Yeast
Iodine
Magnesium
Manganese
Phosphorous
Coenzyme Q10
Vitamin B5
Vitamin C

Herbs

Chickweed
Chili
Daikon
Dandelion
Ginsengs
Holy Basil
Myrrh
Mexican Wild Yam
Ginger
Green Tea
Gymnema Sylvestre
Yohimbe
Wheatgrass

Foods That Help

Scientific research indicates that people who want to lose weight should head for the ocean. Clams, crabs, and oysters significantly lower serum triglycerides, while the iodine in kelp helps those with weight problems caused by thyroid imbalances.[4]

Other foods that lower triglyceride levels include papaya, fish oils and salmon, artichoke, garlic, onions, tofu, and soy beans. Soy is also a good source of lecithin.

Remember the grapefruit diet of the 1970's? Juicing with grapefruit jump-starts a chemical reaction that helps the weight loss process. Add some kiwi for taste, and chromium, a mineral helpful for controlling weight.

Flaxseed oil and mustard seeds added to foods or taken as a supplement are also metabolism boosters, as is the capsaicin in chili. Members of the algae family, such as spirulina, foster weight loss and are rich in protein, vitamins, minerals, and essential fatty acids.[5]

Nutrients and Herbs That Help

Again, remember that we are trying to incorporate healthful products that supplement our vitamin and mineral intake, increase the body's basal metabolic rate, and process glucose properly. A multivitamin is good general protection, and individual supplements of specific nutrients target and enhance weight loss activity. The mineral chromium helps reduce the body's craving for sweets and improves the body's metabolism of glucose, a factor that prevents storage of excess fat. Brewer's yeast is our best source of chromium.

Iodine can help when hypothyroidism is the cause of your weight gain. Magnesium, manganese and phosphorus are other minerals that have been known to reduce weight. It turns out that 52% of obese people are deficient in the coenzyme Q10, so taking foods high in Q10 and supplements can accelerate weight loss.[6]

Thermogenesis *(see "Glossary")*, a process that helps burn calories, is the reason vitamin B5 is recommended to help obese people lose weight. And vitamin C seems to increase weight loss even when calorie intake is not restricted.[7]

Herbs that help return weight to normal ranges include chickweed, chili, cayenne, daikon, and dandelion. Ginseng, holy basil, myrrh, and

Mexican wild yam lower serum triglycerides levels. Ginger gives thermogenesis, and gymnema sylvestre and wheatgrass are appetite suppressants.

Caffeine is known to increase metabolic rate, but too much caffeine is counterproductive to a healthy diet. Green tea is a healthful compromise; it has less caffeine than coffee or black tea yet enough to increase the process of thermogenesis.[8]

Recipes

Breakfast Reducer

1	Grapefruit
1	Lemon

Grapefruit has a reputation for moderating obesity. It lowers serum cholesterol owing to its richness in pectins and galacturonic acids. Lemon relieves constipation and improves metabolism because of its cleansing effect on the liver. Great as a morning drink.

Appetite Suppressor

6 oz	Celery Juice
1 oz	Wheatgrass Juice
1 oz	Spinach Juice

Wheatgrass juice may be taken straight to suppress appetite or used in this palatable combination. Take it on an empty stomach and you will find that the combination of high chlorophyll, live enzymes, and concentrated nutrition satisfies you like a meal substitute. Spirulina and other algaes also have this effect.

Skinny Thick Shake

2 Tbsp	Oat Bran
1 cup	Soy Milk
½	Papaya, ripe
1 Tbsp	Brewer's Yeast
1 tsp	Soy Lecithin
½ -1 tsp	Vitamin C Crystals
½+ cup	Pure Water

Papaya, soy lecithin and soy milk lower triglyceride levels. Brewer's yeast and soy milk are good sources of pantothenic acid (vitamin B5), which promotes thermogenesis, to increase your metabolic rate. Brewer's yeast is a top source of chromium, which helps reduce cravings for sweets and prevents storage of excess fat. Oat bran keeps the food moving through the intestinal tract and is a proven aid to lowering cholesterol. Vitamin C controls obesity.

Add the ingredients in the order listed, blending after each one. Add only enough water to achieve the desired consistency.

Tighten Up Teas

1 bag or ¼ inch	Ginger Root
1 bag or tsp	Ginseng
1 bag or tsp	Green Tea

These make three separate teas. Ginseng lowers serum triglycerides levels, ginger increases thermogenesis, and green tea has enough caffeine to increase thermogenesis but not spike you up like coffee.

Ginger tea can be made fresh by grating a ¼ inch piece into 1–1½ cups of water. Steep for about 15 minutes. Make plenty and refrigerate the leftover tea to quickly reheat later.

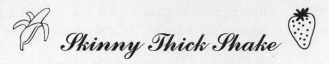

Nature's Finest Healing Foods & Herbs

Only by understanding the wisdom of natural foods and their effects on the body shall we attain the mastery of disease and pain and relieve the burden of mankind.

—William Harvey, M.D. (1578-1657)*

* William Harvey was the English doctor who discovered the concept of blood circulation and the role of the heart in propelling the blood.

Alfalfa & Alfalfa Sprouts

(Medicago Sativa)

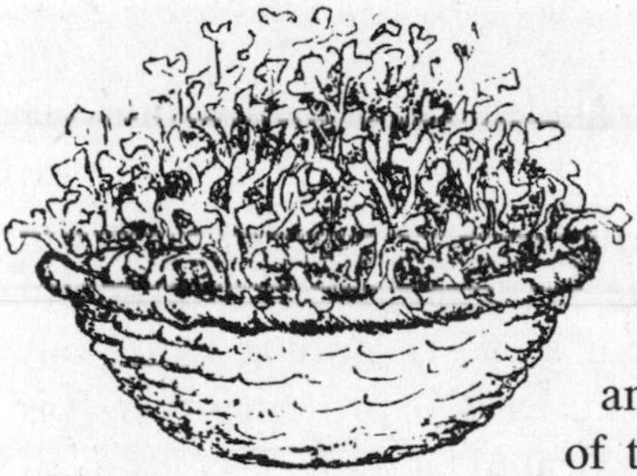

Alfalfa has been farmed for a few thousand years and alfalfa sprouts for only a few decades. Sprouts, however, represent the agriculture of tomorrow. What else can you plant anywhere, at any time of year, regardless of temperature and climate, and harvest in only a week? You don't need to have a green thumb for this kind of gardening nor lots of space. At approximately 50 cents per pound, alfalfa sprouts provide more food value—more nutrients per pound for your dollar than common store bought vegetables. Those muscular 2,000 pound cows and horses don't need a lab report to tell them how nutritious alfalfa is. They determine the nutritive value with their instinct, palate, and olfactory senses.

Health Benefits

Alfalfa sprouts contain concentrated amounts of phytochemicals, plant compounds that can protect us against disease. Canavanine, an amino acid analog in alfalfa, has been shown to help in cases of pancreatic, colon, and leukemia cancers.[1] Plant estrogens are also abundant in sprouts. These increase bone formation and density and prevent bone breakdown or osteoporosis.[2] Other effects of these phytoestrogens decrease human estrogen-related symptoms such as hot flashes, PMS, and fibrocystic breast tumors. Alfalfa sprouts are arguably our finest food source of therapeutic, saponin compounds, which lower bad cholesterol and fat but not the good, high density (HDL) fats. Animal studies have proven their benefit in arteriosclerosis and cardiovascular disease.[3] Saponins also stimulate the immune system by increasing the activity of natural killer cells such as T-lymphocytes and interferon. The saponin content of alfalfa sprouts is 450 times that of the unsprouted seeds. Sprouts also contain an abundance of highly active antioxidants that prevent DNA destruction and protect us from the ongoing effects of aging.[4] It wouldn't be inconceivable to find a fountain of youth here; after all, sprouts exemplify the miracle of birth.

Nutrients

Outdoor alfalfa has roots that reach as deep as forty feet into the earth and deliver a veritable bounty of minerals to this plant. It is so rich in nitrogen (protein) that farmers plant alfalfa just to enrich the soil for other crops! Alfalfa leaf powder is available at most health food stores. By sprinkling some on your salad or adding it to your juices, blended drinks, or dressings, you add a 40% protein green. It is superconcentrated because it is dehydrated. Gram for gram it exceeds the protein levels of heroes such as eggs (13%) and sirloin steak (19%). Alfalfa sprouts, which are 91% water, average 4% protein compared to spinach 3%, romaine lettuce 1.5%, and iceberg 0.8%. Milk is 3.3%. Alfalfa powder is also our greenest vegetable. It contains 2-3% of the vital, blood healing tonic chlorophyll. That is more than any land–grown vegetable. Alfalfa is also one of the rare plant sources of vitamin B12, making it a must for vegetarians.

Now that you know what the animals have known for centuries, you'll want to include alfalfa to your own grazing menu. Sprouts are available from any grocer. Choose sprouts that are brightly colored and firm. Though there have been scares in the past about sprouts contaminated with salmonella, the sprout industry has since developed pasteurization methods to prevent germination of these bacteria. Alfalfa sprouts are one of the best vegetables for juicing because of their high nutrient concentration and low cost per pound. If you like the idea of gardening year round, why not grow them at home. Home sprouting is fun and easy, and you don't need a green thumb. *(The author is the inventor of two home sprouters. "See Resources.")*

Algae

Spirulina, Chlorella, & Blue-Green Algae

You would have to go back to the beginning of life on earth to find the source of these miraculous foods. When all is said and done, it might seem that all we ever needed for survival was here right from the beginning.

Health Benefits

Algae are water-grown greens. Not the more familiar marine macro-algaes such as kelp and nori, but microscopic green plants that grow in water and can be cultivated like vegetables.

Spirulina is an alga that may have descended directly from the first life forms on earth. Although our planet is close to 4.5 billion years old, during its beginning the lack of oxygen and an abundance of nitrogen, carbon dioxide, and water precluded living organisms from flourishing. About 3.6 billion years ago, a cyano-bacterium developed that used solar energy to manufacture the first food carbon compounds, which released oxygen into the environment. A breath of fresh air! Fossils of these earliest life forms resemble spirulina. Today, spirulina is cultivated on "water farms" and is harvested like vegetables. It has millions of years of successful evolutionary wisdom encoded in its DNA, and, in fact, it is its resemblance to DNA's spiral structure that gives spirulina its "spiral" name.

Spirulina has a soft cell wall made up of proteins and polysaccharides (complex sugars) instead of cellulose. It is rich in the essential fatty acid GLA (gamma linolenic acid) and contains lots of easily absorbed iron. At 200 mcg/100g, this food is superior to liver (80mcg) and all other animal foods (cheese is 2mcg) as a source of vitamin B12. At an astonishing 60% protein content, spirulina is arguably the highest protein food on the planet.

There's a good reason why antioxidants and phyto-nutrients have become buzz-words among nutrition circles: they have the power to normalize, repair, and rejuvenate. Spirulina is full of these powerful compounds: phycocyanin, chlorophyll, glycolipids, and sulfolipids, as well as an abundance of beta carotene and 10 other carotenoids. This is why spirulina has been recommended as an immune system booster.

Grown mostly in artificially formed ponds in Southern California deserts and in Hawaii, spirulina cultivation is one of the most exciting new frontiers in farming technology. Since algae is more responsive to its environment than soil-grown vegetables, farmers can add specific nutrients to enhance the ponds in which it grows. Using this method, they can, for example, increase the selenium content of spirulina, which provides an excellent bio-available form of this mineral. This is not genetic manipulation but advanced, certified organic farming for the new millennium.

Chlorella is the highest in chlorophyll of all the earth's foods, about 2-3%, ergo its name. This single cell plant has the unique capacity for self-reproduction. The Chlorella Growth Factor (CGF) has the potential to help in the repair and regeneration of human tissue. Chlorella is 55-65% protein by weight, and its nucleus contains a wealth of neuropeptides and cell-growth factors such as RNA and DNA, the fundamental stuff needed for the creation of life.

Digestion has always been a concern with chlorella, because its tough cellulose walls make absorption of all these wonderful nutrients difficult. Fortunately, Japanese chlorella growers have found a spray drying process that cracks open the cell walls without damaging the nutrients inside.

Blue-green algae differs from spirulina and chlorella in that it is not cultivated in artificial ponds by "farmers" but harvested from lakes by "fishermen"—but not from just any lake. The largest natural algae lake in the world is Klameth Lake in Oregon. The blue-green algae in this lake is called aphanizomenon flos-aquae, or AFA for short. Commercial companies harvest AFA and market it under other names, such as "Super Blue-Green" and "Klamath Blue-Green." Who, after all, is going to go into their local health food store and ask for aphanizomenon? While spirulina and chlorella are also blue-green algaes and are nutritionally similar, AFA is more well-known as a brain food. It is rich in neuropeptides, whose low molecular weights can pass freely through the blood-brain barrier. There they help strengthen neurotransmitters and improve mental alertness, memory, and concentration.

If you have been interested in adopting a vegetarian diet, but are afraid it would be difficult to get enough protein, think again. Nature's first food may change your mind.

Mercury Detox Deluxe

by Dr. Gabriel Cousens, M.D.

1	Banana, almost ripe
1 Tbsp	Chlorella
1/4 inch	Ginger Root, finely chopped
1/2 tsp	Blue-Green Algae Powder
1/2 cup	Cilantro (optional)
2 cups	Pure Water

Blend all of the ingredients until smooth. The purpose of this drink is to pull mercury out of the brain, nerve tissues, and organs.

Dr. Gabriel Cousens is the Director of the *Tree of Life Rejuvenation Center* in Patagonia, Arizona. He practices a synergy of Ayurvedic, naturopathic, homeopathic, Chinese, Essene, yogic, meditative, and live-food approaches to create optimal health. Dr. Cousens is the author of *Conscious Eating, Spiritual Nutrition and the Rainbow Diet,* and *Sevenfold Peace.* His latest book is *Freedom from Depression: Activating Your Pleasure Centers.* www.treeofliferejuvenation.com

Aloe Vera

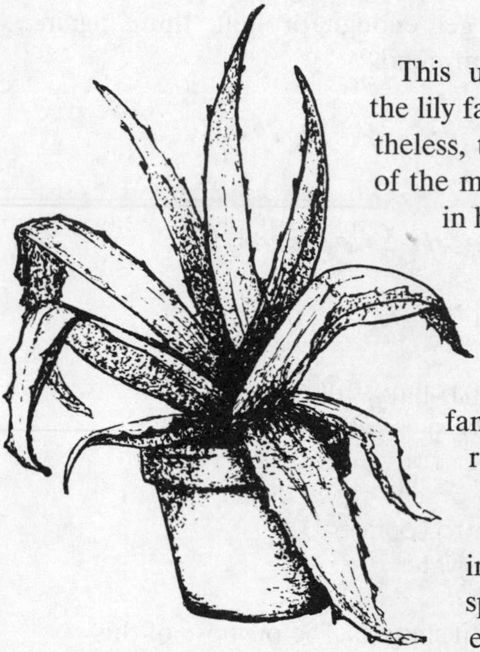

This unassuming cactus-type plant of the lily family is easily overlooked. Nevertheless, this ancient healer stands as one of the most outstanding medicinal plants in history.

Health Benefits

Inside its leaves is a thin, clear, jelly-like material that is famous as a skin salve. Skin healing requires the increase of blood flow to the injured area, and aloe vera dilates capillaries, which increases blood circulation and speeds healing. Aloe vera is an especially effective treatment in cases of frostbite.[1] It helps heal all sores, from canker sores to bed sores, as well as burns, abrasions, herpes lesions, hives, insect bites, stings, scalp itchiness, psoriasis, and sunburn pain.[2] Wounds heal more quickly, and infection and scarring is often prevented.[3] Aloe vera also protects our skin from exposure to ultra-violet radiation.[4] There are even claims that it can eliminate warts.

Aloe vera has amazing anti-inflammatory action in the digestive system. It reduces heartburn, soothes peptic ulcers, eases constipation, and has potential as a treatment for Crohn's disease and ulcerative colitis.[5]

In our immune system, aloe vera juice can reduce tumor mass and inhibit metastasis (spreading) in some types of cancer.[6] It has the ability to stimulate our immune capacity owing to its high content of acemannan, the major carbohydrate in aloe leaves and gel.[7]

Acemannan may even mimic the function of AZT, making it a treatment for AIDS patients. Aloe "shows preliminary signs of boosting AIDS patients' immune systems and blocking the human immunedeficiency virus' spread without toxic side effects."[8] Aloe juice made from both the skin and gel of the plant can also reduce blood sugar and triglyceride levels in diabetes mellitus patients.[9]

Nutrients

Aloe vera juice contains a wealth of vitamins, B1, B2, B3, B6, C, and choline, plus minerals, calcium, chlorine, copper, germanium, iron, magnesium lactate, manganese, potassium, silicon, sodium, and sulfur. But its uniqueness lies in its wealth of phytochemicals such as the organic acids chrysophanic, salicylic, succinic, and uric, polysaccharides such as acemannan, enzymes such as glutathione peroxidase, and various resins.

There is an extra bonus with aloe: you can grow it indoors. No green thumb required. It is attractive and easy to maintain, and when you want to try its magic, just break off a piece and rub the gel on your skin. Or, throw some in your juicer along with your favorite fruits. Aloe vera juice is widely available in health food stores and easy to add to your homemade smoothies or fresh squeezed juices. Look for whole leaf aloe. The juice should be thick and tart.

Apples & Apple Cider Vinegar

(Malus pumila, common apple)

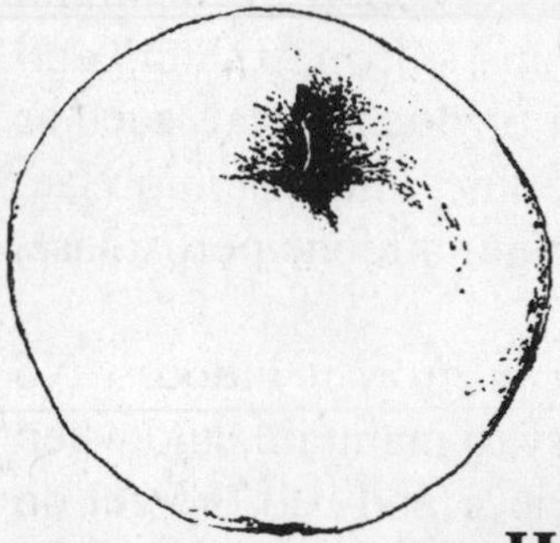

"A rose by any other name would be just as sweet." Considering that all apples come from the rose (rosaceous) family and that there are 7,500 varieties of apples, making it the number 3 fruit crop worldwide, that's saying quite a mouthful.

Health Benefits

Although apples are a wonderful source of vitamins and minerals, they are most notable for their pectin content. Pectin gives fresh apple juice its thick, cloudy appearance. It is also what gives us a healthier digestive system. Pectin forms a gel that breaks down toxins in our intestines, stimulates peristaltic activity, and enhances bowel function. It is also responsible for lowering serum cholesterol levels.[1] Apple cider vinegar (made from fermented apples) is also rich in pectins and malic acid.

Apples are rich sources of ellagic, chlorogenic, quercetin, and caffeic acids (100-130mg/100g). Ellagic acid is an excellent anti-oxidant that protects chromosomes against the cancer-causing activity of certain carcinogens in cigarettes.[2] In one human study of quercetin, people who consumed apple-rich diets had a 46% reduction in their risk of lung cancer.[3] The pectin in apples demonstrated the ability to reduce the incidence of colon cancer.[4]

Apple juice, even the store bottled variety, counteracts virus infections, including the polio virus.[5] Both apple juice and apple cider vinegar stimulate the production of digestive enzymes and hydrochloric acid. This not only stimulates appetite, but also helps relieve diarrhea. And gargling with apple cider vinegar is good for sore throats.

Nutrients

The skins of apples are high in vitamin A, so to enjoy those skins safely, try to juice whole organic apples grown without pesticide sprays. A typical apple contains 7.8mg/100g of vitamin C, significant amounts of potassium (110mg), and some calcium (10mg). But the magic in apples is in its wealth of phytochemicals and enzymes, including peroxidase, laetrile, and bioflavonoids, as well as the organic and phenolic acids, malic, ellagic (101mg), chlorogenic (104mg), and caffeic (100mg) acids. Apples are one of our top sources of soft fiber. Its rich pectins and hemi-celluloses make them arguably our best natural intestinal cleanser. That is why "an apple a day keeps the doctor away." And with 820mg of the complex sugar galactose, that is an easy chore.

No wonder Adam was tempted by this luscious fruit. We are sorry it got him (and Eve) in trouble, but grateful for both his and the apple's prolific progeny.

Bananas

(Musaceae sapientum)

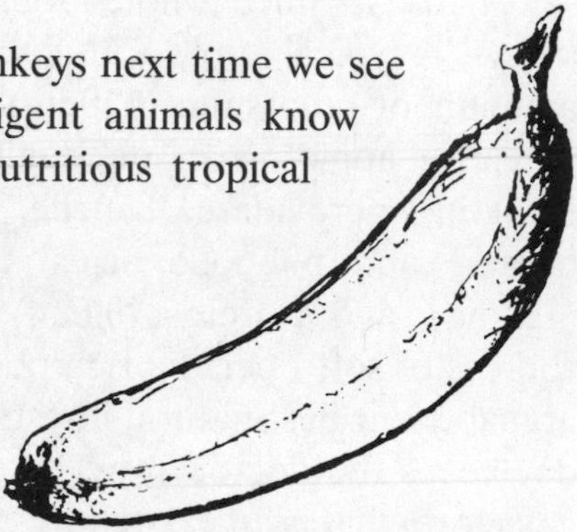

We would be wise to ape the monkeys next time we see them eating a banana. These intelligent animals know well that this is one of the most nutritious tropical fruits.

Health Benefits

Potassium is plentiful in this curvaceous, queen of yellow. Our heart goes out to you dear banana, literally. Potassium treats congestive heart failure, regulates blood pressure, and is a proven remedy for lowering blood pressure in hypertensive patients.[1] Its high pectin content may contribute to the banana's ability to lower cholesterol. Fiber from green, unripe bananas dramatically reduces the bad (LDL) cholesterol and increases the production of good (HDL) cholesterol by up to 30%.[2]

Upset tummy? Eat a ripe banana. This satisfying and stabilizing food soothes digestive disturbances such as constipation and diarrhea. The natural flavonoids in green, unripe bananas and plantains have been used to treat gastric and duodenal ulcers; bananas actually thicken the protective gastric mucosa.[3]

Bananas provide a wonderful source of readily available energy for young and old alike and may reduce fatigue.[4] But if eating a banana is not for you, mash it up and smear it on your skin. The pulp from bananas makes a great facial and a wonderful skin cleanser.

Nutrients

Aside from seaweed and rice bran, dried bananas are superior to all other foods in potassium (1,477mg/100g). With the possible exception of strawberries, no fresh fruit is higher in minerals than bananas. Fresh bananas weigh in at 396mg/100g of potassium, 120mg sulfur, 80mg silicon, 33mg of magnesium, and 26mg phosphorus, along with ample amounts of copper, chromium, iron, fluoride, manganese, selenium, and zinc. Its sodium is delightfully low at 1mg.

Ordinary bananas have a significant amount of vitamin A (190IU), red bananas contain 400IU. For a fruit, its amino acid profile is impressive, with 80.6 mg/100g histidine, 70.6mg leucine, and 47.9mg lysine.

Plantains are a rich source of dietary gums, mucilages, carbohydrates, and minerals (copper, potassium, and selenium), along with vitamins B6, C, and folic acid. They are usually too hard to be eaten raw and are generally baked or fried.

Common bananas are highest in potassium when yellow, but they are most therapeutic for the heart and stomach when green. It is best to buy them green and ripen them at home. Bananas are sacred to smoothie lovers the world over. The sweetest smoothies are made when the bananas mature to a rich yellow with brown speckles.

If our primate friends knew how to use a blender, they would be hanging around the kitchen more than the trees.

Banana Ice Cream

by Dr. Edward Taub, M.D.

2	Bananas, frozen
½ cup	Vanilla Soy Milk
1 Tbsp	Honey (optional)

Place banana into a blender, add soy milk and honey if desired. Blend until creamy or retain some small bits of fruit.

Dr. Edward Taub is a board certified pediatrician and family doctor with over 30 years of experience in Dana Point, California. He has authored 5 books on wellness, including *Balance Your Body, Balance Your Life.*

Ode to a Banana

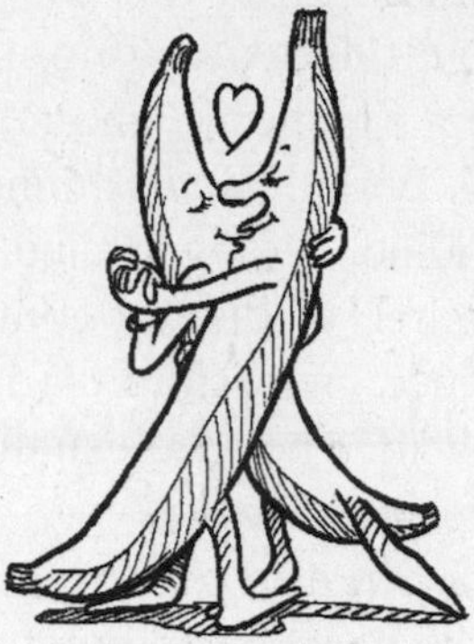

Good morn, sweet, soft, and gentle fruit.
You who glide to earth from high above in thy armour of gold,
thy suit of yellow.
There is no other fruit before me, so handsomely dressed, so
pleasantly curved.
Let me jump into thy crescent and sleep the night away as if the
very moon were in my lap.
And in the day, I bask in your brightness only to be outshown
by the sun itself.
Lend me your finger sweet arch, that I may savor each moment
before thy fall.

Oh, thou phosphorus filled friend, feed me your potassium,
your vitamin A, your sweet fruit sugar.
No other fruit could do the same.
Nay, woulds't I even light upon a lime (too green), a lemon
(too sharp), a logenberry (too tart).
An apple has not the pectin for me!
The breadfruit no bread, the date, no date.
I water not for watermelon.
You are my mango, my papaya,
and I your nut.

Bee Pollen

Propolis & Royal Jelly

Bee pollen is a mixture of bee saliva, plant nectar, and plant pollen. It differs from the sort of pollen that is implicated in allergies. Propolis is collected by bees from flowers, trees and vegetables, then mixed with their own secretions, including beeswax, to form a gummy, resinous substance. Royal jelly is a viscous, honey-like liquid secreted by bees to feed their infants and queen. The queen lives on it her entire life, and it is thought to be the reason for her longevity and larger size. Queen bees live up to five years, whereas the common female worker bees live only forty days. Honey is very healthful and delicious, but is no match for the nutritional potency of its sister bee products.

Health Benefits

Users claim that bee pollen improves their athletic performance and relieves fatigue, and centenarians in Dagestan attribute their longevity to a lifelong practice of eating bee pollen and royal jelly The Swedes and the French, who also eat lots of bee pollen, claim that it makes them look more youthful. It may improve the appearance of our skin and retard wrinkles by increasing the flow of blood to skin cells and by stimulating the growth of new skin tissues.[1]

Bee pollen is an important food for men with enlarged prostate (prostatitis). In double-blind studies and long-term treatments, urological researchers reported that bee pollen reduced enlarged prostates in 53% of men with severe and chronic symptoms of prostatitis.[2]

Bee products can also benefit cancer patients. Lung cancer patients who ate bee pollen lived longer and were better able to tolerate chemotherapy. Propolis has also proven effective in killing liver cancer cells.[3]

The antioxidant and antimicrobial activity of propolis and royal jelly also make them awesome antibiotics. They contain potent antibacterial proteins that make them effective against everything from the common cold to candida albicans, e-coli, salmonella and AIDS.[4]

Nutrients

Bee pollen is 35% protein, including lots of lysine, leucine, and valine—that's more than beef, eggs, or cheese. It contains 2% fat made up of healthy phosphatidylcholine and linoleic acid. Bee pollen also contains a wealth of minerals (1½%), including iron, zinc, potassium, magnesium, calcium, copper, sodium, and selenium, as well as an equal percentage of vitamins (1500mg/100g), especially riboflavin, nicotinic, pantothenic and folic acids, B2, inositol, lots of vitamin C and even some B12. Bee pollen also contains the essential chromosomal nucleic acids DNA and RNA, as well as a whopping 5,000 different healthful enzymes and phytochemicals, including lycopene, quercetin, carotenes, and flavonols. Propolis contains a wealth of polyphenols and royal jelly is high in B vitamins and beneficial fatty acids.

You can put 1-2 tablespoons of bee pollen granules in your smoothies, and a teaspoon of royal jelly is as easy as honey to add to your drinks. Take propolis tablets at the first sign of an infection. Unlike honey, these bee products are only slightly sweet but quite delicious nonetheless. Give them a try and see what all the buzz is about.

Beets

(Beetroot or Beta vulgaris cicla)

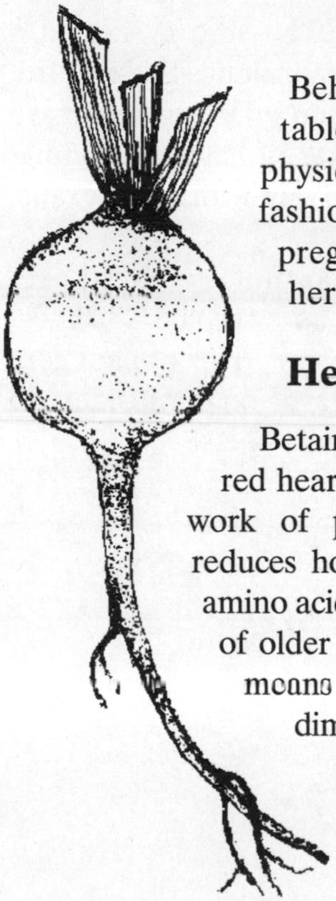

Behold the beautiful beet, the jewel of the vegetable kingdom. One glimpse at her amethyst physique, and we know that this bauble was surely fashioned to tempt! Who could ever resist such a pregnant package, and who would want to once her curative secrets are revealed?

Health Benefits

Betaine is the carotenoid responsible for her ruby red heart. But underneath this pigment lies a vast network of phytochemical activity. Betaine significantly reduces homo-cysteine levels.[1] Homocysteine is a toxic amino acid associated with cardiovascular disease in 30% of older adults. Betaine is also a methyl donor, which means it catalyzes homocysteine into methionine and dimethylglycine (DMG). This means betaine helps our mental functioning. As it lowers homocysteine, it increases another powerful mind enhancer, S-Adenosylmethionine (SAMe). SAMe is a derivative of methionine, normally manufactured by the body, whose supplementation balances moods, improves mental acuity and has been used in the treatment of alcoholic addiction and AIDS.[2]

Betaine is a terrific antioxidant that enhances athletic performance, and improves stamina. It basically optimizes the utilization of oxygen stimulating red blood cell production and lymph activity. It is our liver's best friend. Beets detoxify the liver, improve its function and protect it from excessive alcohol consumption. Beet lovers swear it even adds to their longevity.[3]

Grandma used beets to prevent gallstones and to treat gout and jaundice. Fresh beet juice has a long history as a valuable elixir for anemia and disorders of the bladder and kidney. Today, research suggests using it to treat lung and prostate cancer.[4]

Nutrition

The next time you open your garden gate, be sure to extend a heartfelt greeting to the goosefoot family, which includes Swiss chard, spinach, and beets—what a regal trio! When you juice beets, you are downing a mineral brew that includes the likes of calcium (115mg/100g), potassium, iron, copper, and sodium, along with folic, oxalic, succinic, and fumaric organic acids.

Dried beet juice crystals are a delicious substitute for fresh beet juice and super-nutritious, too. They contain an awesome 2820mcg/100g zinc and 2510mg of potassium *(see Resources)*. This radiant gem is gorgeous on the outside, but even more fantastic on our insides. So throw one in every juice you make. You can't beat beets!

Beet Vitality Cocktail

by Dr. Philip Incao, M.D.

7 oz	Carrot Juice
3 oz	Beet Juice
1 oz	Parsley
1 clove	Garlic, juiced
½ inch	Ginger
½	Lemon, juiced

This vegetable juice is good for supporting vitality and is used for detoxification and strengthening liver function. As an alternative to fresh beets, use one heaping tablespoon of beet powder or crystals.

Dr. Philip Incao, M.D. practices anthroposophical medicine at the Gilpin Street Holistic Center in Denver. He is currently writing *"The Healing Flame: How to Raise a Healthy Child in the 21st Century."*

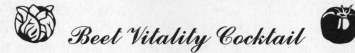

Bran

Oat, Wheat, & Rice Bran

Oat: Avena Sativa, Wheat: Tritcum, Rice: Oryza Sativa

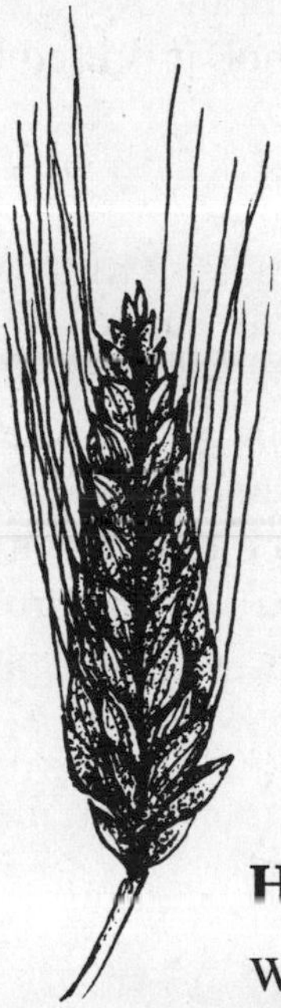

Bran is one of those unfashionable foods–neither hip nor hot, neither tasty nor tantalizing. But when you have to get things moving, who do you call? Not the stylish noni; not the famous echinacea; not the mighty garlic. It's "bring on the bran" and watch your troubles glide away.

Oh, the lowly bran, so fabulously functional, yet not even a food unto itself. The distinguished grains, oat, wheat, and rice, divest themselves of their flak. They throw off that outer husk and reveal the glorious kernel within. Indeed, grains are grand, but what about this casing, this jacket disrobed?

Health Benefits

Woe is the threat of toxins to our health. But for every evil foe, there is a counter-force. Bran to the rescue. Our digestive tracts generate toxins every day in the form of bacteria, fungi, waste products, and non-digestible substances like pesticides. These invaders pitch camp in our colons and sneak rides in our bloodstream. We have become the ultimate bed and breakfast, forever feeding unwanted guests! The result can be diseases of the liver, stomach, colon, thyroid, and pancreas as well as a debilitated immune system. Because of its water-soluble fiber, bran grabs hold of these microbial toxins like a sponge. But this "sponge" is like a locomotive. Once onboard, there is no getting off. Next stop, Niagra Falls. With bran on your side, even the typically tenacious colon cancer has met its match.[1]

Does bran rest after such a journey? Not this indefatigable hero. It's onward to the heart valve and everywhere cholesterol lurks. Bran knocks down the bad LDL cholesterol and cranks up the good HDL cholesterol.[2] From there, it is off to the kidneys to prevent the formation of stones.[3]

The secret is out. Wheat bran has a fondness for women. As little as 10-20 grams per day lowers elevated estrogen levels, which are implicated in many cases of breast cancer.[4] And rice bran loves men. As the richest food source of the lipid gamma oryzanol, it is used by bodybuilders to stimulate muscle growth.[5]

Nutrients

Bran may not be glamorous, but it is a nutritional superstar. It repeatedly takes top position in many of our most fundamental vitamins and minerals, including iron (19.5mg/100g), potassium (1495mg), silicon (643mg), chromium (38mcg), and folic acid (195mcg). And it is the #2 food source of these three crucial nutrients: niacin (29.8mg), magnesium (490mg), and phosphorous (1276mg). In addition, all of the brans are good sources of B-complex vitamins.

Thank you, bran; there is no better coat than thee.

Brewer's Yeast

(Saccharomyces cerevisiae)

There are several types of yeasts. Baker's yeast contains the active cultures needed to release the carbon dioxide that leavens bread. Torula yeast is a type of dietary yeast that is nutritionally similar to brewer's yeast, but it does not contain selenium or chromium (GTF). Brewer's yeast is a dietary yeast produced as a by-product of beer fermentation. Although it is famously nutritious, it is also bitter. Different versions of brewer's yeast made specifically for the health food industry, may be labeled "de-bittered," "good tasting," or "nutritional yeast." Nutritional yeast and yeast "flakes" are similar to brewer's yeast except they are lower in chromium. In any case, you won't have to come up with a lot of dough to get the nutritional benefits of yeast.

Health Benefits

First of all, brewer's yeast does not exacerbate candida albicans. Nutritional and brewer's yeasts are entirely unrelated to yeast infections and do not contain live organisms. It is baker's yeast and the wheat products made from it that candida patients should avoid. If anything, brewer's yeast helps by strengthening the immune system and improves our resistance to infectious diseases.[1] It even has a 'skin respiratory factor' that allows it to be applied topically to accelerate the healing of wounds.[2] Brewer's yeast is so high in chromium (as GTF) that just adding it to the diet of elderly people was enough to normalize their blood sugar levels.[3]

Nutrients

If there were nutrition awards, brewer's yeast would collect an armful. It is one of the top protein foods on the planet (35-47%) and our finest source of chromium, the glucose tolerance factor (112mcg/100g). It vies with spirulina as the leading source of nucleic acids

RNA and DNA (12%) and is arguably our best food for B vitamins—folic acid (2,022mg/100g), vitamin B3 (37mg), B1 (15.6mg), biotin (200mcg) as well as the vegetarian vitamin B12. It is also the food highest in phosphorus (1,753mg), our highest land source of potassium at 1,700mg (only sea vegetables are higher), and has a whopping 424mg of calcium (milk has 119mg).

Start adding brewer's yeast to all your smoothies. It is sure to get a rise out of you.

Yeast Feast

1 cup	Apple Juice
1 Tbsp	Brewer's Yeast
2 Tbsp	Sunflower Seeds
1 Tbsp	Lecithin Granules

Blend all ingredients together until smooth. If you like chewy drinks, add the sunflowers last and only "chop" them in the blender. Brewer's yeast can be added to most smoothies. Although yeast may be slightly bitter, one tablespoon is not enough to significantly alter the flavor of most drinks. The nutritional benefits of yeast far outweigh any changes in taste.

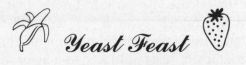

Broccoli & Broccoli Sprouts

(Brassica oleracea italica)

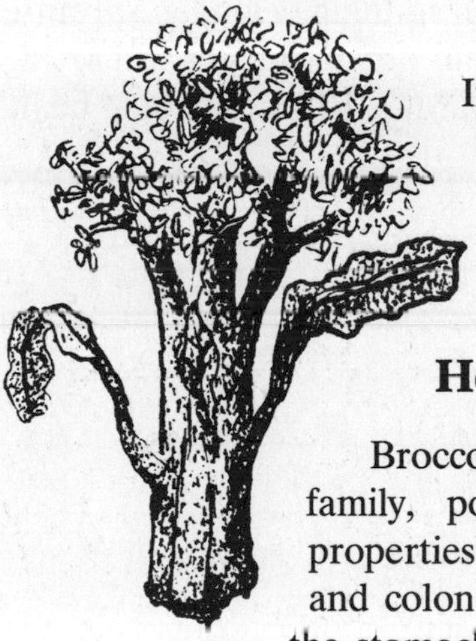

If the steady trickle of positive findings from the health community has not convinced you to get serious about eating a regular diet of broccoli, then listen to this.

Health Benefits

Broccoli, like all of its cousins in the cabbage family, possesses dramatic cancer preventative properties. It is especially effective against breast and colon cancer, but also helps deter cancers of the stomach, esophagus, lung, and ovaries. Its efficacy against breast and ovarian cancer is attributed to its abundance of indoles, compounds that increase the secretion of estrogen hormone co-factors linked to reducing breast cancer risk. Broccoli also contains glucosinolates, which enzymes convert to isothiocyanates. One isothiocyanate, sulforaphane, is the strongest natural inducer of our body's own protective enzymes against carcinogens.[1]

Broccoli sprouts contain 20 to 50 times more sulforaphane than the average adult broccoli plant. Rats given modest daily doses of sulforaphane from sprouts for five days developed significantly fewer and smaller tumors despite a diet of potent carcinogens. It "demonstrate(s), unequivocally, that this compound can substantially reduce the incidence, rate of development, and size of tumors."[2] In three days, you can raise a crop of sprouts containing as much sulforaphane as an acre of broccoli would yield in a year.

Nutrients

Broccoli is an excellent source of vitamin C (110mg/100g), calcium (103mg), phosphorous (78mg), and the essential amino acids valine (170mg), leucine (163mg), lysine (147mg) and arginine (192mg).

The American Cancer Society recommends eating broccoli at least three times a week. If this sounds like a bit much, get out your juicer and set up your sprouter. A pound of the mature broccoli may be hard to eat, but it distills into 2-3 ounces of nutritionally concentrated juice. For potency and economy, however, nothing beats the sprouts. They are fun and easy to grow. So, visit your organic grocer and break out the sprouting seeds for your kitchen garden. Broccoli should be in everyone's diet.

Cabbage

(Brassica oleracea capitata)

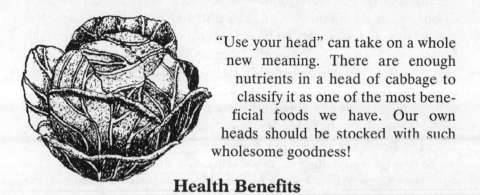

"Use your head" can take on a whole new meaning. There are enough nutrients in a head of cabbage to classify it as one of the most beneficial foods we have. Our own heads should be stocked with such wholesome goodness!

Health Benefits

The most remarkable attribute of cabbage is its power to cure ulcers. A study conducted in the 1940s proved that a seven-day regimen of cabbage juice–one quart per day–works wonders on peptic ulcers. Of the 65 patients who participated in the study, 63 were cured![1] Even the best of today's pharmaceutical treatments cannot claim such success. Duodenal, jejuna, and gastric ulcers all show remarkable improvement with cabbage juice.

Cabbage is highly promoted by the American Cancer Society. Packed with both nutrients and phytochemicals, cabbage belongs in the first line of defense against cancer. It boosts our anti-oxidant defense mechanisms and stimulates production of antibodies. It improves the metabolism of estrogen, inhibits cancer development, and tumor growth, and it blocks the reaction of cancer-causing compounds in cases of breast, colon, liver, lung, and ovarian cancers.[2]

Cabbage is also a super food for your digestive system. It stimulates the flow of bile, alleviates constipation, and cleanses the intestines. It enhances our natural detoxification.

Nutrition

High levels of the minerals potassium, iron, calcium, sulfur, phosphorus, and iodine are found in cabbage, plus the vitamins A, B1, B2, B6, C, E, K, and folic acid. Vitamin A aids in tissue nutrition and rejuvenation. B1 improves nerve function, the absorption of oxygen, and the metabolism of carbohydrates. B2 assists cellular chemical action. Cabbage has an abundance of the sulfur based phytochemicals glucosinolates and isothiocyanates, the most famous of which is sulforaphane. They protect our cells from invasion by carcinogens. It is a rich source of indoles and coumarins, which also block the reactions of cancer causing substances. Its chlorophyll combats anemia along with its high levels of the basic amino acid histidine (105mg/100g), a component of hemoglobin. Histidine also treats allergies and regulates the T-cells in our immune systems.

To best take advantage of these wonderful nutrients, try to eat cabbage raw. Since raw cabbage is too hard for some people to digest, the best way to get your cabbage is to juice it. Also try cabbage sprouts. The sprouts are delicate and easier to digest, and they contain higher levels of nutrients. You can put them in the juicer machine, too.

Carrots

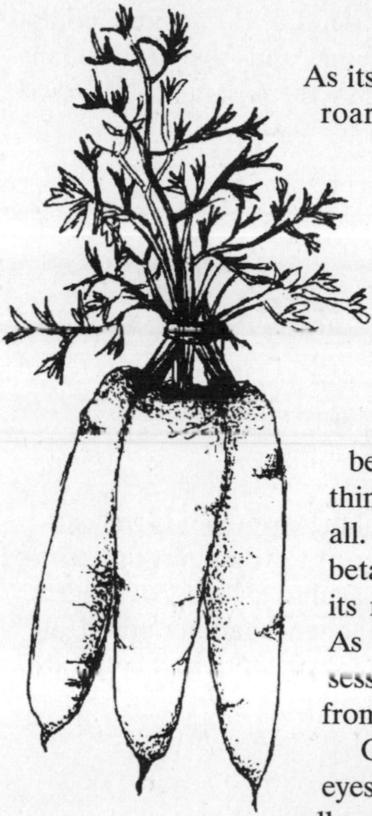

As its strong orange stalk disappears into the roar of the juice machine, you can almost hear it shouting, "You'll never find a better juicing vegetable than me!" As far as juicing goes, this bold member of the parsley family is pretty much king—and a carotenoid king, at that.

Health Benefits

Alpha-carotene, lutein, lycopene, beta-carotene, gamma-carotene, zeaxanthin, and xanthophyll—carrots have them all. They are all nutritional marvels, but beta-carotene has stolen the spotlight with its numerous cancer preventing properties. As a powerful anti-oxidant, carotenes possess life extension properties that protect us from the toxic effects of free radicals.

Carrots are best known for helping our eyes. Beta-carotene, lutein, and zeaxanthin all concentrate in the retina of the eye. And carrots enhance the overall function of our immune system by increasing the production and performance of our white blood cells.[1] The pectin in carrots lowers serum cholesterol levels.[2] Carrots are beneficial for dry skin problems such as psoriasis. They protect the respiratory system from infection and even the bad effects of smoking.[3] Carrots also reduce the risk of stroke, counter arthritis and rheumatism, and stimulate the appetite when eaten 20 minutes before meals.

Nutrients

Since the body converts beta-carotene to vitamin A, carrots are a primary dietary source of pro-vitamin A (28,129IU/100g). They also excel as a source of glutathione, the sulfur-containing amino acid (75mg/100g), which has life extension potential. B-vitamins, potassium, phosphorous, magnesium, vanadium, and the anti-oxidant coenzyme Q10 are all found in carrots. Buy them organically grown and juice it up.

Carotenoid Cocktail

7 oz	Carrot Juice
3 oz	Spinach Juice
2oz	Tomato Juice

Beta-carotene is the most famous of all the carotenoids and carrots are a superb source of it. It is a precursor to vitamin A that stimulates the immune system and protects us against a variety of cancers. Tomatoes have beta-carotene as well as lycopene, another powerful antioxidant carotenoid. Spinach has chlorophyll, alpha and beta-carotene, and the carotenoids lutein and zeaxanthin.

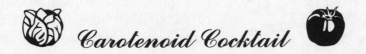

Celery

(Apium graveolens)

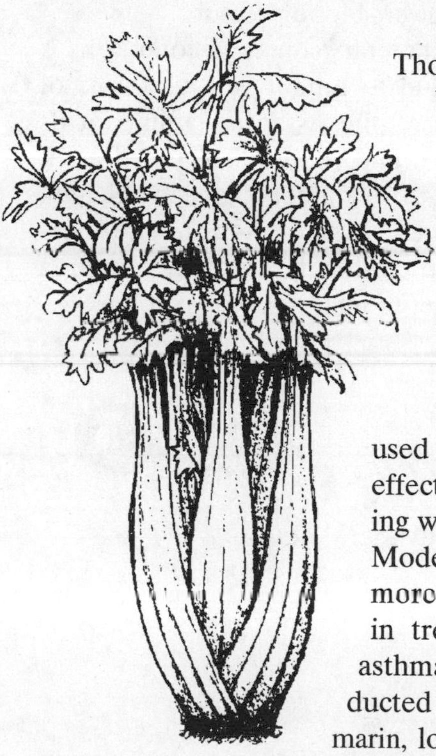

Though it towers over all other vegetables, this juicy giant is sadly underconsumed. Mostly, we chop it into pieces and bury it in soup. Like its cousin parsley, our modern palate has shunned it. But the lofty stalk did not always go unrecognized.

Health

During the middle ages, celery was used as a diuretic and laxative. It was also effective for breaking up gallstones, healing wounds, and soothing irritated nerves. Modern science has discovered a few more valuable benefits. Celery juice aids in treating such respiratory ailments as asthma and bronchitis. In studies conducted on people, its active constituent, coumarin, lowered blood pressure by up to 14% in patients with hypertension. One hypertensive patient experienced a reduction from 158/96 to 118/82 after one week of eating ¼ pound of celery per day.[1]

Celery is also effective in helping prevent colon and stomach cancers.[2] Kidney and liver disorders respond well to celery juice treatments. Gout, rheumatoid arthritis, and rheumatism are all eased by celery, and it has been used successfully to stimulate a weak sexual drive. Celery juice taken before a meal also curbs appetite and is, therefore, a natural diet aid. And because of its calming effect on the central nervous system, celery makes a great night-time tonic for insomniacs.

Nutrients

Let's dispel the ugly rumor that celery is too high in sodium. It's not! The form of sodium found in celery is organic and vital to all of our major organs. It is the table salt that we overuse, not the naturally balanced, sodium-rich organic foods. Because it is also rich in potassium, celery is a perfect post-workout tonic. It replaces lost electrolytes, tones the vascular system, and lowers blood pressure.

Celery and celery seeds are our best dietary source of coumarins, a flavonoid compound with the potential to inhibit various forms of cancer. Celery also contains plenty of the essential amino acids methionine (1,300mg/100gms), cystine, and tryptophan, plus lots of vitamin A, B-complex, and C. Celery is also a great source of calcium, phosphorus, iron, magnesium, manganese, iodine, and copper. Celery does not have many uses in American cuisine, but there is one area where it excels—juice. And don't forget to include the leaves!

Phytonutrient Power Drink

by Dr. Mitchell Gaynor, M.D.

4 oz	Celery
4 oz	Carrots
1 oz	Beet
1 oz	Watercress
1	Apple, cut & cored
1-2 Tbsp	Green Foods Powder

Juice first five ingredients, then stir in your favorite green foods powder. *Phytonutrient Power Drink* is loaded with nutrition, helps to detoxify the system, and is a powerful aid in preventing cancer.

Dr. Mitchell Gaynor practices medicine at the *Strang Cancer Prevention Center* in New York City. He is the author of *Healing Essence—A Cancer Doctor's Practical Program for Hope and Recovery* and *Dr. Gaynor's Cancer Prevention Program*. www.drgaynor.com

Citrus Fruits

Lemon, Orange, Grapefruit

Health Benefits

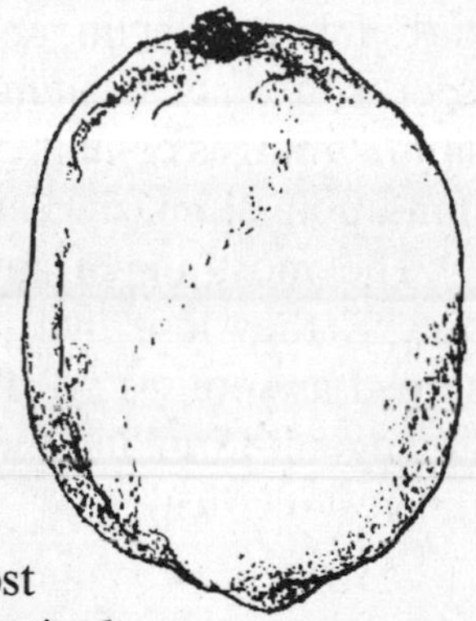

If you thought it was only the vitamin C in citrus fruits that make them such a healthy choice, listen up. Deep inside the white rind and membranes of these fruits lies a miraculous group of plant compounds—bioflavonoids, citric acids, and pectins. So make sure you dig deep into the rind when juicing citrus.

Of all the citric fruits, lemon is the most potent detoxifier. It kills some types of intestinal parasites such as roundworms, and dissolves gallstones.[1] Limonene, the volatile oil responsible for the distinctive lemon aroma, even helps treat some forms of cancer such as breast cancer.[2] If taken in the morning, lemon juice is known to improve liver function and has been used to help eliminate kidney stones. The organic acids in all citrus fruits stimulate digestive juices and relieves constipation.

Oranges are great protectors against colds, flu, bruising, heart disease, and strokes. The alkaloid synephrine found in the orange's peel can reduce the liver's production of cholesterol.

Grapefruit juice eases constipation and improves digestion by increasing the flow of gastric juices. It can also save you pounds. Research shows the pectin content of grapefruits reduces appetite by slowing the emptying of the stomach.[3] Grapefruit pectin also reduces the accumulation of atherosclerotic plaque in patients afflicted with atherosclerosis and strengthens blood vessels and capillaries.[4] In an animal study conducted in Copenhagen, pectin even halted the metastasis of prostate cancer.[5] Owing to its significant stores of the bioflavonoid naringenin, grapefruit arrests the spreading of breast cancer cells and prevents the metastasis of melanoma.[6] In the battle against colds, grapefruit juice helps reduce fever and soothes coughs and sore throats. Consumed at night, grapefruit juice promotes sleep and alleviates insomnia.

Nutrients

Lemons are highest, by far, in both vitamin C (80mg/100gs) and citric acid (6,500mg). They also offer the valuable limonene lipid, the carbohydrate pectin, and calcium and magnesium. Grapefruits are a good source of vitamin C (38mg), calcium, phosphorus, and potassium. Oranges contain 50mgs of vitamin C as well as B-complex vitamins, potassium, zinc, and phosphorus.

The most important thing to know about citrus fruits is how quickly they lose their potency. Once opened, they should be consumed as soon as possible. So before you next get the sniffles, start juicing and drinking the nectar of these citrus healers. Prevention is the best medicine.

Cucumber

(Cucumis sativus)

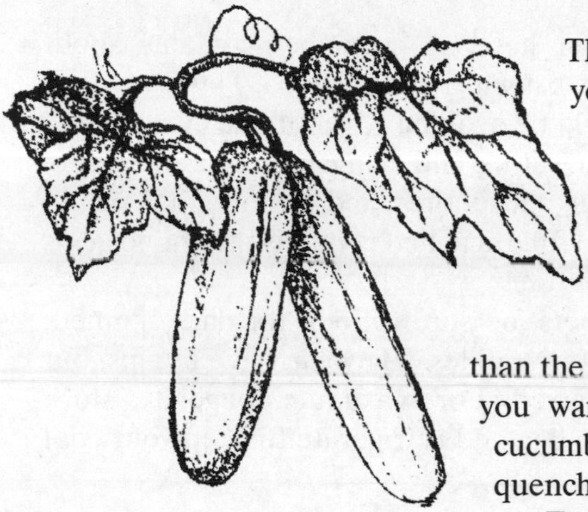

The next time someone tells you that he or she is "cool as a cucumber," you should be impressed. That person is claiming to be about 20 degrees cooler than you are. That's how much cooler a cucumber is inside than the air outside is on a hot day. If you want to be cool, too, grab a cucumber and snack on its thirst-quenching properties.

For a vegetable that's mostly water, this one is pretty impressive. First of all, the water itself is naturally distilled, making it superior to ordinary water. Second, the composition of that water makes it one of the best natural diuretics there is. Third, the cucumber's high water content helps regulate body temperature. Most impressive, perhaps, is the cucumber's role in cell hydration, waste removal and the dissolution of kidney stones.

What about that waxy skin? It is hard to wash off and it could get in your juice. Buy organic cucumbers or kirby cukes—the kind used for pickles. Neither are waxed. Try not to peel cukes, because you'll lose out on the high quantities of silica found there. This wondrous mineral strengthens the connective tissue that basically keeps us from falling apart! Tendons, muscles, cartilage, bones, ligaments, they all love silica. It even adds elasticity to our skin and is great for the complexion. This is why it is an ingredient in so many beauty creams. If you are treating eczema, psoriasis, hair loss, splitting nails, or acne, put cucumbers on your list.

Cucumber juice reduces the high uric acid content that causes rheumatic ailments leading to inflammation or degeneration of joints, muscles, ligaments, or tendons. Cucumber juice also normalizes blood pressure and, because of its temperature regulating properties, makes a great drink when you have a fever.

Nutrients

The skin is also important here. A cucumber contains about 250mg of vitamin A, which is mostly lost when peeled. This is another reason why waxed cukes should be avoided. Overall, the cucumber is valuable for its high potassium, sulfur, and manganese content. It also contains lime, sodium, calcium, phosphorus, and chlorine. It is rich in vitamins A, B-complex, C, and folic acid and contains the amino acids methionine and tryptophan.

When purchasing cucumbers, be sure to look for dark skinned, firm ones with no soft spots or wrinkles. They can have bumps, but otherwise should not be scarred. For maximum longevity, store them in a breathable produce bag and refrigerate to keep your cool cukes cool.

Echinacea

(Echinacea angustifolia, pallida, and purpurea)

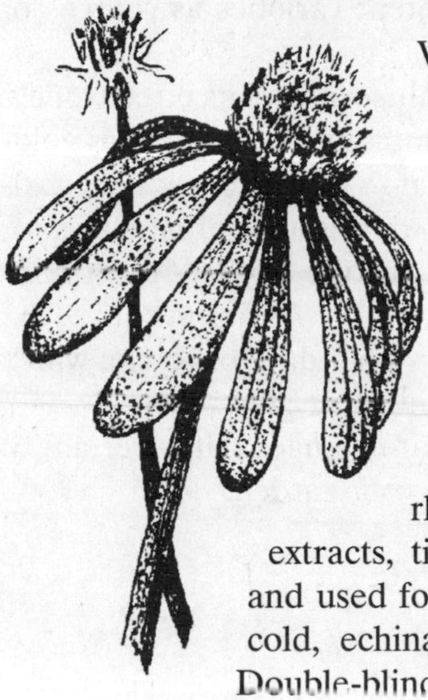

Want some echinacea for that oncoming cold? It might even be right outside your door. Native to North America, purple coneflower, rudbeckia, black samson, or Missouri snakeroot, are all echinacea in disguise.

Health Benefits

What a healer this perennial herb is! Every part of it is therapeutic. The roots, rhizomes, and leaves are made into fluid extracts, tinctures, tablets, and capsules, or dried and used for tea. As a defense against the common cold, echinacea has become a botanical celebrity. Double-blind studies prove that it works.[1] What might not be so well known is that it also successfully treats everything from canker sores, to Crohn's disease, gingivitis, ear infections, and candida. How does it do it? Probably because it can enhance many aspects of our immune system. Echinacea stimulates the production of interleukin-1, an immune protein that activates T-cells and macrophages (bacteria fighters). It stimulates stem cells in the lymphatic system as well as lymphokines (from lymphocytes), which form antibodies for infection control. All of these functions increase the body's capacity to ward off various viruses and bacteria and even to fight tumors.[2]

Cancer research has focused on echinacea's ability to stimulate tumor necrosis (or killing) factor.[3] Echinacea also activates the macrophages (the cells that digest foreign substances) and stimulates NK lymphocytes and phagocyte production in patients with AIDS and chronic fatigue syndrome.[4]

Nutrients

Echinacea contains vitamins A, C, B2 and E. Its mineral content includes copper, potassium, iron, sulfur, selenium, chromium, cobalt, manganese, and zinc. But echinacea gets the most attention for its wealth of polysaccharides and phytochemicals—echinacin, echinacin B, echinacoside, and echinacein. Echinacea angustifolia and echinacea pupurea are considered the most potent varieties as sources of these compounds.

Tea is one of the best ways to enjoy echinacea, and its effectiveness can be enhanced by combining it with compatible herbs such as goldenseal. If you are using a supplement because of a cold or flu, herbalists recommend high doses of echinacea during the initial stages of treatment, for example, 40 drops of the tincture or 400-500mg capsules taken every two hours for one to two days. As a preventive, the maximum effect is achieved with a 4 days on/3 days off cycle, which prevents the immune system from becoming over-stimulated.

No matter how you decide to take your echinacea, it is certain to benefit your body as much as it beautifies your garden.

Flaxseed

(Also known as Linseed)

Flaxseeds present two gifts to humankind—their oil and their fiber. These prizes are beneficial to our heart and digestion, and they help fight breast and prostate cancers.

Health Benefits

Flax is tops in fiber. It is our highest dietary source of plant lignans, containing much more than any other plant. Lignans are a type of plant fiber whose affects in the human body is similar to that of estrogen. We need these lignans, which are often called phytoestrogens. We produce them in the colon (mammalian lignans), but only with the help of friendly bacteria along with the plant lignans contained in foods such as flax. It is the husk of the flaxseed that contains the lignans. Inside the seed lies the oil.

While human estrogen is a powerful and complex hormone, lignans are simpler and lack their side effects. Lignans play a role in cancer prevention by counteracting the secretion of enzymes that nourish cancer cells. Researchers have observed that, with the use of flaxseed supplements, breast tumors get smaller and melanomas recede.[1]

Flaxseed is also number one in oil. Flax contains more of the essential fatty acid alpha linolenic acid (ALA), than any other plant source. ALA is an omega-3 oil that our body uses to create EPA (eicosapentaenoic acid). EPA keeps triglycerides in check, lowers blood pressure, and prevents heart disease. Since plants don't produce EPA, those who are vegetarians must eat precursor foods such as flax to get the building blocks—ALA. (Fish oils are the best nonvegetable source of EPA.)

Diets high in ALA oils are sometimes called "Mediterranean diets," which, along with flaxseed, will lower your blood pressure and help prevent heart disease.[2] Flaxseeds (50 grams per day) will also lower your total cholesterol (by 9%), specifically the bad (LDL) cholesterol (by up to 18%).[3]

Flaxseed oil is very egalitarian. It helps women with breast cancer and men with enlarged prostate. Men with BPH (benign prostatic hyperplasia) saw their dribbling and nighttime urination problems decrease, their urine stream become stronger and their libido increase while taking flaxseed oil.[4]

And flax oil is easy to take. Unlike fish oil, flax does not smell fishy! Fish oil is also easily damaged by oxygen, whereas flax oil is more stable. It can easily be mixed in your salad or taken in soft gel capsules.

Perhaps the most famous use of flaxseed is for constipation. Flax swells in water to form a mucilage that slips and slides its way through your intestinal tract, clearing the track like a sweeper locomotive. There are other mucilaginous seeds, too. Chia is delicious, but not as effective as flax. Psyllium is not very palatable, and it is so absorbent that people often become uncomfortably bloated.

Blend your seeds into a meal or purchase the meal (powder) in your health food store. Blend about 2 tablespoons in 8 ounces of water. Whatever proportions you use, be sure to wait ten minutes until the seeds have fully swelled. By allowing the seeds to swell outside your body, you can avoid bloating inside. You can flavor your drink by using the various flaxseed recipes in this book. *(See "Colon Problems" and "Constipation.")*

Garlic

(Allium sativum)

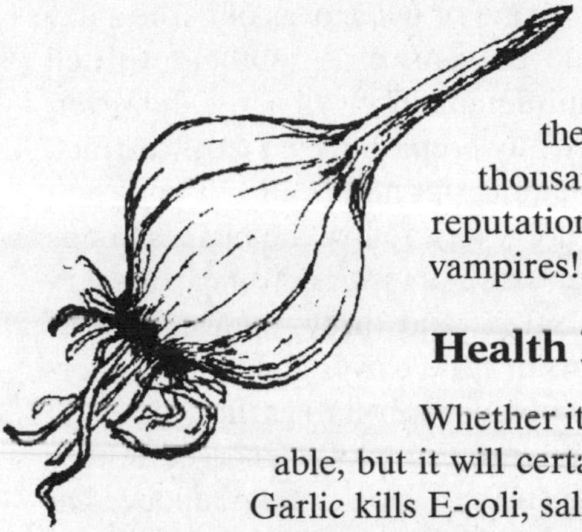

Civilizations have known about the medicinal properties of garlic for thousands of years. So potent was its reputation that it was even used to ward off vampires!

Health Benefits

Whether it will shoo away monsters is debatable, but it will certainly help you fight germ-warfare. Garlic kills E-coli, salmonella, fungi, and yeasts. It suppresses helicobacter pylori (which causes ulcers) and inhibits shigella and candida. Even the common cold is helped by adding garlic to your diet.

Garlic can even help in the war against AIDS. In one double-blind study, garlic was shown to stimulate the ability of lymphocytes to destroy antigens after only 3 weeks of a regimen using aged garlic extract. One hundred percent of the patients had normal levels of their NK lymphocytes restored in just 12 weeks.[1]

Garlic is also a powerful agent in the war against cancer. It reduces the incidence of bladder cancer (in mice) and prevents both prostate and breast cancer in vitro.[2] Garlic fights leukemia and inhibits the proliferation of liver and skin cancer cells. In studies conducted on animals, it reduced the incidence of colon cancer by up to 75%.[3] Finally, in research conducted on people who ate an average of 7 cloves of garlic a day, the incidence of stomach cancer was 10 times lower than those who did not eat garlic.[4]

How is all of this possible? On the preventive front, it is believed that garlic facilitates the liver's ability to detoxify carcinogens before they can harm other parts of the body. It is believed that garlic suppresses a growth factor for cancer cells (thymidine), preventing it from infiltrating into the DNA. Whatever magic is at work here, it is clear that garlic belongs in any cancer preventive/treatment regimen.

But that's not all. Garlic has been shown to lower blood sugar levels in diabetics, eliminate lead and other heavy metals, reduce the levels of the so-called bad (LDL) cholesterol, and lower the incidence of blood clotting.[5]

Some holistic healers believe that one or two cloves of garlic a day is sufficient for both medicinal and preventive use. Others will tell you that three cloves a day is the minimum. They all agree, however, that ingesting raw garlic or the specially prepared aged garlic extract, instead of cooked, is vital to maintaining optimal health. If you can't imagine eating so much raw garlic every day, follow the recipes in this book and sneak them into your juices and dressings. You can also try garlic sprouts. Add them to your salads and throw them into your juicer. They grow like alfalfa sprouts or little chives and add the therapeutic and breath control benefits of chlorophyll to garlic.

When you buy garlic, look for plump, firm cloves encased in uniformly smooth skin. There should be no soft spots and no mildew. Do not refrigerate garlic. Keep it in a cool, dry place. Old, hardened garlic should be disposed. You don't have to string garlic around your neck to ward off the threats to your health.

Ginger

(Zingiber Officinale)

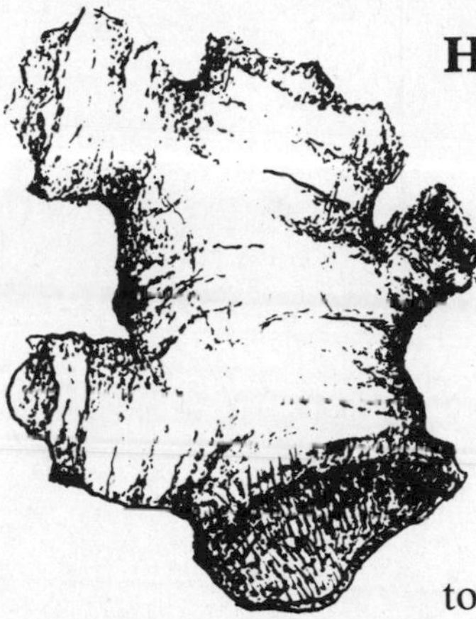

Health Benefits

It may look gnarly and stubby, but it's got talent! Ginger is the classic tonic for the digestive tract and a staple of traditional Chinese medicine for more than 2,500 years. Classified as an aromatic bitter herb, it stimulates digestion, keeps the intestinal muscles toned, relieves ab-dominal bloating, vomiting, and diarrhea, and it may serve to protect the stomach lining against such irritants as alcohol and non-steroidal anti-inflammatory drugs. It effectively combats nausea associated with morning sickness, motion sickness, chemotherapy, and anesthesia.

The medicinal qualities of ginger are found in the underground stem (rhizome) of this perennial herb. About 1-4% of the dried rhizome is made up of volatile oils, and though research is inconclusive as to how ginger acts to combat nausea, the pungent constituents in the volatile oils, gingerol and shogaol, are believed to be the anti-nausea and anti-vomiting agents.

Ginger also possesses anti-inflammatory properties. It is potent as an inhibitor of prostaglandin and thromboxane formation and has strong antioxidant properties similar to that of bromelain for inflammation.[1] In one clinical study, daily doses of ginger were prescribed to seven patients suffering from rheumatoid arthritis. Conventional drugs had offered little relief, but after the ginger treatments each patient reported substantial improvement in pain relief and joint mobility, and a decrease in swelling and morning stiffness.[2]

Ginger supports a healthy cardiovascular system, too. Like garlic, ginger makes blood platelets less sticky. This action reduces a major risk factor for atherosclerosis.[3]

Don't refrigerate fresh ginger. Instead, store it as you would garlic; in a cool, dry place. Grab your cookbooks and start adding this potent and delicious herb to your daily diet. Follow the recipes under the different health ailments in this book for making therapeutic ginger tea. Your stomach will thank you.

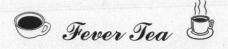

Fever Tea

by Donald W. Novey, M.D.

4 inch piecc	Ginger
1	Cinnamon Bark Stick
1 quart	Water
To Taste	Honey

Drink it as much as you can for muscle pain, soreness, malaise, and fatigue when sick with fever or virus. Do not use if you cannot tolerate spicy foods.

Take a large piece of fresh ginger, about four inches long. Slice it into disks about the thickness of a quarter. Add it to a quart of water along with a cinnamon stick (the bark, not the candy). Bring to a boil and cover for at least 30 minutes. It will turn a golden color.

Dr. Donald W. Novey, M.D., practices medicine at the *Center for Complementary Medicine* in Park Ridge, Illinois. He is author and editor of *Clinicians Complete Reference to Complementary /Alternative Medicine.*

Ginkgo

(Ginkgo biloba)

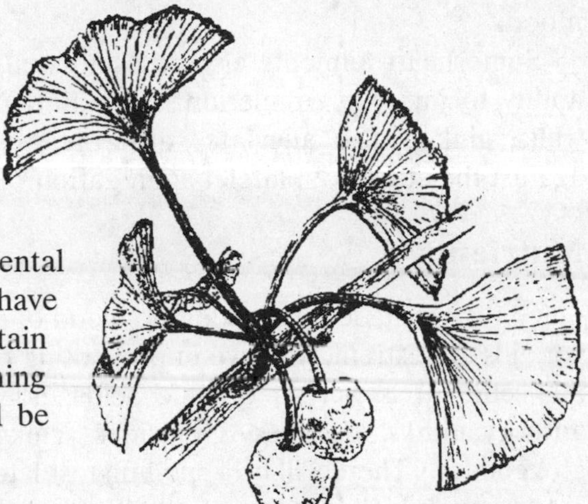

Do you have grandparents who are still sharp as a tack? God bless them, they are the exceptions. Most of us lose memory and mental acuity as we age. We have been searching for a fountain of youth since the beginning of time, and it may well be under the ginkgo tree.

Health Benefits

Aging is no fun. It takes its toll on our eyes and ears. Ginkgo can help. Ginkgo eases age-related hearing loss by improving blood circulation to the ears. It may help relieve tinnitus, which causes people to hear background noises as they age.[1] It may also prevent age-related macular degeneration by protecting the retinas from the effects of free radicals. And it reduces the susceptibility of the eyes to edema and cellular lesions.[2]

Now that we can see and hear better, what about our mental faculties? Normal aging causes the receptors in our brains to diminish in quantity and efficiency. Ginkgo biloba slows this process and actually increases the number of receptors (5-HT1A).[3] Ginkgo is famous for improving memory, but how does it work? For one, it increases the brain's alpha waves and decreases the theta rhythms, effectively increasing alertness.[4] Its ability to improve blood circulation may also be a factor, since this increases oxygenation to the brain. Ginkgo is one of the most effective substances for boosting circulation to the capillaries.[5] Ginkgo nourishes our brain's neurotransmitters and expands the number of receptors for acetylcholine. This improves concentration, attention span, learning ability, and memory.[6]

Ginkgo is especially helpful for Alzheimer's sufferers. After three months of supplementing with ginkgo at 240mg per day, Alzheimer patients improved their attention span, mental function, memory, and mood.[7]

Some heart ailments also respond well to ginkgo because of its ability to improve circulation. By maintaining the flexibility of cell walls, ginkgo also alleviates atherosclerosis and protects arteries against the effects of platelet aggregation.[8]

Nutrients

Ginkgo is made up of a unique blend of phytochemicals. Its bioflavonoids are extremely active in preventing free radicals from destroying cells.[9] It is rich in organic acids, polyphenols, quercetin, proanthocyanidins, flavones, glycosides, ginkgolic acid, lactones, and ginkgolides. (There will be a spelling test later.)

Although ginkgo leaves are available as a loose, dried herb, most health food resources sell it in the form of tablets, capsules, and extracts. Extracts taste good enough to squirt into any fruit juice. A typical therapeutic dosage would be 40mg 3 times per day. For Alzheimer patients, the dosage is doubled. Ginkgo is completely non-toxic even at higher doses. It generally takes from 3 to 6 months of continued use to achieve desired results.

So, when you are feeling fatigued, dazed, or forgetful, let ginkgo help you remember to take your ginkgo.

(For more on memory, see "Longevity" and "Power Drinks for the Mind.")

Ginseng

(Panax Araliaceae)

We bow in gratitude to the great Chinese gods who brought us the amazing ginseng. Don't be confused by the fact that there are several different kinds. The important thing is that they all provide similar health benefits and that they are well worth remembering. In fact, ginseng may even help you remember to take ginseng.

Health Benefits

It is believed that the numerous health benefits of ginseng may be attributed directly to its enhancement of the hypothalamus, the region of the brain that controls things like sleep, body temperature, appetite, and other autonomic nervous system responses. Research proves that ginseng alleviates insomnia and improves coordination, stamina, and endurance. Asiatic ginseng (true ginseng cultivated in Asia) heightens athletic performance by reducing the production of lactic acid and increasing oxygen absorption.[1]

Ginseng enhances cognitive function by measurably increasing blood circulation to the brain. It can increase mental alertness in the elderly, accelerate learning, improve concentration, and increase short and long term memory.[2] Ginseng contains ginsenoside, which prevents the death of neurons and stimulates the growth of axons in the cerebral cortex.[3] Because ginseng also enhances the metabolism of serotonin, it helps in the treatment of stress and depression.[4]

Ginseng, especially Asiatic ginseng, is good for the heart. It stimulates the production of hemoglobin, which improves blood circulation and anemia. It can strengthen the heart muscle, reverse hypertension, fight atherosclerosis, and reduce cholesterol.[5]

Ginseng is a valuable detoxification agent that protects the liver from alcohol and the toxic effects of chemotherapy and radiation.[6]

As an immune system stimulant, ginseng has become an important adjunct therapy for patients afflicted with AIDS and cancer.[7] Ginsenosides increase white blood cells, stimulate interferon production, increase the activity of lymphocytes, and lower the incidence of tumor formation. Ginsenosides are capable of normalizing cancerous human liver cells, and they have also been effective in treating colon, lung, ovarian, pancreatic, and stomach cancer.[8]

All ginseng varieties possess antioxidant properties and enhance the body's production of energy. In women, ginseng reduces PMS symptoms, and some say it even improves fertility. Long before the US drug Viagra appeared on the scene, ginseng was used to increase sexual desire in cases of male impotence.[9]

Diabetes mellitus type 2 sufferers may want to consider a daily dose of 100-200mg of ginseng. Scientific research conducted on diabetics found that it corrects many of the side effects of the illness. It improves control of blood sugar, enhances the release of insulin from the pancreas, and increases the energy levels of patients.[10]

Nutrients

Ginseng can either be "true" ginseng varieties, those in the Panax family, or they may be called Siberian or Eleuthero. American and Asiatic ginseng are true ginsengs and share a very similar chemical makeup. The main difference is that American ginseng contains more ginsenosides than Asiatic ginseng, whereas only Siberian ginseng contains eleutherosides. Although eleuthero gingsengs are not part of the panax family, they have similar therapeutic effects.

Ginseng contains the minerals calcium, cobalt, germanium, iodine, manganese, magnesium, potassium, sodium, copper, iron, phosphorus and sulfur. Their vitamin content includes biotin, folic acid, vitamins A, B1, B2, B12, C, and E.

Ginseng comes in teas, extracts, tablets, pills, capsules, or loose, dried roots. Not all ginsengs are equal, so try to find brands that are standardized in terms of their ginsenoside content. No matter how you decide to incorporate ginseng into your diet, be assured that your body will appreciate it from head to toe.

Grapes

(Vitus vinifera)

Health Benefits

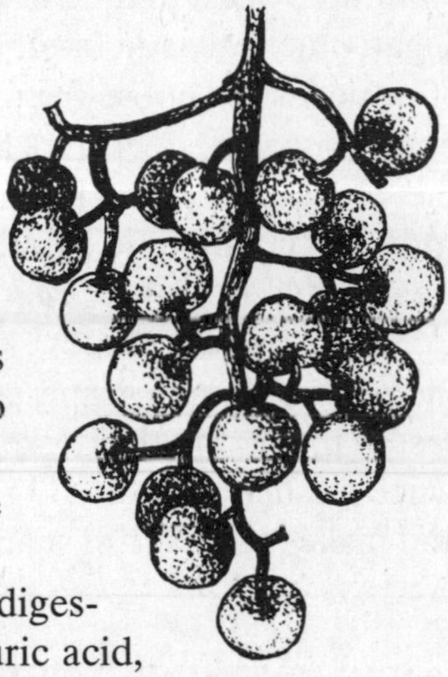

Grapes–seeds and all–are valuable little pearls in the trove of natural food treasures. Dieters and those with a slow metabolism will especially enjoy fresh squeezed grape juice because it stimulates metabolic rate. Grapes are known to improve circulation, prevent blood clotting, and increase blood pressure in those with hypotension (low blood pressure).

Grapes are excellent for treating indigestion, relieving constipation, eliminating uric acid, improving urinary flow, and cleansing the liver. Grapes and wine made from aged grapes are valuable to our immune systems. They kill some forms of bacteria and deactivate some viruses including herpes.[1]

Grape seeds contain protective flavonol compounds called oligomeric proanthocyanidins (OPC's) that scavenge free radicals and promote the growth and repair of connective tissue. They also have numerous benefits for the cardiovascular system, including treatment for such disorders as varicose veins and atherosclerosis.[2] Because these flavonols are also found in the capillaries of the eye, grape seed extract has been used to treat a host of eye problems, including night blindness, retinal disorders, and general vision improvement.[3]

Nutrients

Grapes are a wonderful source of vitamins A, B1, B2, C, and niacin, and a fertile source of minerals—potassium, iron, calcium, chlorine, copper, fluorine, manganese, silicon, sulfur, magnesium, phosphorus and sodium. Grape skins are loaded with the carotenoids beta-carotene and lycopene as well as other valuable plant substances such as ellagic acid, phytosterols (resveratrol), and sulfur compounds (isothiocyanates).They also contain a lot of fruit sugar (fructose), so be careful if you have sugar sensitivities such as diabetes, hypoglycemia, and candida.

Grapes are a unique taste experience, because they combine acids, sugar, mucilage, and bitter and astringent compounds. There are over 50 varieties to choose from including seedless green Thompsons, dark blue Concords, deep red Emperors, and bright red Cardinals. Juice the seeds and skin, too. But since commercial grapes are highly sprayed, buy organic wherever possible or wash them with a natural cleanser. *(See "Power Drinks Basics–How to Wash Fruits & Vegetables.")*

When buying grapes, look for plump, firm grapes that cling to their stems. Green grapes are best when they have a slightly yellowish cast to them, and the darker grapes should have a rich, uniform color. Once washed and dried, grapes keep in the refrigerator for a week and make a wonderful snack.

Green Tea

(Camellia sinensis)

Do you drink green tea? If not, consider this: Certain cancers are almost unheard of in regions where people drink lots of this ancient Asian brew.

Health Benefits

The link between green tea and the reduced incidence of breast, colon, liver, lung, pancreatic, and stomach cancers has been well documented. The tea polyphenol "epigallo-catechin-gallate" (EGCG) in green tea prevents breast cancer in animal studies. Epidemiological evidence indicates that regions with the highest consumption of green tea have the lowest rates of colon and pancreatic cancers.[1]

Green tea also contains catechins like epicatechin gallate (ECG), which along with the polyphenols protect the liver, lungs, esophagus, and stomach from cancer. 1,000mg of green tea daily help the liver counter the toxic effects of alcohol and hepatitis and protect current and former tobacco smokers from lung cancer. Why is green tea such an impressive cancer fighter? The answers are still being researched but the polyphenols in green tea prevent the conversion of nitrates and nitrites into carcinogenic nitrosamines. Also its high EGCG content obstructs the synthesis of tumor cells. Epidemiological studies demonstrate that those who drink green tea at least once a week show a lower risk of contracting cancer.[2]

As if its potent anti-cancer properties were not enough, green tea also benefits cardiac health. Because of its high ninhydrin content, green tea hinders the production of thromboxane, a chemical involved in abnormal blood clotting.[3] When consumed immediately after meals, it significantly lowers blood pressure in people afflicted with hypertension.[4] And those who consume more than 5 cups of green tea per day reduce by five times their risk of stroke.[5]

Green tea possesses an abundance of antioxidants—six times more than black tea. They are 20 times more potent than those in vitamin E, making it a super free-radical scavenger that easily subdues hydrogen peroxide, singlet oxygen, and superoxides.[6]

As a dental aide, green tea helps prevent gingivitis and plaque, increases the resistance of tooth enamel, and blocks streptococcus mutans in the mouth.[7]

Finally, green tea is becoming an important asset in the fight against skin cancer. It obstructs the development of melanoma and helps prevent squamous cell carcinoma.[8]

In order to benefit from the tannins (EGCG and ECG) in green tea, it is essential to drink it without milk. Adding milk causes the tannins to bind to the milk proteins, rendering them unusable. Green tea can be purchased as loose tea leaves for drinking, or you can buy tablets and capsules that are standardized to contain from 23% to 83% polyphenols. The optimal dosage of tea polyphenols is 200mgs a day—equivalent to 5-10 cups of tea per day. The next time you turn on your teapot, reach for green tea.

Kale & Collards

(Brassica oleracea acephali)

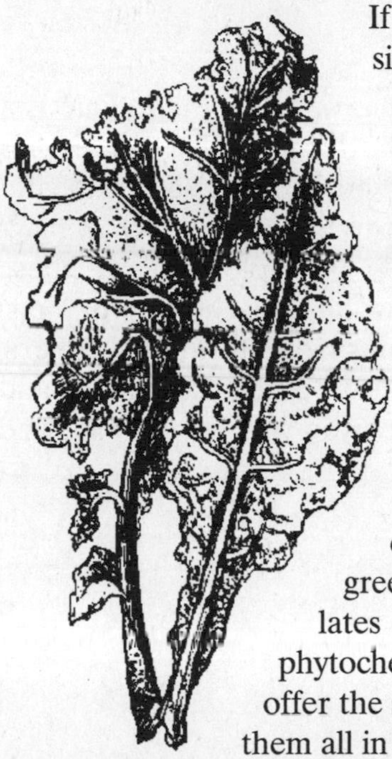

If your experience of kale is wilted leaves sitting in a soup, then be prepared for a new taste experience with one of the most nutritious greens in the garden.

Both kale and its cousin collard greens are important foods in the illustrious category of vegetables known as crucifers, or brassicas. This large family of vegetable healers includes red and green cabbage, Chinese cabbage, bok choy, savoy, cauliflower, broccoli, collard greens, kohlrabi, kale, and the mustard family, which includes watercress, radish, brussels sprouts, and turnip greens. They are all rich sources of glucosinolates and isothiocyanates, a group of potent phytochemicals that protect us from cancer. They offer the same benefits as kale and collards, so use them all in your diet and as often as you please.

Health Benefits

Kale and collards are an especially outstanding source of calcium. A cup of either surpasses the calcium content found in a glass of milk and, because it contains an unusually high ratio of calcium to phosphorus, the calcium found in them is absorbed far more successfully. Calcium is known to fight osteoporosis, and is crucial to nerve conduction, muscle contraction, heartbeat, blood coagulation, energy production, and immune function maintenance. These crucifers are good sources of dietary calcium that according to epidemiological studies, lowers the risk of colorectal cancer.[1]

Because of its large stores of the potent cancer protective compounds indoles, glucosinolates, and isothiocyanates, kale and collards help to prevent breast and lung cancers.[2] The high content of the carotenoids lutein and zeaxanthin in kale also helps prevent age-related macular degeneration of the eyes.[3] As a rich source of chlorophyll, these vegetables oxygenate the blood, improve red blood cell counts, and aid the fundamental processes of cell circulation and respiration.

Nutrients

In addition to its high calcium and chlorophyll content, kale is a significant source of provitamin A in the form of the carotenoids alpha and beta-carotene, lutein, and zeaxanthin. It is also rich in vitamins C, E, B6, K, and folic acid. The minerals iron, potassium, magnesium, phosphorus, zinc, and sodium are plentiful in these vegetables. With today's idolization of low-fat, low-cholesterol diets, you will be happy to know that kale contains virtually none of either.

What's the best way to get this goldmine of precious nutrients and phytochemicals? Turn off the stove, put away your frying pan, and pull out your juice machine.

Licorice

(Glycyrrhiza glabra)

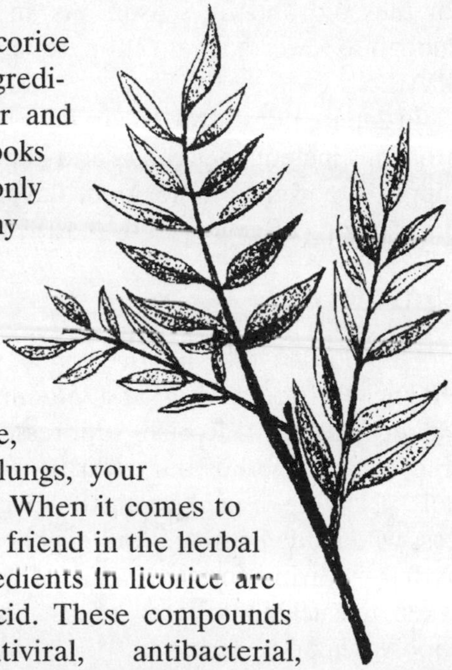

If you think you're getting licorice at the candy store, read the ingredients. In fact, it is mostly sugar and molasses. The real licorice looks like a root "cigarette" and is only slightly sweet. But this earthy stick is what you need to beat away the winter bugs.

Health Benefits

When you think of licorice, think of your stomach, your lungs, your liver, and your immune system. When it comes to ulcers, you cannot find a better friend in the herbal treasure chest. The active ingredients in licorice are glycyrrhizin and glycyrrhetic acid. These compounds are anti-inflammatory, antiviral, antibacterial, anti-allergenic, and anti-asthmatic. The Chinese, for whom licorice is a traditional healing herb, believe that it absorbs stomach acid, promotes pH balance, and coats and soothes the stomach to relieve spasms. Licorice has proven to be an effective healing agent in gastric, duodenal, and peptic ulcers. In one study, 2300mg per day caused a reduction in gastric ulcer size in 78% of subjects and caused complete healing in 44% of the people tested.[1]

If you have rheumatism and arthritis, think licorice. Licorice is an effective anti-inflammatory, because glycyrrhizin activates cortisol, our own bodies anti-inflammatory hormone.[2]

Because of the propensity for glycyrrhizin to act like a steroid, prolonged use of large doses can elevate blood pressure and cause water retention in sensitive people. For this reason, hypertensive patients are advised to use deglycyrrhizinized licorice (DGL), which does not cause these side effects.

Licorice is famous for its ability to heal asthma and bronchitis. In Europe, it is the most often recommended treatment for respiratory ailments, including chronic coughs, allergies, and sinus infections. Its antiviral and antibacterial properties make it an effective prophylactic for the cold and flu season. As an immune builder, it is powerful enough to lower a fever (antipyretic) and to be used in the treatment of AIDS.[3]

In Japan, pure glycyrrhizin licorice extract is widely used for liver problems including cirrhosis and hepatitis B.[4] Licorice contains a rich supply of powerful antioxidant flavonoids that protect the liver from the oxidizing effects of LDL (bad) cholesterol.[5]

Nutrients

One doesn't take licorice for its vitamins, although it has biotin, choline, PABA, inositol, and vitamin E. You take it for its fabulous phytochemicals. Licorice suppresses our coughs, decongests our sinuses, and soothes our arthritis with its quercetin, rutin, polyphenols, glycyrrhetic acid, liquiritin, glycosides and flavonoids. The goddess who made licorice is quite a chemist. Licorice has been a proven herbal medicine for thousands of years. In modern times, we have taken to sucking tobacco sticks. Should you get the urge to lick, choose a licorice stick.

Noni

(Morinda citrifolia)

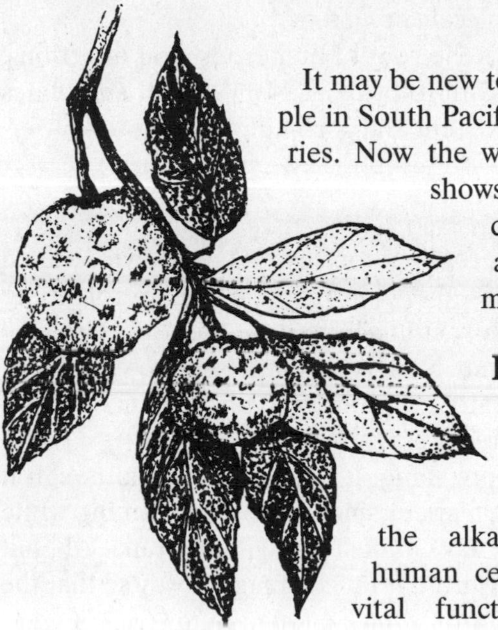

It may be new to us, but Noni has been a staple in South Pacific medicine chests for centuries. Now the word is out. Recent research shows us what South Pacific medicine men have known all along: Noni is one of nature's most remarkable healing gifts.

Health Benefits

In the early 1950s, Dr. Ralph Heinicke, the father of noni research, identified the alkaloid xeronine in healthy human cells. Xeronine performs two vital functions: it activates various enzymes and strengthens the structure of proteins. According to Heinicke, "Xeronine is so basic to the functioning of protein, we would die without it." His research proved that although our own bodies produce xeronine, foods that contain its precursor pro-xeronine are essential. Noni contains pro-xeronine in substantial quantities.[1]

In traditional medicine, noni is best known as a pain reliever. Xeronine promotes endorphin responses in the pituitary gland. These hormones control not only physical pain but also contribute to a sense of emotional well-being. Noni binds very efficiently with serotonin, the "mood hormone," alleviating conditions such as depression, anxiety, sleep disorders, and migraine headaches. Menstrual cramps, sprains, injuries, and arthritis are soothed by the analgesic effects of this plant.[2]

Certain bacterial invaders such as staphylococcus, salmonella, fungi, yeast, and E-coli appear to be restrained by noni juice. This may be due to its caprylic and caproic acid content. These acids also aid digestion and contribute to a healthier intestinal tract. The root of the noni plant contains a miraculous compound called damnacanthal, which can turn precancerous cells into normal, healthy cells significantly extending the life of lung cancer victims.[3]

Decreased T-cell function is the root of numerous viral infections, cancer, arthritis, hepatitis, and fibromyalgia. Noni extract stimulates T-cell activity of our immune system and is completely non-toxic.[4]

Nutrients

Besides the alkaloid pro-xeronine, noni carries an enzyme called pro-xeronase, which facilitates the conversion of pro-xeronine to xeronine. Take noni on an empty stomach to have the best chance of activating this important enzyme. Noni is rich in selenium, vitamins C and B3, caprylic and caproic fatty acids, and the phytochemical damnacanthal.

Noni is famous for one more thing: it stinks! Indeed, although it comes from a lovely tree with a sweet smelling, ever-blooming white flower, the raw fruit and juice have a most repugnant aroma. Ah, but the mavens of marketing have juiced it up in a magical way so that the bottles you find in health food stores have a tang reminiscent of cranberry juice. Thank goodness, because noni is too important to miss.

Noni Juice Cocktail

6 oz	Noni Juice
2 oz	Cranberry Juice
2 oz	Black Cherry Juice
2 oz	Apple Juice

Mix these delicious juices together and experience the pain-relieving power of the marvelous noni juice.

Parsnips

(Pastinaca Sativa)

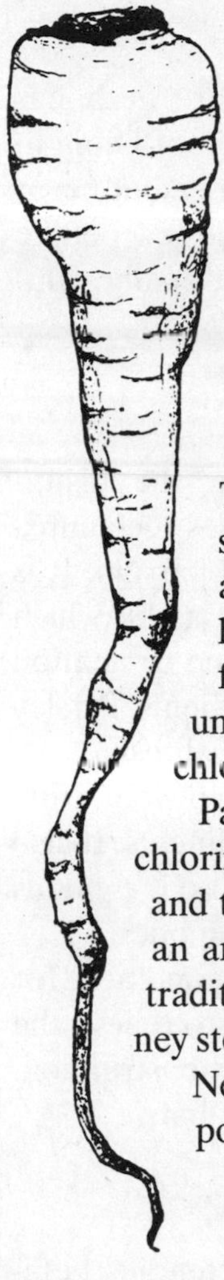

Parsnips are from the same family as carrots and surprisingly just as sweet. In fact, they even look like white/yellow carrots. Parsnips are another low profile vegetable that deserves to be taken out of the soup kettle and put in your juicer.

Health Benefits

Parsnips could be nick-named "the beauty drink." They possess the rare distinction of being wonderfully sweet but very low in calories, so they make a great addition to juices for weight loss. They also strengthen hair and nails and improve skin quality. Those who suffer from acne or other skin disorders will appreciate its unique balance of potassium, phosphorus, sulfur, silicon, chlorine, and vitamin C for their skin flattering benefits.

Parsnips are beneficial for the vital organs, as well. Their chlorine and phosphorus levels improve function in the lungs and the bronchial tubes. They have been used as a diuretic, an anti-arthritic agent, and for detoxifying. In some herbal traditions, parsnip juice is used to help dissolve gall and kidney stones.

Next time you buy carrots for juicing, mix it up. Add a pound of parsnips and enjoy its sweet nutrition.

Parsley

(Petroselinum Sativum Umbelliferae)

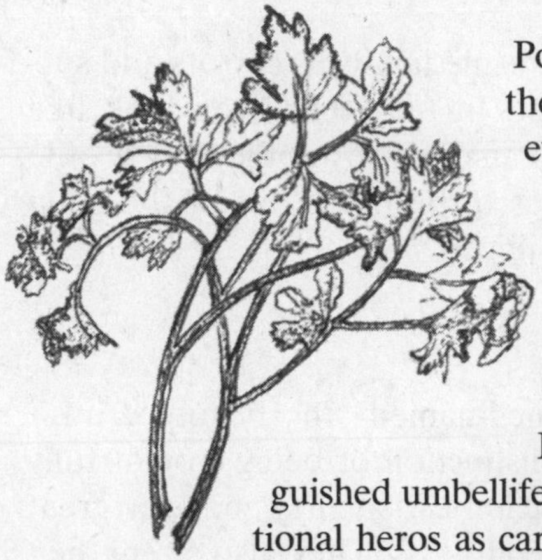

Poor parsley. This culinary herb has the ignominious distinction of being in every restaurant in America but never eaten! It is a pity that so few people know just how nutritionally valuable this "garnish" is.

Health Benefits

Parsley is the head of the distinguished umbelliferae family, which includes such nutritional heros as carrots, celery, fennel, and parsnip. It is perhaps our best source of the volatile oil apiol, which improves appetite and digestion by increasing blood circulation to the digestive tract thereby enhancing absorption of nutrients. Parsley juice also alleviates flatulence and improves bad breath (halitosis).

Parsley is famous as a diuretic, helping keep a healthy flow of urine and preventing kidney stones and various urinary tract ailments. It also helps the adrenals (which sit on top of the kidneys) because it contains nutritional precursors for the manufacture of adrenal hormones.

Parsley is a good source of histidine, the essential amino acid for growth and tissue repair. Herbalists recommend parsley to relieve the symptoms of goiter and rheumatism, and facilitate menstruation. Folklore has it that parsley even promotes the growth of hair.

Nutrition

Parsley is one of nature's finest sources of the carotenoids beta-carotene and chlorophyll, and is a healthy source of calcium (260mg/100g), iron (6.2mg), vanadium (80mcg), and manganese. Go ahead, decorate with it, but don't forget to gobble the garnish!

Peppermint

(Mentha Peperita)

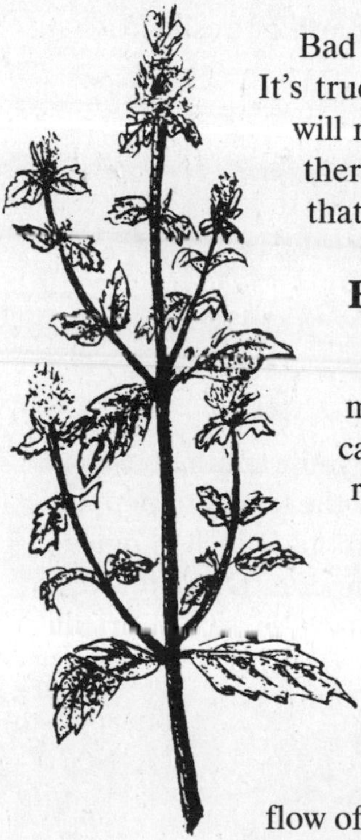

Bad breath? Have no fear, peppermint is here. It's true, a drop of peppermint oil on your tongue will make halitosis go away–and hiccups, too–but there are many more ways to use peppermint that will make you breathe easier.

Health Benefits

Volatile oils arc the secret to peppermint's power. Its potent mentholated oil calms the stomach in cases of nausea, diarrhea, and after regurgitation. It is your best friend for travel nausea and morning sickness. Officially classified as a carminative, reach for peppermint first for flatulence and cramps from intestinal gas.

In addition to calming an upset stomach, peppermint also stimulates digestion and prevents dyspepsia.[1] It stirs the flow of bile from the gall bladder to help digest fats. Enteric coated capsules of peppermint oil release in the colon and ease the symptoms of irritable bowel syndrome.[2] As a tea, peppermint is a tonic for the intestines and is one of the best remedies you can use to calm your infant's symptoms of colic.[3]

Peppermint's high menthol content also soothes respiratory problems. Inhale peppermint oil vapors directly into the nose from tea or from a few drops of the oil in simmering water. Use it for bronchitis, congested sinuses, headaches, and even migraines or just as aromatherapy to perk up the blahs.

Peppermint is a 300-year-old hybrid of spearmint and water mint. You can use spearmint in a similar way, but it is less potent. The aromatic peppermint oil is used in various therapeutic treatments. It makes up 1-4% of this herb, and menthol is the oil's dominant compound, making up more than half of it. Peppermint is available as a loose herb and in tea bags, and as tablets, capsules, and a fluid extract. All are effective.

Whether you inhale it via aromatherapy for enhanced energy or sip it for a soothed tummy, peppermint is a breath of fresh air.

Tummy Tea

10	Peppermint Leaves, crushed
¼ inch	Ginger Root, grated

You can use tea bags of these herbs, but if you want the best results, make this tea from fresh herbs. Crush the leaves of peppermint and steep along with the ginger. Grate about ¼ inch of ginger root into 1–1½ cups of water. Steep for 5+ minutes. Drink this tea hot. Heat can be beneficial to digestion because it increases circulation to the stomach.

Red Pepper

(Capsicum Frutescens)

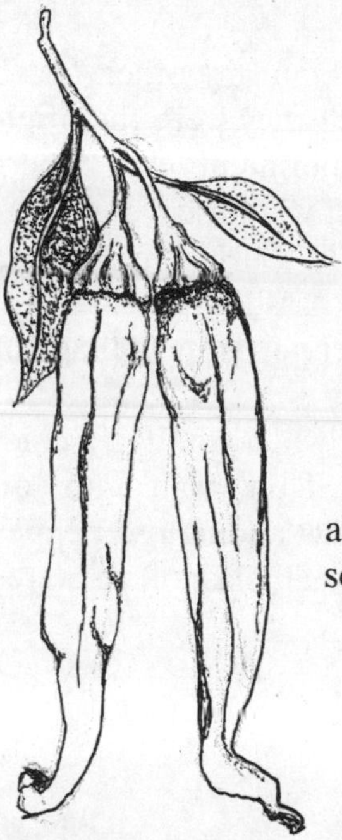

By any name, cayenne, chili pepper, hot pepper, capsicum, Tobasco pepper, or paprika (milder)—this is one hot item!

Health Benefits

Much of what's good about hot peppers is attributable to their capsaicin content. This is what gives chilies that well-known burning sensation. This miracle alkaloid prevents abnormal blood clotting, inhibits the absorption of dietary cholesterol, lowers total serum cholesterol and blood pressure, reduces bad (LDL) cholesterol, and the incidence of abnormal heart rhythms (ventricular fibrillation).[1]

In the digestive system, capsaicin protects the gastric mucosa against alcohol and aspirin-induced damage and reduces both the frequency and severity of peptic ulcers.[2] It also seems to be bacteriostatic against some types of detrimental bacteria, including a strain of streptococcus that causes ulcers.[3] Many symptoms of the common cold are helped by hot peppers, since capsaicin thins the mucous in the lungs and facilitates the expectoration of excessive mucous.[4]

There are numerous topical ointments employing capsaicin for its analgesic properties. They are used for sore muscles and joints, osteoarthritis, tendinitis, and arthritis and to reduce te pain and itching of shingles (herpes zoster). In double-blind studies, nasal sprays of capsaicin have even prevented cluster headaches.[5]

The "heat" of hot peppers induces perspiration (diaphoretic), which helps excrete waste matter from the skin, tissues, lymph, and blood. Chilies also fight fatigue and facilitate weight loss in obese patients.[6] If you have asthma or bronchitis, use hot peppers to keep the respiratory passages open.[7] As anyone who has ever eaten a chili pepper whole can tell you, it also relieves sinusitis.

Nutrients

Red hot peppers contain more vitamin C than any other "raw" food after acerola berries (369mg/100g). In fact, they were the original source of the vitamin used in the experiments by Albert Szent-Györgyi, the Nobel prize-winning inventor who discovered vitamin C. It is also the #2 source of vitamin A (77,000IU/100g) and is among our best food sources for niacin, iron, potassium, and sodium. But the premiere therapeutic compound in pepper is its 700mgs of capsaicinoids.

If you ever drank red pepper and honey tea when you had a cold, you already know its powerful curative effects. Don't wait until you get sick. Follow the recipes in this book and start adding red pepper or a pinch of cayenne powder to your drinks. You'll blast off to better health.

Radish

(Raphanus Sativus)

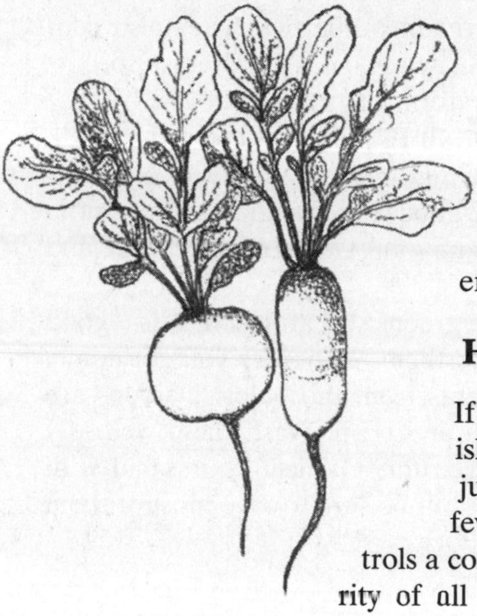

You can find them as red, white (daikon), horseradish, or wasabi (Japanese). Or you can sprout radish seeds. Whichever you choose, they are all nutritional superstars of the cabbage (cruciferous) family.

Health Benefits

If you have a cold, pull out the radishes and get your juicer. Radish juice soothes sore throats, reduces fever, clears the sinus cavities, controls a cough, and helps to restore the integrity of all mucous membranes. Historically, horseradish was used to treat catarrh, an excessive secretion of thick phlegm from the sinuses.

Radishes are a general tonic for the digestive tract. They are the best dietary source of the enzyme diastase, one of the enzymes that helps break down grains and starchy foods. They have also been known to alleviate diarrhea. Radishes can stimulate appetite and help dissolve fat deposits imbedded in body tissue. Because of their high alkali content, they improve kidney and bladder function and may aid the elimination of kidney and gallstones.

Poultices made from radish seeds have even been applied directly on the breasts of cancer patients to mitigate some of the symptoms of breast cancer and the seeds made into a strong tea are said to reduce the incidence of stomach cancer.[1] Poultices made from crushed radishes (with lots of juice) have been used for frostbite and to accelerate the healing of bruises. It has even been used to control body odor by applying it to armpits and feet. Try using it for insect bites and stings. When mixed with ice shavings and placed on burns, it is one of our finest natural anesthetics.

Nutrients

Radishes are an excellent vegetable source of sulfur, which possesses anti-inflammatory and antioxidant properties. They also contain lots of potassium, sodium, iodine, and magnesium. Radish sprouts contain an abundance of the plant form of provitamin A (391 IU/100g) compared to a garden radish (10 IU). That is more than milk (126 IU). The sprouts also have 29mg/100g of vitamin C, which is more than a pineapple. Radishes are good sources of important amino acids: valine (30mg/100g), tryptophane (5mg), threonine (59mg), and lysine (34mg).

When you find radishes with the greens still attached, it is a good sign of freshness. Be sure to remove them as soon as you get home, however, because they drain nutrients from the bulbs. Daikons are long and white and should be firm and crisp. Wash them well, dry them, and keep them in the refrigerator. Garnish your salad with these colorful ornaments if you like, but be sure to save most of them for your juicer.

Soy

Soybeans, Soy Milk, & Soy Products

(Glycine Max)

Western diets are rich in animal proteins. Asian diets are rich in plant proteins, and soy is their number one protein food. Westerners suffer from heart disease and cancer—our top two killers. These diseases are linked to the fat and cholesterol in meat. Asians have only a fraction of these problems. Could it be the soy protein in their diet?

Health Benefits

Soy can completely replace meat in the diet. It contains almost all of the essential amino acids, and it is rich in protein, low in fat, and completely free of cholesterol. In addition to whole soybeans, foods derived from soy include tofu, tempeh, soy milk, textured vegetable protein (a meat substitute known as TVP), soy flour, miso, and soy sauce. Many protein powders on the market are soy-based. It is the perfect meat substitute and you should never have to worry about running out. Soy is the most widely grown legume crop in the world.

It's official: soy protein lowers cholesterol. For over eighty years, soy protein has been researched for its ability to lower cholesterol, and the results have been published in leading medical journals. In 1999, the U.S. Food and Drug Administration gave their blessing by allowing a health benefit statement on the label of soy protein foods. Considering that we have long been a society devoted to animal protein, this was a real milestone. Soy protein reduces the rate of hypercholesterolemia and atherosclerosis. It also thins thick blood (lowers hematocrit levels) and reduces triglyceride levels.[1]

Soy harbors other miracles besides protein. It is one of the highest sources of isoflavones, which behave like plant estrogens, offering the benefits of estrogen without the side effects of taking the hormone.

The isoflavones in soy foods and soy milk reduce hormone dependent breast, prostate, uterine, and endometrial cancers.[2] For the highest levels of soy isoflavones, reach for soy milk, roasted soy nuts, tofu, tempeh, and soy protein isolates.

As we age, we tend to lose bone density. The plant sterols in soybeans help to prevent osteoporosis and can actually increase bone density. This is especially good news for pre– and post-menopausal women.[3]

Nutrients

Soybeans contain most of the essential amino acids. It has 649mg/100g of isoleucine, 935mg leucine, 759mg of lysine, 638mg valine, 2101mg of glutamine, 594mg phenylalanine, plus arginine, tryptophan, methionine, and others. Soybeans are rich in the essential alpha-linolenic, linoleic, and oleic fatty acids, and it is our finest source of the fat-buster lecithin. Its wealth of plant compounds includes polyphenols, isoflavonoids, saponins, phytosterols, and phytoestrogens.

Soy Smoothie

by Dr. Julian M. Whitaker, M.D.

2–3 cups	Favorite Fruit
2 Tbsp	Soy Protein Powder, unsweetened
2 Tbsp	Green Foods Powder
1–2 cups	Pure Water and Ice
Pinch	Stevia

Blend all ingredients together. Add more water or ice to achieve the desired consistency. Serves two.

Dr. Julian M. Whitaker is President and Founder of *Whitaker Wellness Institute* in Newport Beach, California.

Spinach

(Spinacia oleracea)

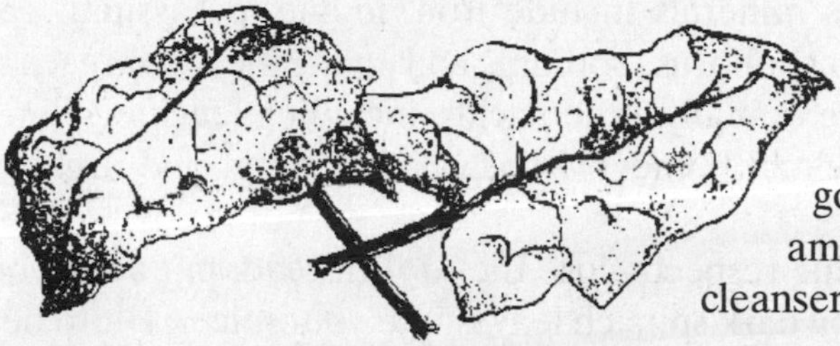

Popeye was a lot smarter than we thought. This green goddess really is an amazing body builder, cleanser, and regenerator.

Health Benefits

Spinach contains nearly twice as much iron as most other greens. Iron enables our red blood cells to carry more oxygen, which strengthens all cells but especially those of the brain and the respiratory system. Because of its high iron content, spinach is a valuable food for the treatment of anemia, circulatory weaknesses, and cholesterol diseases such as hypertension and stroke.[1]

Spinach also contains an abundance of two important carotenoids, zeaxanthin and lutein, which help prevent age-related macular degeneration and retard the development of cataracts.[2]

Like other vegetables high in chlorophyll and carotene, spinach plays a significant role against cancer. In one epidemiological study, women who consumed spinach regularly had a lower incidence of cervical cancer.[3]

The high fiber content of spinach makes it an excellent intestinal tract cleanser and regenerator. The combined cleansing and building properties of spinach make it a good choice for those suffering with constipation, colitis, poor digestion, or ulcers.

The minerals found in spinach are highly alkaline, which helps our bodies fight uric acid buildup and the symptoms of aging that go along with it. But spinach is also high in oxalic acid, which interferes with calcium absorption. Raw spinach enables us to metabolize this acid better than the cooked variety.

Nutrients

The xanthophyll carotenoids, lutein and zeaxanthin, account for 80-90% of the carotenoid content of spinach, while alpha and beta-carotenes account for the rest. Spinach has more protein than most vegetables (2-3%), and is a good source of vitamins A, B complex, C, K, and folic acid. Its minerals include iron, iodine, potassium, calcium, magnesium, phosphorus, sodium, and manganese. Spinach is also a valuable source of many amino acids, including leucine 176mg/100g, glutathione 166mg, lysine 142mg, valine 126mg, and arginine 116mg.

Popeye: with all due respect—lose the *can*! Instead, put a nice big handful of fresh, crisp, dark spinach leaves into your juicer. Bluto better watch out.

Juice For the Eyes

by Dr. Deborah E. Banker, M.D.

7 oz	Carrot Juice
5 oz	Celery Juice
2 oz	Endive Juice
2 oz	Parsley Juice
6 oz	Spinach Juice
1/4 inch	Ginger

This juice is loaded with nutrients that are known to promote eye health. Endive is thought to be helpful with cataracts and celery with inflammation. Spinach is high in lutein, an element necessary to prevent macular degeneration. Juice all ingredients together.

Dr. Deborah E. Banker, M.D. practices medicine at the *Malibu Life Center* in Malibu California, where she leads workshops on eye health.

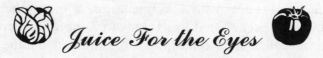

Tomato

(Lycopersicum esculentum)

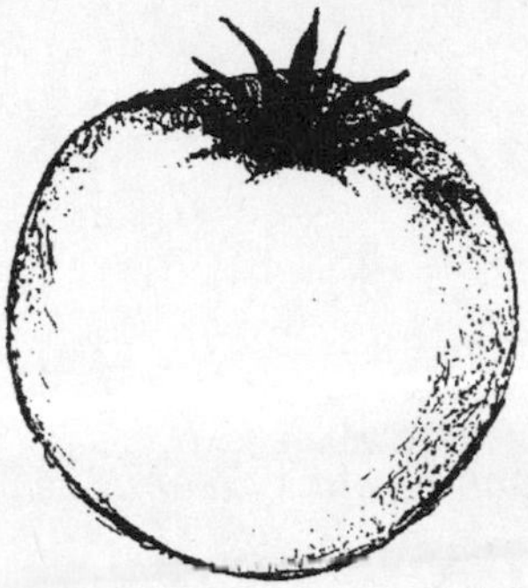

Americans are in love with the tomato. So soft and succulent, so plump and perky, its ruby red, velvet skin holds us in a trance until the spell is broken by a wave of juice that crashes against our taste buds firing one neurotransmitter after another until we rise up and sing—another tomato please!

Health Benefits

How can you even consider buying anything but a vine-ripened tomato! They contain four times the beta-carotene found in green tomatoes and offer more than 50% of the (RDA) recommended daily allowance of vitamin C. Hand on the Bible: Have you been drinking canned tomato juice? Cooked tomatoes have a high amount of oxalic acid, which acidifies the blood and draws minerals from teeth, bones, and tissue. Not so with our fresh and vine-ripened tomatoes. They are alkaline and actually contribute to the absorption of calcium and other minerals.

But nature is so wondrous in its mysteries. There, in the cooked tomato is an abundance of the carotenoid lycopene, which is absorbed more effectively from cooked and/or processed foods than from raw foods.[1] Lycopene is a powerful antioxidant. It concentrates in the cells of the heart and helps prevent heart attacks.[2] Lycopene is also in the pancreas, kidneys, spleen, adrenal glands, liver, testicles, and skin. It reduces our risk of cervical cancer,[3] and protects us against the onslaught of colon, stomach, esophageal, mouth, and pharynx cancers, and pancreatic cancer.[4] It also inhibits the proliferation of cancer cells involved in lung cancer and endometrial (uterine) cancer.[5] Tomatoes have made front page news as numerous studies demonstrate that lycopene reduces the risk of prostate cancer.[6]

Nutrients

These rosy globes are a superb source of the amino acid lysine, organic citric and malic acids, vitamin C (22mg/100g), provitamin A (623IU), potassium (222mg), in addition to the carotenoids lycopene (3.1mgs) and beta-carotene.

Ode to a Tomato

Plump, soft and mellow, the Queen of Red.
Castle? Nay, just a vine divine.
A scrumptious wonder whose bounty is every connoisseur's dream.
Covet her gently, but do not squeeze.
Feel her tenderness, but carefully caress.
Gaze at her design, perfection of shape sublime.
Armour of red crowned by leaves of green.
Stem of stature standing straight and strong.
All in perfect contrast to a richness of red resulting
from a daily diet of nourishing light.
Hot is the colour, but not the taste.
Ripeness is a term this Queen defined.
Uh Oh . . . careful not to tear, for therefrom gushes a
river of juice uncompared. Be prepared.
Like a weakness breached. A birth bursting of flavour and fluid.
Napkins are but a feeble barricade against its eminent stream.
There is no similitude, no peer, no plump contender nor one more slender.
God gave roses aroma, but this red's the best.
Just plant the seed, she'll do the rest.
In tastebud heaven we are ever blessed
Long live the Q u e e n.

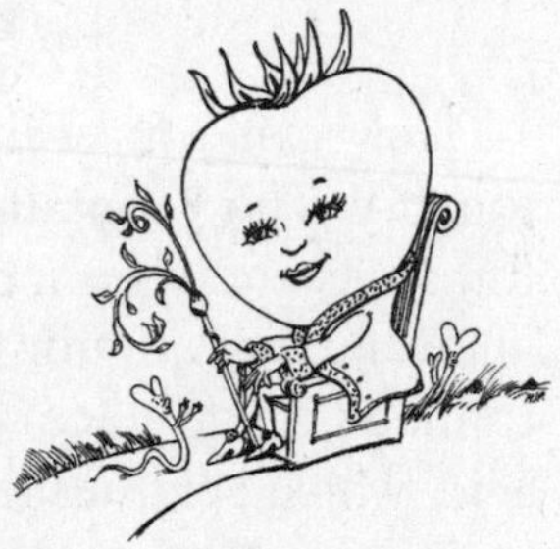

Tropical Fruits

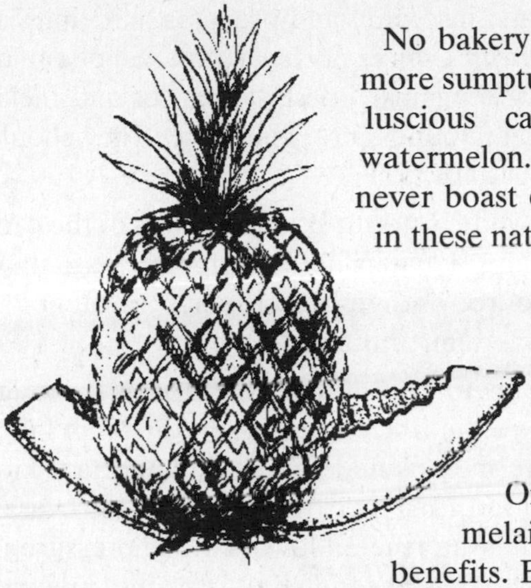

No bakery has ever turned out a treat more sumptuous than a ripe pineapple, a luscious cantaloupe, or a succulent watermelon. Even if they did, they could never boast of the health benefits found in these natural desserts.

Health Benefits

Pineapples are a veritable warehouse of valuable minerals and enzymes. One enzyme in particular, bromelain, is renown for its health benefits. Bromelain helps digestion by breaking down protein into more easily digestible amino acids. Since the mid-1950s, over 200 research documents have been published to promote bromelain's therapeutic effects. In addition to its digestive properties, it is also credited with reducing swelling due to arthritis, sports injuries, and trauma, promoting the healing of wounds, soothing sore throats, treating laryngitis, relieving sinusitis, curbing appetite, and promoting absorption of antibiotic medications.[1]

Pineapple helps prevent and treat cardiovascular diseases. Bromelain alleviates angina, helps prevent and treat atherosclerosis, and may inhibit the abnormal blood clotting that causes second heart attacks.[2] Another enzyme found in pineapple, peroxidase, increases the production of cytokines, an immune system component that stimulates cells to protect themselves against cancer.[3]

Juice only plump, golden, heavy, and sweet smelling pineapples. Tug on the leaves. If they come off easily, it is a sign of ripeness. Remove only the spiny leaves on top, wash the outer skin well, then cut and feed it into the juicer, skin and all.

Cantaloupes are another dynamo in the tropical fruit family, especially when you juice them whole. Much of its valuable nutrition is in the flesh and rind and juicing is the only way to get it. Cantaloupes contain a nucleoside called adenosine, which may prevent angina attacks and deters abnormal blood clotting. The lipid myoinositol in cantaloupes relieves anxiety and insomnia and prevents hardening of the arteries. Finally, the *American Cancer Society* recommends cantaloupes as a natural preventative against intestinal cancer and melanoma.[4] When shopping for cantaloupes, use your nose. They should smell sweet and be firm but not hard.

Honeydew melons are the white, smooth skinned sisters of the cantaloupe. Also known as casaba, Persian, and winter melons, their sweet, green flesh is a good source of digestive enzymes, carotenoids, vitamin C, pro-vitamin A, potassium, and zinc.

Watermelons are second only to cantaloupes in nutritional ratings and, along with cranberries, are the finest diuretics in the plant kingdom. The zinc content of watermelons make them an important kidney and bladder cleanser and, in fact, contributes to overall urogenital and prostate health. Watermelon lowers blood pressure in hypertension patients, eliminates toxins, and stimulates the appetite. When you juice the rind and seed, you release a veritable 'fountain of youth' of therapeutic plant compounds. It becomes a "free-radical scavenger that re-oxygenates cells, counteracts the peroxide dying cells emit, and acts effectively as an anti-aging agent."[5]

Papaya is a yellow and green orb of unrivaled tropical delight. Papayas contain the valuable digestive enzyme, papain, which equals bromelain in its digestive prowess. Papain is so effective that it is the main ingredient used in meat tenderizers. These proteolytic enzymes also facilitate the break down of excess fibrin in the blood, avoiding potential heart attacks. Papayas inhibit several types of bacteria, lower serum triglyceride levels, calm indigestion, and make a great cleanser for the kidneys, liver and intestines.[6]

Nutrients

These are all very important foods, and with a juicing machine you can claim their full value, including the nutritional benefits of the skin and pulp.

Aside from the important bromelain content, pineapples are also a wonderful source of potassium, chlorine, sodium, phosphorus, magnesium, sulfur, calcium, iron, and iodine. They are also rich in provitamin A, vitamin B-complex, and vitamin C.

Cantaloupes are high in vitamin C (25mg/100g), alpha and beta-carotene. potassium (320mg), and for a fruit, contain good amounts of the trace minerals copper, zinc, and iron. This beautiful orange-red gourd is considered by some to be one of the most nutritious fruits we have.

Watermelons rank right behind cantaloupes in nutrition. When you include the rind and seeds, you will get the famous antioxidants beta carotene (pro-vitamin A) and lycopene (4.1mg), and the cancer protective isothiocyanates; plus potassium (120mg), iron, zinc, and the B-vitamins family including folic acid (3mcg).

While papayas are most famous for their digestive enzymes, they are also sky high in beta-carotene (1,012mg/100g). Add to that potassium, calcium, and vitamin C and you have one of the most nutritious smoothie ingredients on earth. Green, unripe papayas yield the highest amount of papain. They can be juiced, blended, or dried for a snack.

So, push away that gooey pastry and reach for a taste of tropical splendor. Your taste buds will swoon and your body will thank you.

Cantaloupe Cooler

by Dr. Rudolph Ballentine, M.D.

¼	Cantaloupe, ripe
1 small	Banana, ripe
½ -1 cup	Soy Milk, Vanilla flavor

Cut one medium ripe banana and an equal amount of ripe cantaloupe into chunks. Add a good tasting soy milk and blend all together. Great as a summer cooler and a light meal in a glass. Kids love it.

Dr. Rudolph Ballentine directs the *Center for Holistic Medicine* in New York City where he practices transformative medicine using herbs, homeopathy, yoga, and meditation. He is the author of *Radical Healing.* www.radicalhealing.com

Watercress

(Nasturtium officinale)

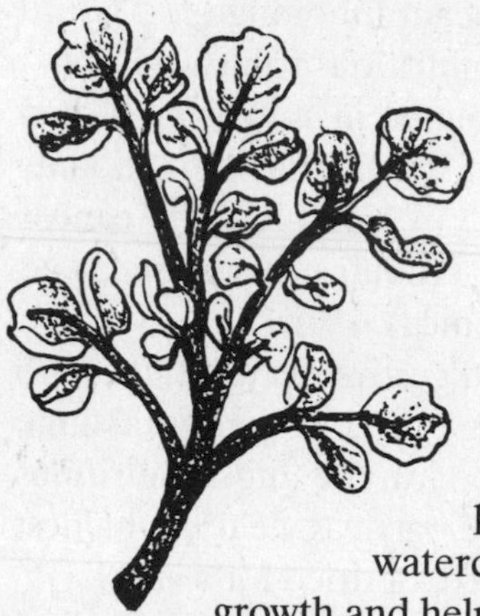

One taste of this peppery, pungent green and you'll wonder if it is as powerful in the body as it is to the taste. It is!

Health Benefits

Watercress combines the acid- forming minerals chlorine, phosphorus, and sulfur to build healthy intestinal walls and improve liver metabolism. The amino acids in watercress (2,900mgs/100g) promote healthy hair growth and help prevent its loss.

Its sulfur bearing glucosinolates and isothiocyanates arrest many common carcinogens including those linked to lung cancer.[1] Blood circulation and oxygenation are helped by its high chlorophyll content, and because it speeds the metabolism of fat into energy, it is excellent for dieters.

Nutrients

Watercress is also high in vitamin A, folic acid, biotin, nicotinic acid, pantothenic acid, vitamin B1, and lots of vitamin C (60mg/100g). In the mineral department, there are significant amounts of potassium (310mg), calcium (220mg), iron and only horseradish contains as much sulfur. Iodine plays an important role in thyroid function and in clearing mucus from our breathing passages. Watercress provides a readily available source of iodine, and this valuable mineral is released most effectively in watercress juice.

Put an ounce of watercress juice in your next drink and taste the kick of its chlorophyll.

Wheatgrass & Barley Grass

(Triticum & Hordeum)

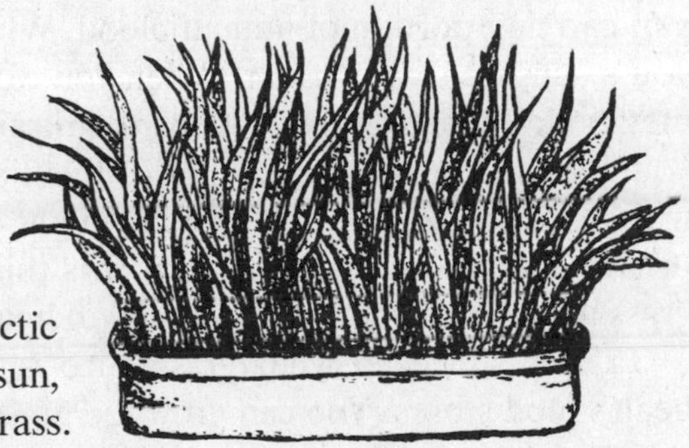

Grass is the world's most ubiquitous vegetation. There are over 9,000 species of grasses. From the outback "down-under" to the one-inch arctic tundra, wherever there is sun, water, and soil, there is grass. All grasses begin as grains such as wheat, barley, oat, rye, and rice. Four of the world's top five crops are grasses. For centuries, farmers have noticed how livestock health improves when they feed on the young grasses of early spring.

In the 1970s, Dr. Ann Wigmore popularized the use of indoor-grown, freshly squeezed grass juice to treat cancer patients who had been pronounced "incurable" after conventional medical treatment. Wigmore had saved her own gangrenous legs from amputation by using her grass treatments and eventually ran in the Boston marathon. Today, wheatgrass juice is available both as a dry powder and as freshly squeezed juice in juice bars and health food stores everywhere.

Health Benefits

As a source of nourishment, grass is a complete food containing all known nutritional elements. People with wheat allergies, by the way, have nothing to fear from this wheat food. Although the grass is grown from grain, it metamorphoses completely into a vegetable with none of the allergic proteins common to glutenous grains. Grass is non-toxic in any dose, but you may react to the results of its detoxifying power. Grass is a powerful purgative for the liver, and too much can release too many poisons too quickly.

Wheatgrass also cleanses and heals the large intestine, another collection point of toxins in the body. But it is, perhaps most famous as a blood purifier. Grass is one of the planet's best sources of high quality chlorophyll. Ultimately, all food on the planet, whether animal or vegetable, comes directly or indirectly from chlorophyll. Even more amazing is that this "blood of plants" is a chemical cousin to hemin. Hemin is a component of hemoglobin, the red, iron-rich, oxygen-carrying portion of human blood. Wheatgrass juice literally gives you a sunshine transfusion. When you drink it, this enzyme-rich and metabolically-active, fresh, living food transfers its high vibration into your system. A one-ounce shot of this liquid chlorophyll leaves you with a "buzz." Eastern philosophy might say it raises your kundalini, or chi, giving you a natural high. It is this energetic lift that enables grass to enhance your body's ability to heal.

Freshly squeezed wheatgrass juice is available at juice bars and health food stores. You can grow the grass at home and juice it yourself, but only certain machines will extract the liquid from its woody pulp *(see "Juicers, Blenders, and Water Purifiers")*. If you don't want to grow it yourself, you can purchase professionally grown grass, which makes it a lot easier. And if you do not want to buy a juicer, you're in luck, since you can buy it frozen, freeze dried, or powdered in most health food stores.

Barley and wheat belong to the same family. As grain or grass, they are difficult to distinguish, and nutritionally they are also similar in many ways. Asians consume more barley than wheat. The Japanese medical doctor and researcher Yoshihide Hagiwara pioneered the use of barley grass and invested much of his profits in scientific research. Universities in Japan and the U.S. have researched the leaf extract from barley grass and discovered a broad range of chemicals that support the immune system, including anti-oxidants, cellular growth factors, anti-inflammatory and anti-ulcer agents, and DNA repair factors. In one 1998 study, barley grass leaf extract dramatically restricted the growth of human prostate and breast cancer cells grown in tissue culture.[1]

Nutrition

Fresh wheatgrass juice is 95% water and 2% protein. Dried wheat or barley grass juice (about 7% water) ranges from 25-45% protein. Grass has 11 times the calcium of cow's milk, 5 times the iron of spinach, 4 times the vitamin B1 of whole wheat flour, 7 times the vitamin C in oranges, as well as an abundance of the elusive vegetarian vitamin B12 (80mcg/100g).[2] Researchers also found unidentified growth factors that enabled animals to survive on a 100% grass diet, while they failed on a diet of carrots, broccoli, cabbage and spinach.[3]

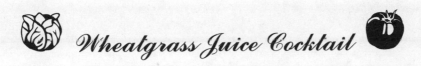

Wheatgrass Juice Cocktail

by Dr. Leonard Smith, M.D.

12 oz	Carrots
1-2 oz	Wheatgrass
1-2 oz	Kale
1 clove	Garlic

This juice helps people achieve optimum health because of its antioxidant and detoxification properties. Fresh wheatgrass juice cleanses the colon, enriches the blood and purges the liver. I have personally experienced the ability of wheatgrass juice to raise blood platelet levels in anemic patients.

Dr. Leonard Smith is a general and gastrointestinal surgeon with 25 years experience in both traditional and alternative medicine. He practices in Gainsville, Florida.

Nutrient Sources

Values are stated in milligrams (mg) per 100 grams except where indicated. Generally, only the top 12 foods are listed per nutrient. In some cases, deference is given to those foods that can be used for juices, blended drinks, and teas. This information has been compiled primarily from data published by the USDA (Department of Agriculture) and, in the cases of specialty foods, form certified nutritional analyses provided by manufacturers.

Acetylcholine

Lecithin 3430, Liver 2170, Beef 600, Wheat Germ, Brewer's Yeast.

Alanine

An Amino Acid. Vegetables: Alfalfa, Carrot, Celery, Dandelion, Lettuce, Cucumber, Turnip, Green Pepper, Spinach, Watercress. Fruits: Apple, Apricot, Avocado, Grapes, Olive, Orange, Strawberry. Nuts: Almond.

Alpha-Linolenic Acid

% of Alpha-Linolenic Acid (LNA) Flaxseed Oil 55, Chia Oil 30, Candlenut Oil 29, Hemp Seed Oil 19, Blackcurrant Seed Oil 16, Canola Oil 10, Soybean Oil 7, Pumpkin Seed Oil 7, Wheat Germ Oil 5.

Arginine

An Amino Acid. Vegetables: Alfalfa, Green Vegetables, Carrot, Beet, Cucumber, Celery, Lettuce, Radish, Parsnip.

Aspartic Acid

An Amino Acid. Vegetables: Carrot, Celery, Cucumber, Parsley, Radish, Spinach, Tomato, Turnip Greens, Watercress. Fruits: Bee Pollen , Lemon, Grapefruit, Apple, Apricot, Pineapple, Watermelon. Nuts: Almond.

Bioflavonoids

Citrus Fruits, Rose Hips, Black Currants, Prunes, Parsley, Apricots, Plums, Cherries, Walnuts.

Bromine

A Trace Mineral. Watermelon 26.20, Celery 17.60, Cantaloupe 9.45, Turnip Greens 4.25, Cucumber 4.00, Asparagus 2.02, Tomato 2.00, Lettuce 1.90, Mushroom 1.90, Carrot 1.40.

Calories—Energy

In calories per 100 grams. Seed and vegetable oils average 800-900, Pecan 687, Coconut, dried 662, Almond 598, Pistachio Nut 594, Sesame Seed, whole 582, Peanut with Skin 564, Cashew Nut 561, Sunflower Seed 560, Pumpkin & Squash Seed 553, Soybean, dried 403, Wheat Germ 363.

Carbohydrates

Banana, dried 88.6, White Rice 80.4, Raisin 77.4, Brown Rice 77.4, Wheat 75.4, Date 72.9, Prune, dried 67.4, Fig, dried 69.1, Lima Beans 64, Bran 61.9.

Citric Acid

Lemon Juice 6.08, Lime Juice 2.02, Blueberry 1.56, Cranberry 1.46, Grapefruit 1.40, Red Raspberry 1.30, Strawberry 1.00, Orange .95, Pineapple .80.

Calcium

Sesame Seed 1160, Kelp 1093, Spirulina 700, Brewer's Yeast 424,Wheat Grass 321, Collard Leaves 250, Kale Leaves 249, Turnip Greens 246, Almond 234, Soybean, dried, 226, Flaxseeds 210, Parsley 203, Alfalfa Sprouts 200, Bee Pollen 158, Orange Peel 161.

Chromium

In mcg per 100 grams. Egg Yolks 183, Molasses 121, Brewer's Yeast 112, Beef 57, Wheat Bran 38, Honey 29, Potato 24, Wheat Germ 23, Capsicum 19, Apple 14, Parsnip 13, Butter 13, Banana 10.

Coenzyme Q10

Sardines 6.4, Peanuts 2.7, Sesame Seeds 2.3, Pistachio 2.0, Walnuts 1.9, Spinach 1.0, Broccoli .86.

Copper

Oysters 14, Brewer's Yeast 3.3, Brazil Nuts 2.1, Sunflower Seeds 1.8, Olives 1.6, Almonds 1.4, Walnuts 1.4, Wheat Bran 1.34, Pecan Nuts 1.2, Spirulina 1.2, Beef Liver 1.1, Wheat Germ .9, Chocolate 0.7, Tomato puree .53, Parsley .52, Apples 0.5.

Cystine

An Amino Acid. Vegetables: Alfalfa, Carrot, Beet, Cabbage, Cauliflower, Onion, Garlic, Kale, Horseradish, Brussels Sprouts. Fruits: Apple, Currants, Pineapple, Raspberry. Nuts: Brazil-Nut, Hazelnut, Filbert.

Fats

Seed & Vegetable Oils 100, Macadamia Nut 71.6, Pecan 71.2, Coconut, dried 64.9, Almond 54.2, Pistachio Nut 53.7, Sesame Seed, hulled 53.4, Sesame Seed, whole 49.1, Peanut with skin 47.5, Sunflower Seed 47.3, Pumpkin & Squash Seed 46.7, Cashew Nut 45.7, Olive, ripe mission 20.1.

Fatty Acids

Total fatty acids, essential and non-essential. Coconut Meat, dry 56, Coconut Milk 22, Peanut Oil 18, Sesame Oil 14, Olive Oil 11, Peanut 10, Pumpkin & Squash Seed 8, Cashew Nut 8, Sunflower Seed 6, Pecan 5.

Folic Acid

In mcg per 100 grams. Brewer's Yeast 2,022, Wheat Germ 305, Beef Liver 295, Soybeans 225, Wheat Grass, Spirulina, Wheat Bran 195, Kidney Beans 180, Mung Beans 145, Lima Beans 130, Navy Beans 125, Chick Peas 110, Lentils 105, Walnuts 77, Spinach 75, Kale 70, Pumpkin Seeds 57.5, Peanuts 56, Almonds 45.

Glutamic Acid

Vegetables: String Beans, Brussels Sprouts, Carrot, Cabbage, Celery, Beet Greens, Dandelion, Parsley, Lettuce, Spinach. Fruits: Papaya, Bee Pollen.

Glycine

An Amino Acid. Vegetables: Carrot, Dandelion, Turnip, Celery, Parsley, Spinach, Alfalfa, Okra, Garlic, Spirulina 3200, Potato. Fruits: Fig, Orange, Huckleberry, Raspberry, Pomegranate, Watermelon. Nuts: Almond.

Histidine

An Amino Acid. Vegetables: Horseradish, Radish, Carrot, Beet, Celery, Cucumber, Endive, Leek, Garlic, Onion, Dandelion, Turnip Greens, Alfalfa, Spinach, Sorrel. Fruits: Apple, Pineapple, Pomegranate, Papaya.

Iodine

In micrograms per 100 grams. Kelp 1500, Swiss Chard 9.9, Turnip Greens 7.6, Summer Squash 6.2, Watermelon 4.0, Cucumber 3.7, Spinach 3.6, Asparagus 3.0, Kale 2.6, Turnip 2.5.

Iron

Kelp 100.0, Wheat Grass 24.9,Rice Bran 19.4, Brewer's Yeast 17.3, Pumpkin Seeds 14.9, Wheat Bran 14.9, Bee Pollen 14, Alfalfa Sprouts 12, Pumpkin & Squash Seed 11.2, Sesame Seed, whole, 10.5, Wheat Germ 9.9, Soybean, dried, 8.4, Hot Red Pepper 7.8, Flaxseeds 7.7, Pistachio Nut 7.3, Sunflower Seed 7.1, Lentil, dried, 6.8.

Isoleucine

An Amino Acid. Fruits: Papaya, Avocado, Olive. Nuts: Coconut; all nuts except: Peanut, Cashew, Chestnut, Sunflower Seed. Spirulina 3500.

Leucine

An Amino Acid. Fruits: Papaya, Avocado, Olive. Nuts: Coconut; all nuts except: Peanut, Cashew, Chestnut, Sunflower Seed. Spirulina 5400.

Linoleic Acid

Percent of linoleic acid. Safflower Oil 75%, Evening Primrose Oil 72%, Grape Seed Oil 71%, Sunflower Oil 65%, Corn Oil 59%, Hemp Seed Oil 55%, Soybean Oil 50%, Sesame Oil 45%, Borage Seed Oil 37.5%, Rice Bran 35%, Peanut Oil 29%, Canola Oil 25%, Flaxseed Oil 14%

Lysine

An Amino Acid. Vegetables: Carrot, Beet, Cucumber, Celery, Parsley, Spinach, Dandelion, Turnip Greens, Alfalfa, Soybean Sprouts, Spirulina 2900. Fruits: Papaya, Apple, Apricot, Pear, Grapes, Bee Pollen.

Magnesium

Kelp 760, Pumpkin Seeds 535, Wheat Bran 490, Alfalfa Sprouts 410, Spirulina 400, Flaxseeds 380, Almond 270, Wheat Germ 270, Cashew Nut 267, Soybean, dried, 265, Brewer's Yeast 231, Peanut 206, Sesame Seed, whole 181, Lima Bean, dried, 180, Pea 180, Millet 162.

Malic Acid

Plum 2.48, Rhubarb 1.77, Prune .44, Sweet cherry .93, Grapes .65, Apple .71, Cauliflower .39, Banana .37.

Manganese

Tea 120, Spirulina 5, Hops 4, Pecans 3.5, Pumpkin Seeds 3.0, Brazil Nuts 2.8, Wheat Grass 2.5, Bee Pollen 1.8, Barley 1.8, Buckwheat 1.3, Split Peas 1.3, Spinach 0.8, Broccoli 0.15, Swiss Cheese 0.13, Peaches 0.10.

Methionine

An Amino Acid. Vegetables: Brussels Spouts, Cabbage, Cauliflower, Dock, Kale, Horseradish, Chive, Garlic, Watercress. Fruits: Pineapple, Apple. Nuts: Brazil Nut, Filbert.

Niacin Vitamin B-3

Brewer's Yeast 37, Rice Bran 29.8, Wheat Bran 21.0, Peanut with skin 17.2, Spirulina 14, Hot Red Pepper, dry, 10.8, Wheat Grass 8.3, Wild Rice 6.2, Kelp 5.7, Sesame Seed 5.4, Sunflower Seed 5.4, Peach 5.3, Brown rice 4.7, Bee Pollen 4.38, Wheat Germ 4.2, Almond 3.5, Apricot, dried 3.3.

Nucleic acids

Bee Pollen, Brewer's Yeast, Spirulina, Chlorella, Blue-Green Algae, Fish.

Oxalic Acid

Spinach 89.2, Swiss Chard 64.5, Rhubarb 50, Cocoa 25, Beetroot 25, Parsley 25.

Phosphorus

Brewer's Yeast 1753, Wheat Bran 1276, Pumpkin Seeds 1174, Wheat Germ 1118, Sunflower Seed 837, Spirulina 800, Flaxseeds 700, Sesame Seed, whole, 616, Wheat Grass 575, Soybean, dried, 554, Almond 504, Pistachio Nut 500, Pinto Bean, dried, 457, Peanut, no skin, 409.

Potassium

Wheat Grass 3225, Dulse 8060,Kelp 5273, Brewer's Yeast 1700, Soybean, dried, 1677, Lima Bean, dried, 1529, Rice Bran 1495, Banana, dried, 1477, Spirulina 1400, Hot Red Pepper, dry, 1201, Wheat Bran 1121, Pea, dried, 1005, Pinto Bean, dried, 984, Wheat Germ 950, Alfalfa Sprouts 890.

Protein

In percent of total content. Spirulina 61, Blue-Green Algae 61, Chlorella 57, Brewer's Yeast 35, Barley Grass 35, Soybean, dried 34.1, Wheat Germ 26.6, Peanut with skin 26.0, Wheat Grass dried 25, Lentil, dried 24.7, Pumpkin Seeds 24.5, Sunflower Seed 24.0, Almond 18.6.

Phenylalanine

An Amino Acid. Vegetables: Carrot, Beet, Spinach, Parsley, Tomato. Fruits: Pineapple, Apple.

Proline

Vegetables: Carrot, Beet, Lettuce, Dandelion, Turnip, Cucumber. Fruits: Apricot, Cherry, Avocado, Fig, Raisin, Grapes, Olive, Orange, Pineapple. Nuts: Coconut, Almond, Brazil Nut.

Quercetin

Wine, Grapes, Apples, Grapefruit, Hawthorn Berries, Passion Flower, Black Tea Broccoli, Onions, Squash, Kale, Fennel.

Serine

Vegetables: Horseradish, Radish, Leek, Garlic, Onion, Carrot, Beet, Celery, Cucumber, Parsley, Spinach, Cabbage, Alfalfa. Fruits: Papaya, Apple, Pineapple.

Selenium

Brazil Nuts, Peanuts, Wheat Germ, Brewer's Yeast, Pumpkin Seeds 5.6, Wheat Bran, Spirulina, Bilberry, Echinacea, Stevia, Celery, Garlic, Onions, Radish.

Silicon

Lettuce: Boston, Bibb 2400, Lettuce: Iceberg 1464, Parsnip 960, Asparagus 950, Rice Bran 885, Horseradish, raw, 818, Onion 810, Spinach 810, Cucumber 800, Strawberry 783.

Sodium

Kelp 3007, Olive, green pickled, 2400, Olive, ripe Sevillano 828, Hot Red Pepper, dry, 373, Swiss Chard 147, Celery, 126, Horseradish 96, Kale, 75, Spinach 71, Beet 60.

Sulfur

Kale 8600, Watercress 5390, Brussels Sprouts 3530, Horseradish 1984, Cabbage 1710, Cranberry 1420, Turnip 1210, Cauliflower 1186, Raspberry 1150, Spinach 1130.

Threonine

Vegetables: Carrot, Alfalfa, Green leafy vegetables. Fruits: Papaya.

Thyroxine

Vegetables: Dulse, Kelp, Sea Lettuce, Carrot, Celery, Lettuce, Spinach, Turnip, Tomato. Fruits: Pineapple.

Tryptophane

Vegetables: Carrot, Beet, Celery, Endive, Dandelion, Fennel, Snap Bean, Brussels Sprouts, Chive, Spinach, Alfalfa, Turnip.

Tyrosine

Vegetables: Alfalfa, Carrot, Beet, Cu-cumber, Lettuce, Dandelion, Parsnip, Asparagus, Leek, Parsley, Green Pepper, Spinach, Watercress. Fruits: Ba-nana, Strawberry, Apricot, Cherry, Fig Apple, Watermelon, Almond Yoghurt.

Valine

Vegetables: Bee Pollen, Carrot, Turnip, Dandelion, Lettuce, Parsnip, Squash, Celery, Beet, Parsley, Okra, Tomato. Fruits: Apple, Pomegranate. Nuts: Almond.

Vitamin A

In international units IU per 100 grams. Spirulina 230,000, Hot Red Pepper, dry, 77000, Carrot 11000, Apricot, dried, 10000, Kale 10000, Collard Greens 9300, Sweet Potato 8800, Parsley 8500, Spinach 8100, Turnip 7600, Swiss Chard 6500, Chive 5800, Parsley 5200, Mango 4800.

Vitamin B-1 Thiamine

Brewer's Yeast 15.6, Spirulina 3.5, Rice Bran 2.26, Wheat Germ 2.01, Sunflower Seed 1.96, Peanut with skin 1.14, Soybean, dried, 1.10, Sesame Seed, whole, .98, Pecan .86, Pinto Bean, dried .84, Pea, dried, .74, Pistachio Nut .67.

Vitamin B-2 Riboflavin

Wheat Grass 16.9, Brewer's Yeast 4.3, Spirulina 4, Hot Red Pepper, dry, 1.33, Almond .92, Wheat Germ .68, Wild Rice .63, Bee Pollen .62, Mushroom .46, Turnip Greens .39, Chestnut, dried, .38, Kelp .33, Collards .31, Pea, dried, .29, Parsley, .26.

Vitamin B-3 *see Niacin*

Vitamin B-5 Pantothenic Acid

Brewer's Yeast 12, Chicken Liver 6, Pork Liver 4.6, Peanuts 2.8, Wheat Bran 2.4, Wheat Germ 2.0, Soybeans 1.7, Pecans 1.7, Sunflower Seeds 1.4, Royal Jelly.

Vitamin B-12

In micrograms per 100 grams. Spirulina 218, Chlorella, Blue-Green Algae, Brewer's Yeast, Wheat Grass 80, Beef Liver 80, Kelp, Chicken Liver 25.

Vitamin C – Ascorbic Acid

Acerola Juice 1600, Hot Red Pepper, raw 369, Wheat Grass 215, Black Currants 200, Kale 186, Parsley 172, Collard Leaves 152, Orange Peel 136, Parsley 133, Broccoli 113, Lemon w/Peel 77, Orange w/Peel 71, Strawberry 59, Papaya 56.

Vitamin D

In international units IU per 100 grams. Halibut Liver Oil 27600, Spirulina 12000, Cod Liver Oil 8400, Bee Pollen 1735, Sunflower Seeds 92.

Vitamin E

Wheat Germ Oil 200, Soybean Oil 87, Sunflower Oil 55, Safflower Oil 34, Corn Oil 31, Peanut Oil 22, Cod Liver Oil 20, Peanuts 12, Shrimp 6.6, Nuts & Seeds.

Zinc

Oysters 150, Brewer's Yeast 7.8, Pumpkin Seeds 7.5, Ginger 6.8, Flaxseeds 5.7, Sunflower Seeds 5.1, Wheat Grass 4.9, Brazil Nuts 4.4, Bee Pollen 3.5, Egg Yolks 3.5, Peanuts 3.3, Oats 3.2, Almonds 3.1, Spirulina 3, Buckwheat 2.5, Turnip 1.1.

Food Glossary

This chapter is intended to help you identify some of the foods and terms used in this book. For more information, refer to the individual chapters on foods & herbs.

Acetylcholine

Acetylcholine is a type of neurotransmitter that is the most abundant neurotransmitter in the brain.

Adaptogen

An adaptogen herb has a changeable normalizing effect rather than a specific fixed effect. Thus a person with high blood pressure may be helped by the same herb as a person with low blood pressure.

Adenosine Triphosphate (ATP)

Manufactured by neurons within the brain, ATP provides the brain's energy. Its effects have been linked to increased alertness, creativity and verbal fluency. Supplement dosage is usually 30-90mg/day.

Algae

A group of aquatic plants that contain chlorophyll. Some examples of macro-algaes are kelp, dulse, nori, and hijiki. Micro-algaes are spirulina, chlorella, and blue-green algae. The micro-algaes are not classified as plants, but as microorganisms since they have more in common with bacteria than plants. They are earth's richest sources of protein, vitamin B12, and chlorophyll.

Amino Acids

The building blocks of proteins and peptides. There are more than 100 in nature, but only 22 occur in animals. In humans, eight are defined as essential because the body cannot manufacture them. The eight amino acids that must be provided by the diet are: isoleucine, leucine, lysine, methionine, phenylalanine, threonine, tryptophan, and valine. Some non-essential amino acids, those the body can manufacture, are: alanine, aspartic acid, cystine, glutamic acid, glycine, histidine, proline, serine, tyrosine.

Antioxidants

Friendly foods and chemicals that have the ability to stop free radicals from oxidizing healthy cells. They help delay aging. Beta-carotene is a famous antioxidant. *(See Longevity chapter.)*

Barley Malt *(See Malt)*

Beta-Carotene

Beta carotene is the plant version of vitamin A. Also called provitamin A, it is probably the most famous antioxidant. See vitamin A for sources.

Brewer's Yeast

Brewer's yeast is a type of dietary yeast produced as a by-product of making beer. It is one of our finest sources of B-vitamins and nucleic acids. *(See Brewer's Yeast.)*

Broccoli

A rich source of isothiocyanates. The most effective means of obtaining the health benefits of broccoli is to make broccoli sprouts. Or, juice the vegetable or the fresh sprouts. *(See Broccoli.)*

Chelation

Chelation therapy is a procedure that uses a series of gentle intravenous infusions of the man-made amino acid Ethylene-Diamine-Tetra-Acetate (EDTA) to extract toxic and heavy metals like lead and aluminum and discharge them from the body.

Coenzyme Q10

A type of fat soluble enzyme that is similar to vitamin E with powerful antioxidant properties.

DHA and EPA

Fish oil and algae are our best sources of these special omega-3 oils that keep blood triglycerides low (high triglycerides cause heart disease) and are valuable to normal brain and nervous system function. These oils are non-essential–they can be synthesized in our bodies and those of other animals. Cod liver oil contains large amounts of EPA and DHA. Algae is the best vegetarian source and flaxseed converts some of its abundant ALA into EPA. *(See Power Drinks for the Mind)*

DHEA

Dehydroepiandrosterone (DHEA) is an androgen steroid hormone manufactured primarily in the adrenal glands of both men and women. It is the most abundant steroid hormone in the bloodstream. *(See Power Drinks for Longevity)*

Essential Fatty Acids

These fats are essential to human life but cannot be manufactured by the body. They must be provided by the diet. They are essential for the formation of prostaglandins, hormone regulation, and for breaking up cholesterol deposits. Deficiency symptoms include brittle and dull hair, nail problems, dandruff, allergies, eczema and other skin problems. They are linoleic (omega 6), alpha-linolenic (omega 3), and arachidonic (omega 3) acids. Linoleic acid is found in common vegetable oils but the best sources are evening primrose, soybeans, grapeseed oil, safflower, hemp and maize. The best sources for alpha-linolenic acid are flaxseeds, chia, and hemp oils. Health professionals recommend consuming omega-3 and 6 in a 3:1 ratio.

Folic Acid

Also known as folate or folacin, it is a water-soluble member of the B-vitamin family that contains PABA (Para-Aminobenzoic Acid) and glutamic acid.

Free Radicals

Very aggressive chemicals with an extra oxygen molecule that is one of the causes of aging. Like a pinball machine, they bang into healthy cells and 'oxidize' them. An example of oxidation is metal rusting. So, the more free radicals we consume, the faster we are going to rust. *(See Power Drinks for Longevity)*

Flaxseeds and Flax Oil

Flax, also known as linseed, is our best source of alpha-linolenic acid, also known as vitamin F. This wonderful plant not only gives us this special oil, but also linen. The seed meal provides a mucilage that is a very effective intestinal tract cleanser. *(See Flaxseeds)*

Glutathione

Glutathione is a sulfur-containing, water-soluble protein made up of three amino acids. It is a particularly effective detoxifying agent and provides immune system support especially for AIDS and cancer. It is found in spinach and tomatoes.

Honey

Use raw, unpasteurized buckwheat or clover honey. Heating honey alters its crystalline structure. Honey does not need to be heated or pasteurized for the purpose of extending shelf life. Raw, unfiltered honey is naturally resistant to souring and molding and, in fact, extends the shelf life of the foods to which it is added. *(See Bee Pollen)*

Hormones

Substances produced by plants and animals that regulate metabolism, growth and development. They are frequently peptides or steroids.

Lecithin

A phosphorus-rich fat common in plants and animals. In people, lecithin is found in the liver, nerve tissue, semen, bile, and blood. It is essential for breaking down fats in the body. The best dietary sources are soybeans, egg yolks, and corn. Deficiency leads to liver and kidney disorders, high serum cholesterol levels, and atherosclerosis. It is available as soy lecithin granules. *(See Power Drinks for the Mind)*

Malt (Barley Malt)

Malt is the short name for the sugar found in grains. This sugar, maltose, is commonly derived from barley (barley malt) as a by-product of the brewing industry. Barley malt is boiled until it achieves a dark viscous state. Although similar in consistency to honey, grain malt is darker in color and stronger in flavor.

Miso Paste

Miso is a fermented soybean paste that has been used for centuries in Asian cuisine. The mashed soybeans are aged and cured much like cheese. It is used primarily as a seasoning and in the preparation of sauces. If it is not pasteurized, it contains live "friendly" bacteria cultures. Miso comes in a variety of flavors and colors, much like cheese. Hatcho miso is the strongest and darkest. Blonde miso is light in color, mellow in flavor and low in salt.

Neuropeptides

Peptides are groups of two or more linked amino acids. Neuropeptides behave like hormones and neurotransmitters in that they regulate various brain and nervous system functions, but they effect only local areas. *(See Power Drinks for the Mind)*

Neurons

Neurons are nerve cells. They are the impulse-conducting cells that make up nerves, the brain and spinal column.

Neuropathy

Neuropathy is any ailment of the peripheral nervous system, usually causing numbness. Neuritis refers specifically to an inflammation of a nerve.

Neurotransmitters

Inside neurons are neurotransmitters. They transmit impulses that are received by the receptors of other neurons. This is how the brain, spinal cord and nervous system communicate. Like the electrical wiring in your house, when you press the switch the lights go on. You don't think about the wires or the current flowing from switch to lamp. There are approximately forty different neurotransmitters. Serotonin is a popular neurotransmitter. When you picked up this book, your brain sent a signal to your hands via neurotransmitters.

Nitrosamines

Nitrosamines are extremely toxic carcinogens that can cause cancer in any part of the body. Technically, they are organic oxides of nitrogen that form in the body when nitrites or nitrates in our diet react with our body's supply of amino acids (proteins). Avoid nitrite and nitrate foods such as bacon, salami, frankfurters, hams and other processed meats.

Nucleic Acids

Nucleic acids are also responsible for the production of ATP (Adenosine Triphosphate) which is manufactured by neurons within the brain. ATP increases alertness, provides energy, and has been linked to creativity and verbal fluency. Bee pollen, brewer's yeast, spirulina, chlorella, blue-green algae, and fish are our best food sources.

Omega Fatty Acids

Group classification of the different fatty acids. The three groups are omega 3, 6 and 9. Omega-3's are alpha-linolenic acid, EPA and DHA. Oily fish such as sardines are excellent food sources. Flaxseed oil is the best vegetarian source. Omega-6's are linoleic acid from vegetable oils, gamma-linolenic acid from evening primrose oil, and arachidonic acid from animal foods. Health professionals recommend consuming omega-3 and 6 in a 3:1 ratio.

Peptide

A compound of two or more amino acids linked together.

Phytochemicals

Plant chemicals or compounds that are different from vitamins, minerals, proteins, and fats. There are hundreds of phytochemicals. Some famous phytochemicals are bioflavonoids, beta-carotene, chlorophyll, lycopene, saponins, superoxide dismutase (SOD), pycnogenol, allicin, proanthocyanidins, isothiocyanates, indoles, and isoflavonoids.

Prostaglandins

Hormone-like substances created from essential fatty acids. Unlike most hormones, they are produced in many parts of the body rather than from one organ. Prostaglandins regulate neurotransmitters, help organ muscles contract, control stomach acid, lower blood pressure, and moderate body temperature.

Quercetin

A type of bioflavonoid found in wine, grapes, apples, and grapefruits. Supplementation with quercetin for therapeutic purposes, such as allergies, is usually 1-3 grams per day.

SAMe

SAMe (S-Adenosyl-Methionine) is a natural metabolite of the amino acid methionine. *(See Power Drinks for Longevity)*

Sebaceous Glands

Simple, branched glands that reside in the dermis of the skin and open into the hair follicles of the scalp/skin. There are approximately 100 sebaceous glands per square inch of skin. These glands secrete sebum (type of endogenous oil) onto the surface of the skin through small ducts that lead to the hair follicles.

Serotonin

Serotonin is the neurotransmitter that drugs like Prozac elevate. *(See "neurotransmitters")*

Steroid

A fat-soluble organic hormone-like compound.

Stevia

A non-sugar, non-glucose alternative sweetener. It has no relation to sugar cane or beet sugar. Instead it is a South American herb grown high in the Andes mountains of Brazil. It is 300 times sweeter than sugar and actually helps to lower blood sugar. The herb is green and flavorful. When processed into a white powder, it has a mostly neutral flavor.

Tamari

This is a quality soy sauce made from aged soybeans. Soy sauce is usually made with wheat but tamari is often wheat-free. There are several brands of tamari available at health food stores.

Thermogenesis

Thermogenesis is the term used to describe the burning of calories, usually from fatty tissue. During thermogenesis, the body temperature increases and energy is transferred to the muscles. An increase in thermogenesis means an increase in your metabolic rate.

Triglycerides

Triglycerides are the form in which fatty acids are stored in fat tissue (adipose tissue). Triglycerides provide fuel to all organs of the body except the brain.

Ume or Umeboshi

A sour, pickled plum popular in Japanese cuisine that is good for stomach integrity and digestion. Ume is the Japanese word for plum.

Wheat Germ

Wheat germ is the germination or vitality center of the wheat grain. If the germ is damaged, the grain will not grow. It is an excellent source of Bvitamins, minerals, and essential fatty acids. It comes as granules and is a popular cereal or snack. Wheat germ oil, extracted from the germ, is one of our finest 'health' oils. Wheat germ is highly perishable and should be purchased in vacuum or nitrogen packed jars.

Xylitol

Xylitol is a natural sugar found in raspberries and strawberries. Unlike most carbohydrates, it does not increase blood sugar levels.

Scientific Research Notes

Juices & Drinks vs. Food

1. Krebs-Smith, S.M., Cook, A., Subar, A.F., et al. US Adults' Fruit and Vegetable Intakes, 1989 -1991. A revised baseline for the Healthy People 2000 Objective. *AM J Public Health* 85:1623-1629. 1995.

2. *Journal of Nutrition.* Pgs. 1442-1449, Sept. 28, 1999.

Power Drinks—Medicine Chest

Acne

1. Kugen, A., et al. Oral vitamin A in acne vulgaris. *Arch Dermatol.* 118:891-894, 1982.

2. Dreno, B., et al. Low doses of zinc gluconate for inflammatory acne. *Acta Derm Venereol.* 69:541-543, 1989.

Anemia

1. J.H. Hughes and A.L. Latner. Chlorophyll and Hemoglobin Regeneration After Hemmorrhage. *Journal of Physiology.* Vol.86, #388, 1936 University of Liverpool.

2. Labonia, W. D. L-Carnitine Effects on Anemia and Hemodialyzed Patients Treated with Erythropoietin. *American Journal of Kidney Diseases.* 26(5):757-764, 1995.

3. Yuan, Y., et al. Studies of Rehmannia glutinosa Libosch. f. hueichingensis as a blood tonic. *Chung Kuo Chung Yao Tsa Chih.* 17(6):366-368, 1992.

4. Leonard, P. J., et al. Effect of alpha-tocopherol administration on red cell survival in vitamin E-deficient human subjects. *American Journal of Clinical Nutrition.* 24:388-393, 1971.

Arthritis

1. Zeller, M. Rheumatoid arthritis—food allergy as a factor. *Ann Allerg* 1949;7:200-205, 239.

2. Pujalte, J. M., et al. Double-blind clinical evaluation of oral glucosamine sulphate in the basic treatment of osteoarthritis. *Curr Med Res Opin.* 7:104-109, 1980.

Asthma

1. Hodge, L. Consumption of oily fish and childhood asthma risk. *Medical Journal of Australia.* 164:137-140, 1996.

2. Gong, H., Jr., et al. Bronchodilator effects of caffeine in coffee. A dose-response study of asthmatic subjects. *Chest.* 89(3):335-342, 1986.

3. Okayama, H., et al. Bronchodilating effect of intravenous magnesium sulfate in bronchial asthma. *Journal of the American Medical Association.* 257(8):1076-1078, 1987.

4. Bielory, L., et al. Asthma and Vitamin C. *Annals Allergy.* 73:89-96, 1994.

5. Simon, S. W. Vitamin B12 therapy in allergy and chronic dermatoses. *J Allergy.* 2:183-185, 1951.

6. Collip, P. J., et al. Pyridoxine treatment of childhood bronchial asthma. *Annals of Allergy.* 35:93-97, 1975.

7. Rasmussen, J. B., et al. Reduction in days of illness after long-term treatment with N-acetyl-cysteine controlled release tablets in patients with chronic bronchitis. *Eur Respir J.* 1:351-355, 1988.

Cancer

1. Goldin, B. R., et al. Estrogen excretion patterns and plasma levels in vegetarian and omnivorous women. *The New England Journal of Medicine.* 307:1542-1547, 1982.

2. Zhang, Y., et al. A major inducer of anticarcinogenic protective enzymes from broccoli: isolation and elucidations of structure. *Proceedings of the National Academy of Sciences USA.* 89:2399-2403, 1992.

~ Fahey JW, Zhang Y, Talalay P. Broccoli sprouts: An exceptionally rich source of inducers of enzymes that protect against chemical carcinogens. *Proc Natl Acad Sci USA* 1997 Sep 16;94(19):10367-10372

3. Thomas DA, Rosenthal GA, Gold DV, Dickey K (1986): Growth inhibition of a rat colon tumor by L-canavanine. *Cancer Res.* 46: 2898-2903.

~ Swaffar DS, Ang CY, Desai PB, Rosenthal GA (1994): Inhibition of the growth of human pancreatic cancer cells by the arginine antimetabolite, L-canavanine. *Cancer Res.* 54: 6045-6048.

~ Green MH, Brooks TL, Mendelsohn J, Howell SB (1980): Antitumor activity of L-canavanine against L1210 murine leukemia. *Cancer Res.* 40: 535-537.

4. Takeuchi, S., et al. Benzaldehyde as a carcinostatic principle in figs. *Agric Biol Chem.* 42(7):1449-15

5. Coles, S., & Harris, S. B. Co-enzyme Q-10 and life extension. In: *Advances in Anti-Aging Medicine.* Volume 1. Dr. Ronald M. Klatz (editor), 1996

6. Liao, S., et al. Growth inhibition and regression of human prostate and breast tumors in athymic mice by tea epigallocatechin gallate. *Cancer Letters.* 96:239-243, 1995.

Colds & Flu

1. Shibuya, N., et al. The elderberry (Sambucus nigra L.) bark lectin recognizes the Neu5Ac(alpha 2-6)Gal/GalNAc sequence. *Journal of Biological Chemistry.* 262(4):1596-1601, 1987.

~ Mori, K., et al. Studies on the virus-like particles in Lentinus edodes (Shii-ta-ke), in Mushroom Science IX (Part 1), Proceedings of the *Ninth International Science Congress on the Cultivation of Edigel Fungi.* Tokyo, 1974 (Kiryu, Japan: Mushroom Research Institute, 1976), 541-546.

2. Serkedjieva, J., et al. Anti-influenza virus effect of some propolis constituents and their analogues (esters of substituted cinnamic acids). *Journal of Natural Products.* 55:294-302, 1992.

3. Mossad, S. B., et al. Zinc gluconate lozenges for treating the common cold. *Annals of Internal Medicine.* 125(2):81-88, 1996.

4. Hayek, M. G., et al. Vitamin E supplementation decreases lung virus titers in mice infected with influenza. *J Infect Dis.* 176(1):273-276, 1997.

5. Nakayama, M., et al. Inhibition of the infectivity of influenza virus by tea polyphenols. *Antiviral Res.* 21:289-299, 1993.

6. Sachs, Allan, D.C., C.C.N. *The Authoritative Guide to Grapefruit Seed Extract.* Pages 77-78. Life Rhythm, Mendocino, California, USA, 1997. ISBN: 0-940795-17-5

7. Fujiwara, S., et al. A potent antibacterial protein in royal jelly. Purification and determination of the primary structure of royalisin. *J Biol Chem.* 265(19):11333-11337, 1990.

Colon Problems

1. Imes S, Plinchbeck BR, Dinwoodie A, et al. Iron, folate, vitamin B12, zinc, and copper status in out-patients with Crohn's disease: effect of diet counseling. *J Am Dietet Assoc* 1987;87:928-30.

2. Dvorak AM. Vitamin A in Crohn's disease. *Lancet* 1980;i:1303-4.

Constipation

1 Leng-Peschlow, E. Plantago ovata seeds as dietary fiber supplement: physiological and metabolic effects in rats. *British Journal of Nutrition.* 66:331-349, 1991.

2. Thompson, L. U., et al. Flaxseed and its lignan and oil components reduce mammary tumor growth at a late stage of carcinogenesis. *Carcinogenesis.* 17(6):1373-1376, 1996.

Depression

1. Adams, P., et al. Arachidonic acid to eicosapentaenoic acid ratio in blood correlates positively with clinical symptoms of depression. *Lipids.* 31(Supplement):S157-S161, 1996.

2. Christensen, L., Psychological distress and diet-effects of sucrose and caffeine. *J Applied Nutr.* 40:44–50, 1998.

3. Gelenberg, A. J., et al. Tyrosine for the treatment of depression. *Adv Biol Psychiat.* 10:148-159, 1983.

4. Kleijnen J, Riet GT, Knipschild P. Vitamin B6 in the treatment of the premenstrual syndrome—a review. *Brit J Obstet Gynaecol.* 97:847–52, 1990.

~ Holmes JM. Cerebral manifestations of vitamin B12 deficiency. *J Nutr Med.* 2:89–90, 1991.

~ Coppen A, Chaudrhy S, Swade C. Folic acid enhances lithium prophylaxis. *J Affective Disorders.* 10:9–13, 1986.

5. Wolkowitz OM, et al. Dehydroepiandrosterone (DHEA) treatment of depression. *Biol Psychiatr.* 41:311-8, 1997.

6. Kagan, B. L., et al. Oral S-adenosylmethionine in depression: A randomized, double-blind placebo-controlled trial. *American Journal of Psychiatry.* 147:591-595, 1990.

7. Witte, B., et al. Treatment of depressive symptoms with a high concentration of hypericum preparation - a multicenter placebo-controlled double-blind study. *Fortschr Med.* 113(28):404-408, 1995.

Diabetes

1. Jamal, G. The use of gamma linolenic acid in the prevention and treatment of diabetic neuropathy. *Diabetic Medicine.* 11:145-9; 1994.

2. Snowdon, D. A., et al. Does a vegetarian diet reduce the occurrence of diabetes? *American Journal Public Health.* 75:507-512, 1985.

3. Baskaran, K., et al. Anti-diabetic effects of a leaf extract from Gymnema Sylvestre in non-insulin-dependent diabetes mellitus patients. *Journal of Ethnopharmacology.* 30(3):295-305, 1990.

Diarrhea

1. Rump, J. A., et al. Treatment of diarrhea in human immunodeficiency virus-infected patients with immunoglobulins from bovine colostrum. *Clinical Investigator*, 70(7):588-5.

Ear Infections

1. Uhari M, Kontiokari T, Niemela M. A novel use of xylitol sugar in preventing acute otitis media. *Pediatr* 1998;102:879–84.

2. Sachs, Allan, D.C., C.C.N. The Authoritative Guide to Grapefruit Seed Extract. Pages 77-78. *Life Rhythm,* Mendocino, California, USA, 1997. ISBN: 0-940795-17-5.

3. Melchart D, Linde K, et al. Immunomodulation with Echinacea——a systematic review of controlled clinical trials. *Phytomed* 1994;1:245—54.

~ Melchort D, Walther E, Linde K, et al. Echinacea root extracts for the prevention of upper respiratory tract infections: A double-blind, placebo-controlled randomized trial. *Arch Fam Med* 1998;7:541—45.

Eye Problems

1. Corbe, C., et al. Light vision and chorioretinal circulation: Study of the effect of procyanidolic oligomers (Endotelon). *J Fr Ophtalmol.* 11:453-460, 1988.

2. Bilberry —the Vision Herb. *MediHerb Professional Review.* Number 59. August 1997

~ Jayle, G. E., et al. [Study concerning the action of anthocyanoside extracts of Vaccinium Myrtillus on night vision.] *Ann Ocul* (Paris). 198(6):556-562, 1965.

3. Human lenses. Invest Ophthalmol Vis Sci. 36(13):2756-2761, 1995.

~ Runge P, Muller DP, McAllister J, et al. Oral vitamin E supplements can prevent the retinopathy of abetalipoproteinaemia. *Br J Ophthalmol* 1986;70:166–73.

Fatigue

1. Holmes, G. P., et al. Chronic fatigue syndrome: A working case definition. *Annals of Internal Medicine.* 108:387-389, 1988.

~ Demitrack, M. A., et al. Evidence for impaired activation of the hypothalamic-pituitary-adrenal axis in patients with chronic fatigue syndrome. *Journal of Clinical Endocrinology and Metabolism.* 73:1224-1234, 1991.

2. Hinds G, Bell NP, McMaster D, McCluskey DR. Normal red cell magnesium

concentrations and magnesium loading tests in patients with chronic fatigue syndrome. *Ann Clin Biochem* 1994;31(Pt. 5):459–61.

3. Ellis FR, Nasser S. A pilot study of vitamin B12 in the treatment of tiredness. *Br J Nutr* 1973;30:277–83.

Gingivitis

1. Bliznakov, E. & Hunt, G. L. *The Miracle Nutrient: CoEnzyme Q10.* Thorsons Publishing Group, United Kingdom, 1988:148. The author describes a case report of a patient with advanced gingivitis placed on 30 mg coenzyme Q10 per day. Within one week the patient experienced a reduction in pain (enabling him to brush his teeth) and inflammation. After six months, coenzyme Q10 was ceased and within four days the symptoms of gingivitis reappeared.

2. Sakanaka, S., et al. Inhibitory effects of green tea polyphenols on growth and cellular adherence of an oral bacterium, Porphyromonas gingivalis. Biosci *Biotechnol Biochem.* 60:745-749, 1996.

3. Vogel, R. I.; et al. The effect of folic acid on gingival health. *Journal Periodontol.* 47(11):667-668, 1976.

Headache–Migraine

1. Egger J, Carter CM, Wilson J, et al. Is migraine food allergy? A double-blind controlled trial of oligo-antigenic diet treatment. *Lancet* 1983; II:865-9.

2. Hasselmark L, Malmgren R, Hannerz J. Effect of a carbohydrate-rich diet, low in protein-tryptophan, in classic and common migraine. *Cephalalgia* 1987;7:87-92.

3. Glueck CJ, McCarren T, Hitzemann R, et al. Amelioration of severe migraine with omega-3 fatty acids: a double-blind placebo controlled clinical trial. *Am J Clin Nutr* 1986;43(4):710[abstr].

4. Murphy, J. J., et al. Randomized double-blind placebo-controlled trial of feverfew in migraine prevention. *The Lancet.* 2:189-192, 1988.

5. Fusco B. M., et al. Preventative effect of repeated nasal applications of capsaicin in cluster headache. *Pain.* 59:321-325, 1994.

Heart Disease

1. That's peanuts to you. *All Natural Muscular Development.* 35(2):32, 1998.

2. Gerhardt, A. L., et al. Full-fat rice bran and oat bran similarly reduce hypercholesterolemia in humans. *Journal of Nutrition.* 128(5):865-869, 1998.

3. Breithaupt-Grogler, K., et al. Protective effect of chronic garlic intake on elastic properties of aorta in the elderly. *Circulation.* 96(8):2649-2655, 1997.

~ Bordia, A. Effect of garlic on human platelet aggregation, in vitro. *Atherosclerosis.* 30:355-361, 1978.

4. Wojcicki, J., et al. Clinical evaluation of lecithin as a lipid-lowering agent. *Phytotherapy Research.* 9:579-597, 1995.

5. Seetharamaiah, G. S., et al. Studies on hypo-cholesterolemic activity of rice bran oil. *Atherosclerosis.* 78(2-3):219-223, 1989.

6. Frenkel, E. N., et al. Inhibition of oxidation of human low-density lipoprotein by phenolic substances in red wine. *The Lancet.* 341(8843):454-457, 1993.

7. Loeper, J., et al. The antiatheromatous action of silicon. *Atherosclerosis.* 33:397-408, 1979.

8. Khaw, K., et al. Dietary potassium and stroke-associated mortality. *The New England Journal of Medicine.* 3(16):235-240, 1987.

9. Congestive heart failure and cardiomyopathy update. *Life Extension.* 4(2):35-37, 1998.

10. Op. Cit. #5.

11. Van den Berg M., et al. Combined vitamin B6 plus folic acid therapy in young patients with arteriosclerosis and hyperhomocysteinemia. *Journal Vascular Surgery.* 20(6):933-940, 1994.

12. Gale, C. R., et al. Vitamin C and risk of death from stroke and coronary heart disease in cohorts of elderly people. *British Medical Journal.* 310:1563-6, 1995.

13. Rewerski VW, Piechoscki T, et al. Some pharmacological properties of oligomeric procyanidin isolated from hawthorn (Crataegus oxyacantha). *Arzneim-Forsch Drug Res* 1967; 17:490-1.

14. Keli, S. O., et al. Dietary flavonoids, antioxidant vitamins, and incidence of stroke: The Zupthen study. *Archives of Internal Medicine.* 157:637-642, 1996.

Hemorrhoids

1. Facino, R. M., et al. Anti-elastase and anti-hyaluronidase activities of saponins and sapogenins from Hedera helix, Aesculus hippocastanum, and Ruscus aculeatus: factors contributing to their efficacy in the treatment of venous insufficiency. *Arch Pharm (Weinheim).* 328(10):720-724, 1995.

2. Chlorophyll. *Nature's Green Magic* by Theodore M. Rudolph, Ph.D. Nutritional Research Publishing Company. PO Box 489, San Gabriel, CA. 1957.

Hypoglycemia

1. Shansky, A. Vitamin B3 in the Alleviation of Hypoglycemia. *Drug and Cosmetic Industry.* 129(4):68, 1981.

~ Anderson, R. A., et al. Effects of Supplemental Chromium on Patients with Symptoms of Reactive Hypoglycemia. *Metabolism.* 36:351-355, 1987.

~ Gaby AR, Wright JV. Nutritional regulation of blood glucose. *J Advancement Med* 1991;4(1):57–71.

2. Jiang, J., et al. Effects of general saponin of panax notoginseng and sanchinoside C-1 on blood sugar in experimental animals. *Acta Pharmaceutica Sinica* (Yao Hsueh Hsueh Pao). 17(3):222-225, 1982.

Indigestion

1. Wright, J. V., M.D. The Digestive Failure Theory of Aging II. *Life Enhancement News.* January 1998.

2. Mills SY. *Out of the Earth: The Essential Book of Herbal Medicine.* London: Viking Press, 1991, 448–51

3. Goso Y, Ogata Y, Ishihara K, Hotta K. Effects of traditional herbal medicine on gastric acid. *Biochem Physiol* 1996;113C:17–21.

4. Zimmerman W. Bitter plant compounds in gastroenterology. *Z Allgemeinmed* 1976;54:1178-84 [in German].

Liver Problems

1. Welsh, A. L. Lupus erythematosus: Treatment by combined use of massive amounts of pantothenic acid and vitamin E. *Arch Derm Syph.* 70:181-198, 1954.

2. Vien, C. V., et al. Effect of vitamin A treatment on the immune reactivity of patients with systemic lupus erythematosus. *Clin Lab Immunol (Italy).* 26:33-35, 1988

3. Ferenci, P., et al. Randomized controlled trial of silymarin treatment in patients with cirrhosis of the liver. *J Hepatol.* 9:105-113, 1989.

4. Takeda, S., et al. Effect of gomisin A (TJN-101), a lignan isolated from schisandra fruits, on liver function in rats. *Nippon Yakurigaku Zasshi.* 91(4):237-244, 1988.

Lyme Disease

1. Shahani, K. M., et al. Natural antibiotic activity of Lactobacillus acidophilus and bulgaricus, II, Isolation of acidophilin from L. acidophilus. *Cult Dairy Prod J.* 12:8, 1977.

2. Cavallito, C. J., et al. Allicin, the antibacterial principle of allium sativum. Isolation, physical properties and antibacterial action. *Journal of the American Chemical Society.* 66:1950-1951, 1945.

3. Fujiwara, S., et al. A potent antibacterial protein in royal jelly. Purification and determination of the primary structure of royalisin. *J Biol Chem.* 265(19):11333-11337, 1990.

~ Mirzoeva, O. K., et al. Antimicrobial action of propolis and some of its components: the effects on growth, membrane potential and motility of bacteria. *Microbiol Res.* 152(3):239-246, 1997.

~ Jeddar, A., et al. The antibacterial action of honey. *South African Medical Journal.* 67(7):257-258, 1985.

4. Furukawa, S., et al. Glutamine-enhanced bacterial killing by neutrophils from postoperative patients. *Nutrition.* 13:863-869, 1997.

5. Thurman, R. B., et al. The molecular mechanisms of copper and silver ion disinfection of bacteria and viruses. A paper in the First International Conference on Gold

and Silver in Medicine. *The Silver Institute.* 18(4):295, 299-302, 1989.

6. Stimpel, M., et al. Macrophage activation and induction of macrophage cyto-toxicity by purified polysaccharide fractions from the plant Echinacea purpurea. *Infection and Immunity.* 46:845-849, 1984.

~ Juven, et al. Studies on the mechanism of the antimicrobial action of oleuropein. *Journal of Applied Bacteriology.* 35:559-567, 1972.

7. Cichewicz, R. H., et al. The antimicrobial properties of chili peppers (Capsicum) and their uses in Mayan medicine. Journal of *Ethnopharmacology.* 2(52):61-70, 1996.

Parasites

1. Ghannoum, M. A. Inhibition of Candida adhesion to buccal epithelial cells by an aqueous extract of Allium sativum (garlic). *Journal of Applied Bacteriology.* 68(2):163-169, 1990.

2. Sachs, Allan, D.C., C.C.N. *The Authoritative Guide to Grapefruit Seed Extract.* Page 72. Life Rhythm, Mendocino, California, USA, 1997. ISBN: 0-940795-17-5.

3. Phillipson, J. D. A matter of some sensitivity. *Phytochemistry.* 38(6):1319-1343, 1995.

PMS

1. Werbach MR. Nutritional influences on illness, 2d ed. Tarzana, CA: *Third Line Press,* 1993,540-41 [review].

2. Xu, Xia Ph.D., Kurtzer MS, Dietary Phytoestrogens, News Extract from the *Annual Review of Nutrition*, 17:353-381 1997.

3. Block, E. The use of vitamin A in premenstrual tension. *Acta Obst. Gynec.* Scandinavia. 39:586-592, 1960.

4. London, R. S. Efficacy of alpha-tocopherol in the treatment of the pre-menstrual syndrome. *Journal of Reproductive Medicine.* 32(6):400-404, 1987.

5. Stewart, A. Clinical and biochemical effects of nutritional supplementation on the premenstrual syndrome. *Journal of Reproductive Medicine.* 32(6):435-441, 1987.

6. Böhnert KJ, Hahn G. Phytotherapy in gynecology and obstetrics—Vitex agnus castus. *Erfahrungsheilkunde* 1990; 39:494-502.

7. Qi-bing M, Jing-yi T, Bo C. Advance in the pharmacological studies of radix Angelica sisnensis (oliv) diels (Chinese danggui). *Chin Med J* 1991; 104:776-81.

8. Smith, C. J. Non-hormonal control of vaso-motor flushing in menopausal patients. *Chicago Medicine.* March 7, 1964.

Pregnancy

1. Gold S and Sherry L. Hyperactivity, learning disabilities, and alcohol. *J Learn Disabil* 1984;17(1):3-6.

~ Haglund B et al. Cigarette smoking as a risk factor for sudden infant death syndrome. *Am J Publ Health* 1990;80:29-32.

~ Fenster I et al. Caffeine consumption during pregnancy and fetal growth. *Am J Public Health* 1991;81: 458-61.

2. Tamura T, Goldenberg R, Freeberg L, et al. Maternal serum folate and zinc concentrations and their relationships to pregnancy outcome. *Am J Clin Nutr* 1992: 56; 365-370.

3. Villar J and Repke JT. Calcium supplementation during pregnancy may reduce pre-term delivery in high-risk populations. *Am J Obstet Gynecol* 1990;163: 1124-31.

4. Hibbeln, J. R., et al. Dietary polyunsaturated fatty acids and depression: when cholesterol does not satisfy. *American Journal of Clinical Nutrition.* 62(1):1-9, 1995.

5. Crawford, M. The role of essential fatty acids in neural development: Implications for perinatal nutrition. *American Journal of Clinical Nutrition.* 57:703S-710S, 1993.

6. Gladstar R. *Herbal Healing for Women.* New York: Simon and Schuster, 1993, 176-177.

7. Della Loggia, R., et al. The role of triterpenoids in the topical anti-inflammatory activity of Calendula officinalis. *Planta Medica.* 60(6):516-520, 1994.

8. Badart-Smook, A., et al. Fetal growth is associated positively with maternal intake of riboflavin and negatively with maternal intake of linoleic acid. *Journal of the American Dietic Association.* 97:867-870, 1997.

Prostate Problems

1. Giovannucci, E., et al. A prospective study of dietary fat and risk of prostate cancer. *Journal of the National Cancer Institute.* 85(19):1571-1579, 1993.

~ Marchand, L. L., et al. Animal fat consumption and prostate cancer: a prospective study in Hawaii. *Epidemiology.* 5(3):276-282, 1994.

2. Levy, J., et al. Lycopene is a more potent inhibitor of human cancer cell proliferation than either alpha-carotene or beta-carotene. *Nutr Cancer.* 3(24):257-266, 1995.

3. Sigounas, G., et al. S-allylmercaptocysteine inhibits cell proliferation and reduces the viability of erythroleukemia, breast, and prostate cancer cell lines. (Garlic) *Nutr Cancer.* 27:186-191, 1997.

4. Wright, J. V., Vasquez, A. Treatment of benign prostate hypertrophy with zinc. *Townsend Letter for Doctors & Patients.* April 1996, page 82, 100.

5. Schwartz, G. G., et al. Human prostate cancer cells: inhibition of proliferation by vitamin D analogs. *Anticancer Research.* 14(3A):1077-1081, 1994.

6. Virtamo, J., et al. Beta-carotene, vitamin A and prostate cancer. *Annals of Medicine*

7. Pienta, K. J., et al. Inhibition of spontaneous metastasis in a rat prostate cancer model by oral administration of modified citrus pectin. *J Natl Cancer Inst.* 87:348-353; 1995.

8. Gilad, E., et al. Functional melatonin receptors in human prostate epithelial cells. *Endocrinology.* 137(4):1412-1417, 1996.

9. Murray, M. Saw palmetto extract vs. Proscar. *Am J Natural Med.* 1:8-9, 1994.

10. Kreski, T., et al. Comparison of efficacy and tolerability of two dosages of a combined preparation of extracts of stinging nettle root (UR 102) and Pygeum africanum (PY 102): a double-blind study in 134 patients with benign prostatic hyperplasia. *Clin Ther.* 15:1011-1020, 1993.

11. Barlet, A. Efficacy of Pygeum africanum extract in the medical therapy of urination disorders due to benign prostatic hyperplasia: Evaluation of objective and subjective parameters. A placebo controlled double-blind multicenter study. *J. Wien Klin Wochenschr.* 102:667-73, 1990.

12. Liao, S., et al. Growth inhibition and regression of human prostate and breast tumors in athymic mice by tea epigallocatechin gallate. *Cancer Letrs..* 96:239-243, 1995
.

Skin Cancer

1. Di Pasquale, M. Research Update: Burning questions about sunscreens and skin health. *Muscle Media.* 69:170, 1998.

2. Kuttan, R., et al. Tumor reducing and anticarcinogenic activity of selected spices. *Cancer Letters.* 51:85-89, 1990.

~ Yan, L., et al. Dietary flaxseed supplementation and experimental metastasis of melanoma cells in mice. *Cancer Letters.* 124(2):181-186, 1998.

3. Jang, M., et al. Cancer chemo-preventative activity of resveratrol, a natural product derived from grapes. *Science.* 275(5297)218-220, 1997.

4. Picard, D. The biochemistry of green tea polyphenols and their potential application in human skin cancer. *Alt Med Rev.* 1:31-42, 1996.

5. Murakoshi, M., et al. Inhibition by squalene of the tumor-promoting activity of 12-O-tetradecanoylphorbol-13-acetate in mouse-skin carcinogenesis. *Int J Cancer (USA).* 52:950-952; 1992.

6. Pauling, L., et al. Supplemental ascorbate in the supportive treatment of cancer: Prolongation of survival times in terminal human cancer. *Proceedings of the National Academy of Sciences USA.* 73(10):3685-3689, 1976.

7. Mochizuki, M., et al. Inhibitory effect of tumor metastasis in mice by saponins, ginsenoside Rb2, 20(R)- and 20(S)-ginsenoside-Rg3, of red ginseng. *Biol Pharm Bull.* 18(9):1197-1202, 1995.

Skin Problems

1. Veien NK, Hattel T, Justesen O, et al. Dermatoses in coffee drinkers. *Cutis* 1987; 40:421-2.

2. Naldi, L., et al. Dietary factors and the risk of psoriasis. *British Journal of Dermatology.* 134(1):101-106, 1996.

3. Donadini, A., et al. Plasma levels of Zn, Cu and Ni in healthy controls and in psoriatic patients. *Acta Vitamin Enzy mol.* 1:9-16, 1980

4. Majewski, S., et al. Decreased levels of vitamin A in serum of patients with psoriasis. *Archives of Dermatology Research.* 280:499-501, 1989.

~ Strosser, A. V., et al. Synthetic vitamin A in the treatment of eczema in children. *Annals Allergy.* 10:703-704, 1952.

5. Morimoto S, Yoshikawa K, Kozuka T, et al. An open study of vitamin D3 treatment in psoriasis vulgaris. *Brit J Dermatol* 1986;115:421-9.

6. Ruedemann, R. Treatment of psoriasis with large doses of vitamin B12: 1,000 micrograms per cubic centimeter. *Archives of Dermatology.* 69:738, 1954.

7. Misik, V., et al. Lipoxygenase inhibition and antioxidant properties of protoberberine and aporphine alkaloids isolated from Mahonia aquifolium. *Planta Medica.* 61(4):372-373, 1995.

8. Thurmon, F. M. The treatment of psoriasis with sarsaparilla compound. *New England Journal of Medicine.* 227:128-133, 1942.

9. Muller, K., et al. The anti-Psoriatic Mahonia Aquifolium (Oregon grape) and its active constituents; II. Antiproliferative activity against cell growth of human keratinocytes. *Planta Medica.* 61(1):74-5, 1995

10. Bittiner SB, Tucker WFG, Cartwright I, Bleehen SS. A double-blind, randomized, placebo-controlled trial of fish oil in psoriasis. *Lancet* 1988;I:378-80.

~ Catherine, E., et al. Topical eicosapentaenoic acid (EPA) in the treatment of psoriasis. *British Journal of Dermatology.* 120:581-584, 1989.

Sleep Disorders

1. Levy, M., et al. Caffeine metabolism and coffee-attributed sleep disturbances. *Clin Pharmacol Ther.* 33(6):770-775, 1983.

2. MacFarlane, J., et al. The effects of exogenous melatonin on the total sleep time and daytime alertness of chronic insomniacs: a preliminary study. *Biological Psychiatry.* 30:371-376, 1991.

~ Zisapel, N., et al. Melatonin replacement therapy of elderly insomniacs. *Sleep.* 18:598-603, 1995.

3. Battaglia, S. Essential oil profile: Neroli. Aromatherapy Today. *Quarterly Journal of Clinical and Holistic Aromatherapy.* 3:7-8, 1996.

4. Chauffard, F., et al. Aqueous extract of valerian reduces latency to fall asleep. *Planta Medica.* 144-148, 1985.

Stress

1. Sembulingam, K., et al. Effect of Ocimum sanctum Linn on noise induced changes in plasma corticosterone level. *Indian J Physiol Pharmacol.* 41(2):139-143, 1997.

2. Zhang, S. C., et al. The anti-stress effect of saponins extracted from panax ginseng fruit and the hypophyseal-adrenal system. *Yao Hsueh Hsueh Pao.* 16(11):860-863, 1981.

Tinnitus

1. Tohgi, H., et al. Effect of vinpocetine on oxygen release of hemoglobin and erythrocyte organic polyphosphate concentrations in patients with vascular dementia of the Bingwaner type. *Arzneim Forsch Drug Res.* 40:640-643, 1990.

~ Manconi, E., et al. A double-blind clinical trial of vinpocetine in the treatment of cerebral insufficiency of vascular and degenerative origin. *Curr Ther Res Clin Exp.* 40:702-709, 1986.

2. Shemish, A., et al. Vitamin B12 deficiency in patients with chronic tinnitus and noise induced hearing loss. *Am J Otolarygol.* 14:94-99, 1994.

3. Salerna, G. La cimifuga racemosa nel campo otoiatrico: ricerche sperimentali. *Minerva Otorinolaringologica.* 5(12):140-147, 1955.

4. Holgers, K. M., et al. Ginkgo biloba extract for the treatment of tinnitus. *Audiology [Switzerland].* 33:85-92, 1994.

~ Meyer, B. A multicentre, randomized, double-blind drug versus placebo study of Ginkgo biloba extract in the treatment of tinnitus. *La Presse Medicale.* 15:1562-1564, 1986.

5. Shambaugh, G. E. Interviewed in: *Geriatrics.* 38(4):21, 1983.
~ Shambaugh, G. E. Zinc: An essential trace element. *Clin Ecology.* 2(4):203-206, 1984.

Toothache
1. Kashket, S., et al. In-vitro inhibition of glucosyl-transferase from the dental plaque bacterium Streptococcus mutans by common beverages and food extracts. *Archives of Oral Biology.* 30(11-12):821-826, 1985.

2. Otake, S., et al. Anticaries effects of polyphenolic compounds from Japanese green tea. *Caries Research.* 25(6):438-439, 1991.

3. Murray, M. C., et al. A study to investigate the effect of a propolis-containing mouthrinse on the inhibition of de novo plaque formation. *J Clin Periodontol.* 24(11):796-798, 1997.

4. Losee, F. L. et al. A study of the mineral environment of caries-resistant navy recruits. *Caries Res.* 3:23-31, 1969.

Ulcer
1. Asaka, M., et al. What role does Helicobacter pylori play in gastric cancer? *Gastroenterology.* 113(6 Supplement):S56-S60, 1997.

2. Rydning A, Berstad A, Aadland E, Odegaard B. Prophylactic effect of dietary fiber in duodenal ulcer disease. *Lancet 1982;* ii:736-9.

3. Yudkin J. Eating and ulcers. *BMJ* Feb 16, 1980:483 [letter].
~ Sonnenberg A. Dietary salt and gastric ulcer. *Gut* 1986;27:1138-42.

4. Cheney, G. Healing of peptic ulcers in patients receiving fresh cabbage juice. *California Medicine.* 70:10-14, 1949.

5. Zhang, H. M., et al. Vitamin C inhibits the growth of a bacterial risk factor for gastric carcinoma: Helicobacter pylori. *Cancer.* 80(10):1897-1903, 1997.
~ Sivam, G. P., et al. Helicobacter pylori - in vitro susceptibility to garlic (Allium sativum) extract. *Nutr Cancer.* 27(2):118-121, 1997.

6. Kumar, N., et al. Do chilies influence healing of duodenal ulcer? *British Medical Journal.* 288:1803-1804, 1984.

7. Cooke, W. M., et al. Metabolic studies of deglycyrrhizinised licorice in two patients with gastric ulcers. *Digestion.* 4:264-268, 1971

Urinary Tract
1. Sobota AE. Inhibition of bacterial adherence by cranberry juice: potential use for the treatment of urinary tract infections. *J Urol* 1984;131:1013-6.

2. Axelrod DR. Ascorbic acid and urinary pH. *JAMA* 1985;254(10): 1310.

3. Mori S, Ojima Y, Hirose T, et al. The clinical effect of proteolytic enzyme containing bromelain and trypsin on urinary tract infection evaluated by double blind method. *Acta Obstet Gynaec Jap* 1972;19:147-53.

4. Kodama, R., et al. Studies on the metabolism of d-limonene. *Xenobiotica.* 6:377-389, 1976.

Weight Loss
1. Valentine, G. Thyroid deficiency syndrome. *Life Enhancement.* January 1998, pages 3-6.

2. Suter, P. M., et al. The effect of ethanol on fat storage in healthy subjects. *The New England Journal of Medicine.* April:983-987, 1992.

3. Skov, A. R., et al. The effects of a low-fat, high protein vs. a low-fat, high carbohydrate diet on cardiovascular risk factors in obese subjects. *International Journal of Obesity.* 20(Supplement 4):47 (abstract 03-082-WB2), 1996.
~ Yamamoto, T., et al. Soy Protein and its hydrolysate reduce body fat of dietary obese rats. *Proceedings of the Second International Symposium on the Role of Soy in Preventing and Treating Chronic Disease.* Brussels, Belgium. Pages 55-56, 1996.

4. Childs, M. T., et al. Effect of shellfish consumption on cholesterol absorption in normolipidemic men. *Metabolism.* 36(1):31-35, 1987.

5. Becher EW, Jakober B, Luft D, et al. Clinical and biochemical evaluations of the alga spirulina with regard to its application in the treatment of obesity. A double-blind crossover study. *Nutr Rep Intl.* 33(4):565-573, 1986.

6. Van Gaal, L., et al. Exploratory study of coenzyme Q10 in obesity. In: Biomedical and Research Aspects of Coenzyme Q, Vol 4. Folkers, K., & Yamura (eds.). Elsevier Science Publishers. *Amsterdam,* 1984, pp. 369-373.

7. Naylor, G. J., et al. A double blind placebo controlled trial of ascorbic acid in obesity. *Nutr. Health*

8. Dullo, A. G., et al. Tealine and thermogenesis: Interactions between polyphenols, caffeine and sympathetic activity. *International Journal of Obesity.* 20(Supplement 4):71, 1996.

Nature's Finest Healing Foods & Herbs

Alfalfa

1. Thomas DA, Rosenthal GA, Gold DV, Dickey K (1986): Growth inhibition of a rat colon tumor by L-canavanine. *Cancer Res.* 46: 2898-2903.

~ Swaffar DS, Ang CY, Desai PB, Rosenthal GA (1994): Inhibition of the growth of human pancreatic cancer cells by the arginine antimetabolite, L-canavanine. *Cancer Res.* 54: 6045-6048.

~ Green MH, Brooks TL, Mendelsohn J, Howell SB (1980): Antitumor activity of L-canavanine against L1210 murine leukemia. *Cancer Res.* 40: 535-537.

2. Xu, Xia Ph.D., Kurtzer MS, Dietary Phytoestrogens, News Extract from the *Annual Review of Nutrition*, 17:353-381 1997.

3. Malinow M, et al. Prevention of elevated cholesterolemia in monkeys by alfalfa saponins. *Steroids* 1977;29:105

~ Malinow M, et al. Alfalfa saponins and alfalfa seeds: dietary effects in cholesterol-fed rabbits. *Atherosclerosis* 1980;37:433

4. Cav GH, Sofic E, Prior RL, Antioxidant Capacity of Tea and Common Vegetables. A News Extract from *Journal of Agricultural and Food Chemistry,* 44: (11) 3426-3431 Nov. 1996.

Aloe Vera

1. Miller, K.B., et al. Treatment of experimental frostbite with pentoxifylline and aloe vera cream. *Arch Otolaryngol Head Neck Surg.* 121(6):678-680, 1995.

2. Syed, T,A., et al. Management of psoriasis with aloe vera extract in hydrophilic cream: a placebo-controlled, double-blind study. *Trop Med Int. Health.* 1(4):505-509, 1996.

~ Visuthikosol, V., et al. Effect of aloe vera gel to healing burn wound: A clinical and histological study. *J. Med. Assoc. Thai.* 78(8):403-409, 1995.

3. Davis, R.H., et al. Wound healing. Oral topical activity of aloe vera. *J. Am Podiatr Med Assoc.* 79(11):559-562, 1989.

4. Strickland, F.M., et al. Prevention of ultraviolet radiation-induced suppression of contact and delayed hypersensitivity by aloe barbadensis gel extract. *J Invest Dermatol.* 102(2):197-204, 1994.

5. Vazquez, B., et al. Anti-inflammatory activity of extracts from aloe vera gel. *Journal of Ethnopharmacology.* 55(1):69-75, 1996.

6. Gribel, N. V., et al., Antimetastatic properties of aloe juice. Vopr Onkol. 32:38-40, 1986.

7. Womble, D., et al. Enhancement of aloe responsiveness of human lymphocytes by acemannan (Carrisyn). *International Journal of Immunopharmacology.* 10:967-974, 1988.

8. McDaniel, H Reginald, Aloe Vera May Mimic AZT Without Toxicity, *Medical World News,* December, 1993.

9. Bunyapraphatsara, N., et al. *Phytomedicine.* 3:245-248, 1996.

~Yongchaiyudha, S., et al. *Phytomedicine.* 3:241-243, 1996.

Apples

1. Sablee-Amplis, R. Further studies on the cholesterol-lowering effect of apple in humans: Biochemical mechanisms involved. *Nutr Res.* 3:325-328, 1983.

2. Smart, R.C., Huang, M.T., Chang R.L. et al., Effect of ellagic acid and 3-0-decylellagic acid on the formation of benzo[a]-pyrene in mice. *Carcinogenesis* 7:166-75, 1986.

3. Stavric, B. Quercetin in our diet: from potent mutagen to probable anticarcinogen. *Clin Biochem.* 27:245-248, 1994.

4. Watanabe, K., et al. Effect of dietary alfalfa, pectin, and wheat bran on

azoxymethane- or methylni trosourea-induced colon carcinogenesis in F344 rats. *Journal of the National Cancer Institute.* 63:141-145, 1979.

5. Konowalchuk, J., et al. Antiviral effect of apple beverages. *Applied and Environmental Microbiology.* 36(6):798-801, 1978.

Bananas

1. MacGregor, S. A., et al. Moderate potassium supplementation in essential hypertension. *The Lancet.* ii:567-570, 1982.

2. Usha, V., et al. Effect of dietary fiber from banana (Musa paradisiaca) on cholesterol metabolism. *Indian Journal of Experimental Biology.* 22:550-554, 1984.

3. Best, R., et al. The anti-ulcerogenic activity of unripe plantain banana (Musa species). *British Journal of Pharmacology.* 82(1):107-116, 1984.

~ Lewis, D. A., et al. A natural flavonoid present in unripe plantain banana pulp (Musa sapeintum L. var. paradisiaca) protects the gastric mucosa from aspirin-induced erosions. *Journal of Ethnopharmacology.* 65(3):283-288, 1999.

4. Friedland, J., et al. Potassium and fatigue. *The Lancet.* 2:961-962m, 1988.

Bee Pollen

1. Research on wrinkles by M. Esperrois, French Institute of Chemistry. Reported in *Better Nutrition Magazine.* May 1997, page 62.

~ Broadhurst, C. L. Bee products: Medicine from the hive. *Nutrition Science News.* August 1999.

2. Habib Fouad, K., et al. Identification of a prostate inhibitory substance in a pollen extract. *Prostate.* 26:133-139, 1995.

~ Yasumoto, R., et al. Clinical evaluation of long-term treatment using Cernitin pollen extract in patients with benign prostatic hyperplasia. *Clinical Therapeutics.* 17:82-86, 1995.

3. Furusawa E, et al. Antitumor potential of pollen extract on Lewis lung carcinoma implanted intraperitonally in syngeneic mice. *Phytotherapy Research.* 9:255-259, 1995.

~ Matsuno, T., et al. Preferential cytotoxicity to tumor cells of 3,5-diprenyl-4-hydroxycinnamic acid (artepillin C) isolated from propolis. *Anticancer Research.* 17(5A):3565-3568, 1997.

4. Fujiwara, S., et al. A potent antibacterial protein in royal jelly. Purification and determination of the primary structure of royalisin. *J Biol Chem.* 265(19):11333-11337, 1990.

~ Serkedjieva, J., et al. Anti-influenza virus effect of some propolis constituents and their analogues (esters of substituted cinnamic acids). *Journal of Natural Products.* 55:294-297, 1992.

~ Harish, Z., et al. Suppression of HIV-1 replication by propolis and its immunoregulatory effect. *Drugs Exp Clin Res.* 23(2):89-96, 1997.

Beets

1. Montero Brens, C., et al. Homocystinuria: Effectiveness of the treatment with pyridoxine, folic acid and betaine. *Anales Espanoles de Pediatria.* 39(1):37-41, 1993.

2. Castagna, A., et al. Cerebrospinal fluid S-adenosylmethionine (SAMe) and glutathione concentrations in HIV infection: effect of parenteral treatment with SAMe. *Neurology.* 45(9):1678-1683, 1995.

~ South, J. SAMe - the ultimate nutrient for mood, liver, heart, joint and brain protection. International Antiaging Systems: *Anti-Aging Bulletin.* 3(5):14-19, 1998

3. Barak, A. J., et al. S-adenosylmethionine generation and prevention of alcoholic fatty liver by betaine. *Alcohol.* 11:501-503, 1994.

~ Mann, J. TMG-15: New life-extension breakthrough. *Journal of the MegaHealth Society.* 1984, 1(4):1-2, 1984.

4. Le Marchand, I., et al. Intake of specific carotenoids and lung cancer risk. *Cancer Epidemiology*. 2:183-187, 1993.

~ Wainfan, E., et al. Methyl groups in carcinogenesis: effects on DNA methylation and gene expression. *Cancer Research.* 52(7 Supplement: 2071S-2077S, 1992.

Bran

1. Alabaster, O., et al. Potential synergism between wheat bran and psyllium: enhanced

inhibition of colon cancer. *Cancer Letters.* 75:53-58, 1993.

2. Gerhardt, A.L., et al. Full-fat rice bran and oat bran similarly reduce hypercholesterolemia in humans. *Journal of Nutrition.* 128(5):865-869, 1998.
~ Kashtan, et al. Wheat-bran and oat-bran supplements's effects on blood lipids and lipoproteins. *American Journal of Clinical Nutrition.* 55:976-980, 1992.

3. Ohkawa, T., et al. Rice bran treatment for patients with hypercalciuric stones: Experimental and clinical studies. *Journal of Urology.* 132:1140-1145.

4. Rose, D.P., et al. Effects of diet supplements with wheat bran on serum estrogen levels in the follicular and luteal phases of the menstrual cycle. *Nutrition.* 13:535-539, 1997.

5. Bucci, L. R., et al. Effects of ferulate on strength and body composition of weightlifters. *J Appl Sport Sci Res.* 4:104-109, 1990.

Brewer's Yeast

1. Sinai, Y., et al. Enhancement of resistance to infectious diseases by oral administration of brewer's yeast. *Infec. Immun.* 9:781-787, 1974.

2. Leibovich, S.J., et al. Promotion of wound repair in mice by application of glucan. *Journal of the Reticuloendothelial Society.* 27:1-11, 1980.

3. Offenbacher, E.G., et al. Improvement of glucose tolerance and blood lipids in elderly subjects. *American Journal of Clinical Nutrition.* 33:916, 1980.

Brocolli

1. Verhoeven, D. T., et al. Epidemiological studies on brassica vegetables and cancer risk. *Cancer Epidemiol Biomarkers Prev.* 5(9):733-748, 1996.
~ Zhang, Y., et al. Major inducer of anticarcinogenic protective enzymes from broccoli: isolation and elucidations of structure. *Proceedings of the National Aca-demy of Sciences USA.* 89:2399-2403, 1992.

2. Fahey JW, Zhang Y, Talalay P. Broccoli sprouts: An exceptionally rich source of inducers of enzymes that protect against chemical carcinogens. *Proc Natl Acad Sci USA* 1997 Sep 16;94(19):10367-10372

Cabbage

1. Cheney, G., Rapid healing of peptic ulcers in patients receiving fresh cabbage juice, *Cal Med.* 70:10-14, 1949.

2. Albert, P. M., Physiological effects of cabbage with reference to its potential as a dietary cancer-inhibitor and its use in ancient medicine. *Journal of Ethnopharmacology.* 9:261-272, 1983.

Carrots

1. Brevard, P. B. Beta-carotene affects white blood cells in human peripheral blood. *Nutr Rep Intern.* 40:139-150, 1989.

2. Robertson, J., et al. The effect of raw carrot on serum lipids and colon function. *American Journal of Clinical Nutrition.* 32(9):1889-1892, 1978.

3. Le Marchand, I., et al. Intake of specific carotenoids and lung cancer risk. *Cancer Epidemiology.* 2:183-187, 1993.

Celery

1. Murray, Michael T. *The Healing Power of Foods.* Prima Publishing, Rocklin, California, USA. 1993. pp. 110-111.

2. D'Argenio, G., et al. Butyrate enemas in experimental colitis and protection against large bowel cancer in a rat model. *Gastroenterology.* 110:1727-1734, 1996.

Citrus Fruits

1. Kodama, R., et al. Studies on the metabolism of d-limonene. *Xenobiotica.* 6:377-389, 1976.

2. Crowell, P.L. Mono-terpenes in breast cancer chemo-prevention. *Breast Cancer Res Treat.* 46(2-3):191-97, 1997.

3. El-Shebini, S. M., et al. The role of pectin as a slimming agent. *J Clin Biochem Nutr.* 4:455-262, 1968.

4. Baekey, P. A., et al. Grapefruit pectin inhibits hypercholesterolemia and atherosclerosis in miniature swine. *Clinical Cardiology.* 9(11):597-600, 1988.

5. Pienta, L.J., et al. Inhibition of spontaneous metastasis in a rat prostrate cancer model by oral administration of modified citrus pectin. *J Natl Cancer Inst.* 87:348-353; 1995.

6. Cancer and naringenin and grapefruit. *Science News.* 149(18):287, 1996.

Echinacea

1. Hoheisel, O., et al. Echinagard treatment shortens the course of the common cold: a double-blind, placebo-controlled clinical trial. *Eur J Clin Res.* 9:261-268, 1997.

2. Wacker, A., et al. Virus-inhibition by echinacea purpurea. *J Med Chem.* 15:619-623, 1972.

~ Stimpel, M., et al. Macrophage activation and induction of macrophage cytotoxicity by purified polysaccharide fractions from the plant Echinacea purpurea. *Infection and Immunity.* 46:845-849, 1984.

3. Voaden, D.J., et al. Tumor-inhibitors III. Identification and synthesis of an oncolytic hydrocarbon from American coneflower roots. *Jour Med Chem* 15:(6):619-623, 1972

4. See, D.M., et al. In vitro effects of echinacea and ginseng on natural killer and antibody-dependent cell cytotoxicity in healthy subjects and Chronic Fatigue Syndrome or Acquired Immuno-Deficiency syndrome patients. *Immunopharmacology.* 35(3):229-22-35, 1997.

Flaxseed

1. Yan, L., et al. Dietary flaxseed supplementation and experimental metastasis of melanoma cells in mice. *Cancer Letters.* 124(2):181-186, 1998.

~ Thompson, L. U., et al. Flaxseed and its lignan and oil components reduce mammary tumor growth at a late stage of carcinogenesis. *Carcinogenesis.* 17(6):1373-1376, 1996.

2. De Lorgeril M, Renaud S, Maelle N, et al. Mediterranean alpha-linolenic acid-rich diet in secondary prevention of coronary heart disease. *Lancet* 1994;343:1454-9.

3. Chan JK, Bruce VM, McDonald BE. Dietary a-linolenic acid is as effective as oleic acid and linoleic acid in lowering blood cholesterol in normolipidemic men. *Am J Clin Nutr* 1991; 53:1230-4.

4. Hart JP, Cooper WL. Vitamin F in the treatment of prostatic hypertrophy. Report Number 1, *Lee Foundation for Nutritional Research,* Milwaukee, Wisconsin, 1941.

Garlic

1. Abdullah, T. H., et al. Enhancement of natural killer cell activity in AIDS with garlic. *Deutsch Zietschrift fur Onkologie.* 21:52-53, 1989.

2. Pinto, J., et al. Garlic constituents modify expression of biomarkers for human prostatic carcinoma cells. *FASEB*, 11:A439, 1997.

3. Kuttan, R., et al. Tumor reducing and anti-carcinogenic activity of selected spices. *Cancer Letters.* 51:85-89, 1990.

4. Sivam, G. P., et al. Helicobacter pylori - in vitro susceptibility to garlic (Allium sativum) extract. *Nutrition and Cancer.* 27(2):118-121, 1997.

5. Cha, C. W. A study on the effect of garlic to the heavy metal poisoning of rat. *Journal of Korean Medical Science.* 2(4): 213_224, 1987.

~ Kamanna, V. S., et al. Effect of garlic on serum lipoproteins and lipoprotein cholesterol levels in albino rats rendered hypercholesteremic by feeding cholesterol. *Lipids.* 17(7):483-488, 1982.

Ginger

1. Murray, M.T., N.D. *The Complete Book of Juicing* (Rocklin, CA; Prima Publishing)1992, 1998;pg.155

2. Srivastava KC and Mustafa T, Ginger (Zingiber officinale) and rheumatic disorders, *Med Hypothesis* 29:25-28, 1989.

3. Verma SK, Singh J, et al. Effect of ginger on platelet aggregation in man. *Indian J Med Res* 1994;98:240-2.

Ginkgo

1. Holgers, K. M., et al. Ginkgo biloba extract for the treatment of tinnitus. *Audiology [Switzerland].* 33:85-92, 1994.

2. Pritz-Hohmeier, S., et al. Effect of in vivo application of Ginkgo biloba extract Egb 761

(Rokan) on the susceptibility of mammalian retinal cells to proteolytic enzymes. *Ophthalmic Research.* 26:80-86, 1994.

3. Huguet, F., et al. Decreased cerebral 5-HT1A receptors during aging: reversal by Ginkgo biloba extract (EGb 761). *Jrnl. of Pharmacy & Pharmacology.* 46: 316-318, 1994.

4. Gebner, B., et al. Study of long-term action of a Ginkgo biloba extract on vigilance and mental performance as determined by means of quantitative pharmaco-EEG and psychometric measurements. *Arzneimittel-Forschung.* 35(9):1459-1465, 1985.

5. Jung, F., et al. Effect of ginkgo biloba on fluidity of blood and peripheral micro-circulation in volunteers. *Arzneim-Forsch Drug Res.* 40:589-593, 1990.

6. Krieglstein, J., et al. Neuro-protective effects of ginkgo biloba constituents. *Journal Pharm Sci.* 3:39-48, 1995. Op. cit. #4

7. Kanowski, S., et al. Proof of efficacy of the ginkgo biloba special extract egb 761 in outpatients suffering from mild to moderate primary degenerative dementia of the Alzheimer type or multi-infarct dementia. *Pharmacopsychiatry.* 29(2):47-56, 1996.

8. Auguet, M., et al. Ginkgo biloba extract (Egb 761) and the regulation of vascular tone. In: Cardiovascular Effects of Ginkgo biloba Extract. (Clostre F., DeFeudis, FV, eds) *Elsevier, Amsterdam,* 1994.19-26.

9. Ferrandini, C., Droy-Lefaix, M. T., Christen, Y. (editors). Ginkgo biloba extract (Egb 761) as a free radical scavenger. *Elsevier, Paris.* 1993.

Ginseng

1. Forgo, I. The duration of effect of the standardized ginseng extract G115(r) in healthy competitive athletes. *Notabene Medici.* 9:636, 1985.

2. Petkov, V. D., et al. Effects of standardized Ginseng extract on learning, memory and physical capabilities. *American Journal of Chinese Medicine.* 15(1-2):19-29, 1987.

3. Li, J., et al. Inhibition of apoptosis by ginsenoside Rg1 in cultured cortical neurons. *Chin Med J.* 110(7):535-539, 1997.

4. Fulder, S. J. Ginseng and hypothalamic-pituitary control of stress. *American Jrnl. of Chinese Medicine.* 9(2):112-118, 1981.

5. Chen, X. Experimental study on the cardiovascular effects of ginsenosides. *Chung Hua Hsueh Kuan Ping Tsa Chih.* 10(2):147-150, 1982.

6. Brekham, I.I. Pharmacological investigations of glycosides from ginseng and eleutherococcus. *Lloydia.* 32:46-51, 1969

~ Lee, F.C., et al. Effects of Panax ginseng on blood alcohol clearance in man. *Clinical and Experimental Pharmacology and Physiology.* 14:543-546, 1987.

7. See, D. M., et al. In vitro effects of echinacea and ginseng on natural killer and antibody-dependent cell cyto-toxicity in healthy subjects and Chronic Fatigue Syndrome or Acquired ImmunoDeficiency Syndrome (AIDS) patients. *Immunopharmacology.* 35(3):229-235, 1997.

8. Odashima, S., et al. Induction of phenotypic reverse transformation by ginsenosides in cultured Morris hepatoma cells. *European Journal of Cancer.* 15:885-892, 1979.

~ Yun, T., et al. Preventive effect of ginseng intake against various human cancers: A case-control study on 1,987 pairs. *Cancer Epidemiology, Biomarkers and Prevention.* 4:401-408, 1995.

9. Salvati, G., et al. Effects of Panax Ginseng, C.A. Meyer saponins on male fertility. *Panminerva Medica.* 38(4):249-254, 1996.

10. Zhang, T., et al. Ginseng root: Evidence for numerous regulatory peptides and insulinotropic activity. *Biomed Res.* 11:49-54, 1990.

Grapes

1. Masquelier, J. The bactericidal action of certain phenolics of grapes and wine. *The Pharmacology of Plant Phenolics.* New York: Academic Press, 1959.

~ Konowalchuk, J., et al. Virus inactivation by grapes and wines. *Applied Environmental Microbiology.* 32(6):757-763, 1976.

2. Gomez Trillo, J. T. Varicose veins of the lower extremities: Symptomatic treatment with a new vasculotrophic agent. *Prensa Med Mex.* 38:293-296, 1973.

~ Henriet, J. P. Veno-lymphatic insufficiency: 4,729 patients undergoing hormonal and pro-cyanidol oligomer therapy. *Phlebologie*. 46:313-325, 1993.

3. Corbe, C., et al. Light vision and chorioretinal circulation: Study of the effect of pro-cyanidolic oligomers (Endotelon). *Journal Fr Ophtalmology.* 11:453-460, 1988.

Green Tea

1. Liao, S., et al. Growth inhibition and regression of human prostate and breast tumors in athymic mice by tea epigallocatechin gallate. *Cancer Letters.* 96:239-243, 1995.

~ Kohlmeier, L., et al. Tea and cancer prevention: an evaluation of the epidemiologic literature. *Nutrition and Cancer.* 27(1):1-13, 1997.

~ Ji, B.T., et al. Green tea consumption and the risk of pancreatic and colorectal cancers. *International Journal of Cancer.* 70(3):255-258, 1997.

2. Klaunig, J.E. Chemo-preventive effects of green tea components on hepatic carcinogenesis. *Preventive Medicine.* 21:510-519, 1992.

~ Ohno, Y., et al. Tea consumption and lung cancer risk. A case-control study in Okinawa, Japan. *Japanese Journal of Cancer Research.* 86:1027-1034, 1995.

~ Yu, T.G., et al. Reduced risk of esophageal cancer associated with green tea consumption. *Journal of the National Cancer Institute.* 86(11):855-858.

~ Kono, S., et al. A case-control study of gastric cancer and diet in northern Kyushu, Japan. *Japanese Journal of Cancer Research.* 79:1067-1074, 1988.

~ American Health Foundation. Exploring the chemopreventive properties of tea. Primary Care and Cancer: *American Health Foundation Update.* 15(2):30-31, 1995.

3. Sagesaka-Mitane, Y., et al. Platelet aggregation inhibitors in hot water extracts of green tea. *Chem Parm Bull* (Tokyo). 38:790-793, 1990.

4. Henry, J.P., et al. Reduction of chronic psychosocial hypertension in mice by decaffeinated tea. *Hypertension.* 6(3):437-444, 1981.

5. Keli, S.O., et al. Dietary flavonoids, antioxidant vitamins, and incidence of stroke: The Zupthen study. *Archives of Internal Medicine.* 157:637-642, 1996.

6. Ho, C., et al. Antioxidative effect of polyphenol extract prepared from various Chinese teas. *Prev Med.* 21:520-525, 1992.

7. Sakanaka, S., et al. Antibacterial substances in Japanese green tea extract against streptococcus mutans, a cariogenic bacterium. *Agric Biol Chem.* 53:2307-2311, 1989.

8. Picard, D. The biochemistry of green tea polyphenols and their potential application in human skin cancer. *Alt Med Rev.* 1:31-42, 1996.

Kale and Collards

1. Garland, C et al. Dietary vitamin D and calcium and risk of colorectal cancer: A 19 year prospective study in men. *Lancet*. 1:307-9, 1985.

2. MacLennan, R., et al. Risk factors for lung cancer in Singapore Chinese, a population with high female incidence rates. *International Journal of Cancer.* 20:854-860, 1977.

~ Katdare, M., et al. Prevention of mammary pre-neoplastic transformation by naturally-occurring tumor inhibitors. *Cancer Letters.* 111(1-2):141-147, 1997.

3.Seddon, J., et al. Dietary carotenoids, vitamins A, C, and E, and advanced age-related macular degeneration. *Journal of the American Medical Association.* 272:18:1413-1420, 1994.

Licorice

1. Glick, L. Deglycyrrhizinated liquorice in peptic ulcer. *The Lancet.* 2:817, 1982.

2. Tangri, K.K., et al. Biochemical study of the anti-inflammatory and anti-arthritic properties of glycyrrhetic acid. *Biochem Pharmacol.* 14(8):1277-1281, 1965.

3. Ito, M., et al. Mechanism of inhibitory effect of glycyrrhizin on replication of human Immuno-Deficiency Virus (HIV). *Antiviral Research.* 10:289-298, 1988.

~ Saxen, R.C., et al. Antipyretic effect of glycyrrhetic acid and imiprmine. *Japanese Journal of Pharmacology.* 18(3):353-355, 1968.

4. Fujisawa, K., et al. Therapeutic approach to chronic active hepatitis with glycyrrhizin. *Asian Medical Journal.* 23:745-756, 1980.

5. Vaya, J., et al. Antioxidant constituents from licorice roots: isolation, structure elucidation and anti-oxidative capacity toward LDL oxidation. *Free Radical Biol Med.* 23(2):302-313, 1997.

Noni

1. Heinicke, R.M., Ph.D., "The Pharmacologically Active Ingredient of Noni," *Pacific Tropical Botanical Garden Bulletin,* University of Hawaii, Vol.XV-No.1, 1985.

2. Younos, C., et al. Analgesic and behavioral effects of morinda citrifolia. *Planta Medica.* 56:430-434, 1990.

3. Hirazumi, A., Furusaw, E., Chou, S.C., Hokama, Y., "Anti-cancer Activity of Morinda citrifolia (Noni) on Intraperitonally Implanted Lewis Lung Carcinoma in Syngeneic Mice," *Proc. West. Pharmacol. Soc.*, 37:145-146, 1994.

4. See, Darrly, M.D., Khemka, P., Sah, L, et al, "The Role of Natural Killer Cells in Viral Infections," *Scandinavian Journal of Immunology.* Vol. 46-3. Pp.217-224, Sept. 1997.

Peppermint

1. May B, Kuntz HD, Kieser M, Kohler S. Efficacy of a fixed peppermint/caraway oil combination in non-ulcer dyspepsia. *Arzneim Forsch Drug Res* 1996;46:1149-53.

2. Rees W, Evans B, Rhodes J. Treating irritable bowel syndrome with peppermint oil. *Brit Med J* 1979; ii:835-6.

3. Weizman Z, Alkrinawi S, Goldfarb D, Bitran C. Efficacy of herbal tea preparation in infantile colic. *J Pediatr 1993;* 122:650–52.

Radish

1. Perry, L. J. *Medicinal Plants of East and Southeast Asia.* Massachusetts Institute of Technology Press, Cambridge.

~ Hartwell, J. L. The author claims that fomentation's of radish juice in cooking oil are useful for the treatment of stomach cancer. *Lloydia.* March 1969.

Red Pepper

1. Visudhiphan, S., et al. The relationship between high fibroinolytic activity and daily capsicum ingestion in Thais. *American Journal of Clinical Nutri..* 35(6):1452-1458, 1982.

~ Sambaiah, K., et al. Hypocholesterolemic effect of red pepper and capsaicin. *Indian Journal of Experimental Biology.* 18(8):898-899, 1980.

2. Kumar, N., et al. Do chillies influence healing of duodenal ulcer? *British Medical Journal.* 288:1803-1804, 1984.

3. Cichewicz, R. H., et al. The antimicrobial properties of chili peppers (Capsicum) and their uses in Mayan medicine. *Journal of Ethnopharmacology.* 2(52):61-70, 1996.

4. Cichewicz, R. H., et al. The antimicrobial properties of chili peppers (Capsicum) and their uses in Mayan medicine. *Journal of Ethnopharmacology.* 2(52):61-70, 1996.

5. Fusco B. M., et al. Preventative effect of repeated nasal applications of capsaicin in cluster headache. *Pain.* 59:321-325, 1994.

6. Henry, C. J. K., et al. Effect of spiced food on metabolic rate. Human Nutrition: *Clinical Nutrition.* 40(2):165-168, 1986.

7. Op. Cit. #4.

Spinach

1. Iritani, N., et al. Effect of spinach and wakame on cholesterol turnover in the rat. *Atherosclerosis.* 15:87-92, 1972.

2. Seddon, J., et al. Dietary carotenoids, vitamins A, C, and E, and advanced age-related macular degeneration. *Journal of the American Medical Association.* 272:18:1413-1420, 1994.

~ Hankinson, S. E., et al. Nutrient intake and cataract extraction in women: a prospective study. *British Medical Journal.* 305:335-339, 1992.

3. Marshall, J. R., et al. Diet and smoking in the epidemiology of cancer of the cervix. *Journal of the National Cancer Institute.* 70(5):847-851, 1983.

Soy

1. Anderson, J. W., et al. Meta-analysis of the effects of soy protein intake on serum

lipids. *The New England Journal of Medicine.* 333:276-282, 8/1995.

2. Messina, M., et al. The role of soy products in reducing the risk of cancer. *Journal of the National Cancer Institute.* 83(8):541-546, 1991.

~ Petrakis, J., et al. A clinical trial of the chemo-preventive effect of a soy beverage in women at high risk for breast cancer. Department of Epidemiology, University of California, Ca., and Department of Pharmacology, University of Alabama at Birmingham, Al.

3. Arjmandi, B. H., et al. Dietary soybean protein prevents bone loss in an ovariectomized rat model of osteoporosis. *Journal of Nutrition.* 126:161-167, 1996.

Tomato

1. Stahl, W., et al. Uptake of lycopene and its geometrical isomers is greater from heat-processed than from unprocessed tomato juice in humans. *Journal of Nutrition.* 122:2161-2166, 1992.

2. Burke, E. Lycopene protects against heart attack. *All Natural Muscular Development.* 35(6):32, 1998.

3. Batieha, A. M., et al. Serum micro-nutrients and the subsequent risk of cervical cancer in a population-based nested case-control study. *Cancer Epidemiol Biomarkers Prev.* 4(2):335-339, 1993.

4. Francheschi, S., et al. Tomatoes and risk of digestive-tract cancers. *International Journal of Cancer.* 59:181-184, 1994.

5. Levy, J., et al. Lycopene is a more potent inhibitor of human cancer cell proliferation than either alpha-carotene or beta-carotene. *Nutr. Cancer.* 3(24):257-266, 1955.

6. Clinton, S.K., et al. Cis-trans lycopene isomers, carotenoids, and retinol in the human prostate. *Cancer Epidemiol Biomarkers Prev.* 5(10):823-833, 1996.

~ Giovanucci, E., et al. Intake of carotenoids and retinol in relation to risk of prostate cancer. *Journal of the National Cancer Institute.* 87:1767-1776, 1995.

Tropical Fruits

1. Taussig, S.J., et al. Bromelain, the enzyme complex of pineapple (Ananas comosus) and its clinical application. An update. *Journal of Ethnopharmacology.* 22:191-203, 1988.

2. Felton, G.E. Fibrinolytic and antithrombotic action of bromelain may eliminate thrombosis in heart patients. *Medical Hypotheses.* 6:1123-1133, 1980.

3. Tausig, S.J., et al. Inhibition of tumor growth in vitro by bromelain, an extract of the pineapple plant (ananas comosus). *Planta Medica.* 52:538-539, 1985.

4. Pinski S. L. and Maloney J.D., Adenosine:A new drug for acute termination of spraventricular tachycardia, Clev. *Clinical Journal of Medicine.* 57:383-88, 1990.

~ Altman, R., et al. Identification of platelet inhibitor present in the melon (Cucurbitacea Cucumis melo). *Thrombosis and Haemostatis.* 53(3):312-313, 1985.

5. Jay Kordich, the Juiceman. *The Juiceman's Power of Juicing* by Jay Kordich. Warner Books, New York. 1993.

6. Osato, J.A., et al. Antimicrobial and antioxidant activities of unripe papaya. *Life Sciences.* 53(17):1383-1389,1993.

~ Kumar, A., et al. Effect of feeding Carica papaya (papita) fruits on blood lipid profile of albino rabbits. *Indian Journal of Clinical Biochemistry.* 8(1):47-50, 1993.

Watercress

1. Hecht, S.S., et al. Effect of watercress consumption on metabolism of tobacco-specific lung carcinogen in smokers. *Cancer Epidemiol Biomarkers Preview.* 4(8):877-884,1995.

Wheatgrass

1. *Biochemical Characterization of the Novel Molecule(s) in Barley Leaf Extract That Inhibits Growth of Human Prostate Cancer Cells.* Preliminary report. By M. Badamchian and Allan L. Goldstein, Ph.D, Dept. of Biochemistry and Molecular Biology. George Washington Univ. Medical center.

2. *Young Barley Plant Juice,* by Yoshihide Hagiwara, M.D. pub by The Green and Health Assoc, Tokyo, Japan April, 1980.

3. *Wheatgrass Nature's Finest Medicine. The Complete Guide to Using Grass Foods &*

Juices to Revitalize Your Health by Steve Meyerowitz. Book Publishing Company. 1999. 1-878736-97-3.

Power Drinks for The Physical Body

1. Blomstrand E, Hassmen P, Ek S, et al. Influence of ingesting a solution of branched-chain amino acids on perceived exertion during exercise. *Acta Physiol Scand.* 159:41-9, 1997.

2. From *Wheatgrass Nature's Finest Medicine* by Steve Meyerowitz. Chapter: "Real Stories from Real People." ISBN#1-878736-97-3. 1999.

3. Beiler, J. M., et al. Anti-fertility activity of pisum sativum (pea). *Experimental Medicine and Surgery.* 11:179-185, 1953.

4. Wilson, C. Athletic Super Water Adds More Oxygen to H2O. *USA Today.* July 18, 1997, Section D.

5. Kawata, T., et al. Effect of vitamin B12 deficiency on testicular tissue in rats fed by pair-feeding. *Int J Vitam Nutr Res.* 67(1):17-21, 1997.

6. Op. Cit. #1.

7. Gatnau, R., et al. Effect of excess dietary leucine and leucine catabolites on growth and immune response in weanling pigs. *Journal of Animal Science.* 73:159-165, 1995.

8. Swart, I., et al. The effects of L-carnitine supplementation in plasma carnitine levels and various performance parameters of male marathon athletes. *Nutr Rev.* 17:405-414, 1997.

9. Balsom, P., et al. Creatine supplementation and dynamic high-intensity intermittent exercise. *Scandinavian J Med Sci Sports.* 3:143-149, 1993.

10. Vanfraechem, J. H. P., et al. Coenzyme Q10 and physical performance, in Folkers, K., Yamamura, Y., Eds., *Biomedical and Clinical Aspects of Coenzyme Q.* 3:235-241, 1981.

11. Birkmayer, J. G. D., et al. Reduced coenzyme 1 (NADH) improves pyschomotoric and physical performance in athletes. *White Paper Report,* New York: Menuco Corp., 1996.

12. Fry, A. C., et al. The effects of gamma-oryzanol supplementation during resistance exercise training. *Int J Sports Nutr.* 7(4):318-329, 1997.

13. Dekkers JC, van Doornen LJ, Kemper HC. The role of antioxidant vitamins and enzymes in the prevention of exercise-induced muscle damage. *Sports Med* 1996;21(3):213-38.)

14. Stanko, R. T., et al. Enhancement of arm exercise endurance capacity with dihydroxyacetone and pyruvate. *J Appl Physiol.* 68:119-124, 1990.

15. Bohmen, D., et al. (editors). Treatment of chondropathia patellae in young athletes with glucosamine sulfate. *Current Topics in Sports Medicine. Urban and Schwarzenberg,* Vienna. 1984.

16. Forgo, I. The duration of effect of the standardized ginseng extract G115 in healthy competitive athletes. *Notabene Medici.* 9:636, 1985.

17. Ellison, J. M., et al. Fluoxetine-induced genital anesthesia relieved by ginkgo biloba extract. *J Clin Psychiatry.* 59(4):199-200, 1998.

~ Rowland, D. L., et al. Yohimbine, erectile capacity, and sexual response in men. *Archives of Sexual Behavior.* 26:49-62, 1997.

Power Drinks for the Mind

1. Safford, F., et al. Testing the effects of dietary lecithin on memory in the elderly: An example of social work/medical research collaboration. *Research On Social Work Practice.* 4:349-358, 1994.

~ Little, A., et al. A double-blind, placebo controlled trial of high-dose lecithin in Alzheimer's Disease. *Journal of Neurology, Neurosurgery and Psychiatry.* 48:736-742, 1985.

2. Nodine, J. H., et al. A double-blind study of the effect of ribonucleic acid in senile brain disease. *American Journal of Psychiatry.* 123:1257-1259, 1967.

3. Domingo, J., et al. Citric, malic and succinic acid as possible alternatives to deferoxamine in aluminum toxicity. *Journal of Toxicology - Clinical Toxicology.* 26(1-2):67-79, 1988.

4. Moss, M. C., et al. Oxygen administration enhances memory formation in healthy young adults. *Psychopharmacology (Berlin).* 124(3):255-260, 1996.

5. Crawford, M. The role of essential fatty acids in neural development: Implications for perinatal nutrition. *American Journal of Clinical Nutrition.* 57:703S-710S, 1993.

6. Crook, T. H., et al. Effects of phosphatidylserine in age-associated memory impairment. *Neurology.* 41(5):644-649, 1991.

7. Vernon, M. & Jeffre, M. *Brain Power–A Neurosurgeon's Complete Program to Maintain and Enhance Brain Fitness Throughout Your Life.* P. 139. New York Houghton Mifflin. 1989.

8. Wurtman, R., et al. Choline and lecithin in brain disorders. *Nutrition and the Brain*, Vol 5. Raven Press, New York, NY, USA. 1979.

9. Levy, R., et al. Early results from double blind, placebo controlled trial of high dose phosphatidylcholine in Alzheimer's Disease. *The Lancet.* 1:474-476, 1982.

10. Imagawa, M. Megavitamin therapy (Coenzyme Q10 and vitamin B6) in Alzheimer's disease and senile dementia of Alzheimer type. In: *Basic, Clinical and Therapeutic Aspects of Alzheimer's and Parkinson's Diseases,* Volume 2, by Nagatsu, et al, pages 489-491, Plenum Press, New York, 1990.

11. Neri, D. F., et al. The effects of tyrosine on cognitive performance during extended wakefulness. *Aviation Space Environ Medicine.* 66(4):313-319, 1995.

12. Calvani, M., et al. Action of Acetyl-L-Carnitine in neurodegeneration and Alzheimer's disease. *Annals of the New York Academy of Sciences (USA).* 663:483-486, 1993.

13. Flood, J. F., et al. Dehydroepiandrosterone and its sulfate enhance memory retention in mice. *Brain Research.* 447:269-187, 1988.

14. Leone, M., et al. Melatonin versus placebo in the prophylaxis of cluster headache: A double-blind pilot study with parallel groups. *Cephalalgia.* 16(7):494-496, 1996.

15. Deijen, J. B., et al. Cognitive impairments and mood disturbances in growth hormone deficient men. *In Press.*

16. Zhang, X., et al. Protective effects of nicotinic acid on disturbance of memory retrieval induced by cerebral ischemia-reperfusion in rats. Chin J Pharm Tox. 10:178-180, 1996.

~Niacin improves memory. *Life Enhancement News.* 27:8, 1996.

17. Colombo, M. L., et al. Ascorbic acid in children with Down's syndrome. *The Lancet.* 2(7896):1554, 1974.

18. Pidoux, B. Effects of ginkgo biloba extract on functional activity of the brain. *La Presse Medicale.* 15:1588-1591, 1986.

19. Zyryanova, T. M. Effects of extracts of panax, eleutherococcus and leuzea on blood supply to the brain. *Stimulytory Tsent Nerv Sist.* 37, 1966.

20. Linde, K., et al. St. John's wort for depression - an overview and meta-analysis of randomized clinical trials. *British Medical Journal.* 313(7052) 253-258, 1996.

21. Cheng, D. H., et al. Huperzine A, a novel promising acetylcholinesterase inhibitor. *Neuroreport.* 8:97-101, 1996.

22. Nishiyama, N., et al. Beneficial effects of aged garlic extract on learning and memory impairment in the senescence-accelerated mouse. *Experimental Gerontology.* 32:149-160, 1997.

Power Drinks for Longevity

1. Living Longer by Living Better. *The New England Journal of Medicine.* April, 1998.

2 .Weindruch, R., Sohal, R. Caloric restriction and aging. *The New England Journal of Medicine.* 337(14):986-994, 1997.

3. *Epidemiology* 3[5], 1992: p.389-391.

4. Steffen, C., et al. Enzyme treatment in comparison with immune complex determination in rheumatoid arthritis. *Zeitschrift fur Rheumatologie.* 44:51-56, 1985.

5. Turning on telomerase to stop cell aging: the quest for immortality. *Life Extension.* 4(2):41-46, 1998.

6. St. Leger, A. S., et al. Factors associated with cardiac mortality in developed countries with particular reference to the consumption of wine. *The Lancet.* May 12, 1979.

7. Masquelier, J., et al. Stabilization of collagen by procanidolic oligomers. *Acta Therap* 7:101-105, 1981.

8. Moriguchi, T., et al. Anti-aging effect of aged garlic in the inbred brain atrophy mouse model. *Clin Exp Pharmacol Physiol.* 24:235-242, 1997.

9. Brink, W. Whey protein powder. *Life Extension.* 4(3):21-23, 1998.

10. Loriaux, S. M., et al. The effects of nicotinic acid (niacin) and xanthinol nicotinate on human memory in different categories of age: A double blind study. *Psychopharmacology.* 87:390-395, 1985.

~ Miettinen, et al. Decrease in serum cholesterol by 25 percent and triglycerides by 30 percent in human subjects after two weeks on 3 gms of niacin per day. *Acta Med. Scand,* 186: 247-253, 1969.

11. Ghigo, E., et al. Low doses of either intravenously or orally administered arginine are able to enhance growth hormone response in elderly subjects. *J Endocrinol Invest.* 17(2):113-117, 1994.

12. Enstrom, J. F. Vitamin C intake and mortality among a sample of the United States population. *Epidemiology.* 3:194-202, 1992.

~ Malik, N. S., et al. Vitamins and analgesics in the prevention of collagen aging. *Age and Ageing.* 25:279-284, 1996.

13. Poulin, J. E., et al. Vitamin E prevents oxidative modification of brain and lymphocyte band 3 proteins during aging. *Proceedings of the National Academy of Sciences.* 93:5600-5603, 1996.

14. Allard, J. P., et al. Effects of beta-carotene supplementation on lipid peroxidation in humans. *American Journal of Clinical Nutrition.* 59(4):884-890, 1994.

15. Di Mascio, P., et al. Lycopene as the most efficient biological carotenoid singlet oxygen quencher. *Arch Biochem Biophysics.* 274:532-538, 1989.

16. Kamei, A. Glutathione levels of the human crystalline lens in aging and its antioxidant effects against the oxidation of lens proteins. *Biol Pharm Bull.* 16:870-875, 1993.

17. Orr, W. C., et al. Extension of life-span by over-expression of superoxide dismutase and catalase in Drosophilia melanogaster. *Science.* 263:1128-1130, 1994.

18. Odens, M. Prolongation of the life span in rats. *Journal of the American Geriatrics Society.* 21:450-451, 1973.

19. Baulieu, E. E. Dehydroepiandrosterone (DHEA): a fountain of youth? [editorial]. *J. Clin. Endocrinol. Metab.* 81:3147-51, 1996.

20. Rudman, D., et al. Effects of human growth hormone in men over 60 years old. *The New England Journal of Medicine.* 323:1-6, 1990.

21. Sahelian, R. The promise of pregnenolone. *Life Enhancement.* 36:3-11, 1997.

22. Clinical Application Medicago sativa extracts, by Paul Reilly, N.D. *Journal of Naturopathic Medicine.* Volume 1, No. 1. Pgs 62-65, 1990.

~ Xu, Xia Ph.D., Kurtzer MS, Dietary Phytoestrogens, News Extract from the *Annual Review of Nutrition,* 17:353-381 1997.

23. Levy, R. , et al. Early results from double blind, placebo controlled trial of high dose phosphatidylcholine in Alzheimer's Disease. *The Lancet.* 1:474-476, 1982.

24. Herschler, R. J. Dietary and pharmaceutical uses of methylsulfonylmethane and compositions comprising it. *United States Patent 4514421.* April 30, 1985

25. South, J. SAMe - the ultimate nutrient for mood, liver, heart, joint and brain protection. International Anti-aging Systems: *Anti-Aging Bulletin.* 3(5):14-19, 1998.

26. Huguet, F., et al. Decreased cerebral 5-HT1A receptors during aging: reversal by ginkgo biloba extract (EGb 761). *Jrnl. of Pharmacy and Pharmacology.* 46: 316-318, 1994.

27. Serafini, M., et al. In vivo antioxidant effect of green and black tea in man. *European Jrnl. of Clinical Nutrition.* 50:28-32, 1996.

Resources

Visit your natural foods store for many of these products or contact the companies for more information.

Manufacturers of Juice Related Products

Pines International, Inc. Lawrence, KS 66044. 1-800-MY-PINES, (800-697-4637) Fax: 785-841-1252. www.wheatgrass.com Makers of beet, alfalfa, wheat grass and barley grass powders.

Green Foods Corporation. Oxnard, CA 93030. 800-777-4430, fax 805-983-8843. www.greenfoods.com Makers of barley grass and full line of vegetable juice powders.

The Sprout House. Ramona, CA. 1-800-SPROUTS (800-777-6887) 760-788-4800, fax 760-788-7979. www.SproutHouse.com Distributes fresh wheatgrass, organic seeds, and home sprouting kits designed by the author including the sprout bag used in some recipes.

Wheatgrass Direct. 877-5-JUICED. 610-346-6687, Fax: 610-346-9478. Ottsville, PA 18942. www.wheatgrassdirect.com

Super Food Provisions. Petaluma, CA. 800-544-3657. Tablets and powders of barley and wheat grasses, spirulina and chlorella via mail order.

Earthrise. 800-949-RISE, 707-778-9078, fax 707-778-9028. www.spirulina.com Large producer of spirulina and algae powders.

Greens+. Orange Peel Enterprises, Inc. Vero Beach, FL 32960. 800-643-1210, fax 561-562-9848. www.greensplus.com The original multi-green powder drink.

Cyanotech Corporation. Kailua-Kona, HI 96740. 808-329-4677,Fax: 808-329-4533. www.cyanotech.com Large producer of spirulina algae powders and flakes.

Bio-Nutritional Products. Westwood, NJ 07675. 800-431-2582, fax 201-666-2929. Distributer of beet juice crystals, acidophilus, yeast, and royal jelly products.

Kyo-Green. Wakunaga of America Co. Ltd. Mission Viejo, CA 92691. 800-421-2998. 714-855-2776. Fax 714-458-2764. www.kyolic.com Grasses, chlorella, and aged garlic.

Sonne V.E. Irons. Cottonwood, CA 96022. 800-544-8147, fax 916-347-5921. Makers of *Sonne's #7 Colloidal Bentonite,* for detoxification and intestinal cleansing.

Tahiti Trader Brands. Las Vegas, NV 89101. 800-842-5309, fax 949-362-0128. www.tahititrader.com Manufacturer of superb noni juice.

Wisdom of the Ancients. Tempe, AZ 85281. www.wisdomherbs.com 800-899-9908, fax 602-966-3805. Manufacturer of stevia, an herbal sugar alternative, in several varities.

C.C. Pollen Company. Phoenix, AZ 85018. 800-875-0096, Fax: 602-381-3130. Raw bee pollen, royal jelly, propolis bee products.

Doctor's Preferred. Rockville, MD. 1-877-433-3436. www.defience.com Multi-green juice powder.

San Fransisco Herb & Natural Food Co. 510-770-9021. www.herbspice-tea.com Freemont, CA 94538. Full line of herbs and teas.

Traditional Medicines. Sebastapol, CA. 707-823-8911, fax 707-823-1599. Medicinal teas.

Republic of Tea. Novato, CA. 800-298-4832, 618-478-5520. Green & black teas. www.RepulicofTea.com

Guayaki. San Luis Obispo, CA 1-888-482-9254. www.guayaki.com Yerbe-maté and other rainforest teas.

Source Naturals. Scotts Valley CA 95066. 831-438-1144. Source of liquid grapefruit seed extract and other supplements. www.sourcenaturals.com

NuNaturals. Eugene, OR 97440. 800-753-4372, fax 541-343-0915. Stevia products. www.NuNaturals.com

Juicers & Other Equipment

Miracle Exclusives, Inc. Port Washington, NY 11050. 800-645-6360, fax 516-621-1997. MiracleExclusives.com Full line of juicers and a soy milk-making machine.

Omega Juicers. Harrisburg, PA 17111. 800-633-3401, fax 717-561-1298. Full line of juicers.

Green Power Juicer. 888-254-7336. Downey, CA 90241. www.green-power.com Twin-gear juicers.

L'Equip. Harrisburg, PA 17043. 800-816-6811. 717-730-7100, fax 717-730-7200. Juicers. www.lequip.com

Vita-Mix Corp. Cleveland, OH 44138. 800-848-2649, fax 440-235-3726. www.vitamix.com Blenders.

Multi-Pure Corp. 1-800-689-4199. 206463-1501. Large manufacturer of home water filters.

Waterwise. Leesburg, FL 800-874-9028, 352-787-5008, fax 352-787-8123. www.waterwise.com Large manufacturer of home water distillers.

General

Tree of Life Center. Gabriel Cousens, MD. Patagonia, AZ 85624. 520-394-2520, fax 520-394-2099. www.treeof-liferejuvenation.com Spiritual, eco-retreat center, wheatgrass, and other fresh squeezed juices.

The American Botanical Council. PO Box 201660, Austin, TX 78720. 512-926-4900.

American Holistic Medical Association. McLean, VA 703-556-9728, or fax 703-556-8729. Patient referral directory. www.HolisticMedicine.org

American Holistic Health Association. Anaheim, CA 92817-7400. 714-779-6152. www.AHHA.org

Life Extension. Hollywood, FL 33022. 800-841-5433 or 800-544-4440. www.LEF.org Anti-aging magazine and non-profit organization.

Ailments Index

Foods & Herbs Index

General Index

—A—

—B—

—C—

—D—

—E—

—F—

—G—

—H—

—I—

—J—

—K—

—L—

—Q—

—R—

—S—

—T—

—U—

—V—

Other Books

By Steve Meyerowitz

Wheat Grass—Nature's Finest Medicine
The Complete Guide to Using Grass Foods & Juices to Revitalize
Your Health 1999.

Juice Fasting & Detoxification
Use the Healing Power of Fresh Juice to Feel Young and Look Great 1999.

Food Combining and Digestion
A Rational Approach to Combining What You Eat to Maximize Digestion and Health 1996.

Sproutman's Kitchen Garden Cookbook
Sprout Breads, Cookies, Soups, Salads & 250 Other Low Fat, Dairy Free Vegetarian Recipes 1999.

Sprouts—the Miracle Food
The Complete Guide to Sprouting 1999.

Sproutman's "Turn the Dial" Sprout Chart
A Field Guide to Growing and Eating Sprouts 1998.

Clinician's Complete Reference to Complementary/Alternative Medicine.
Steve Meyerowitz, co-author. Edited by Donald W. Novey, M.D. 2000.

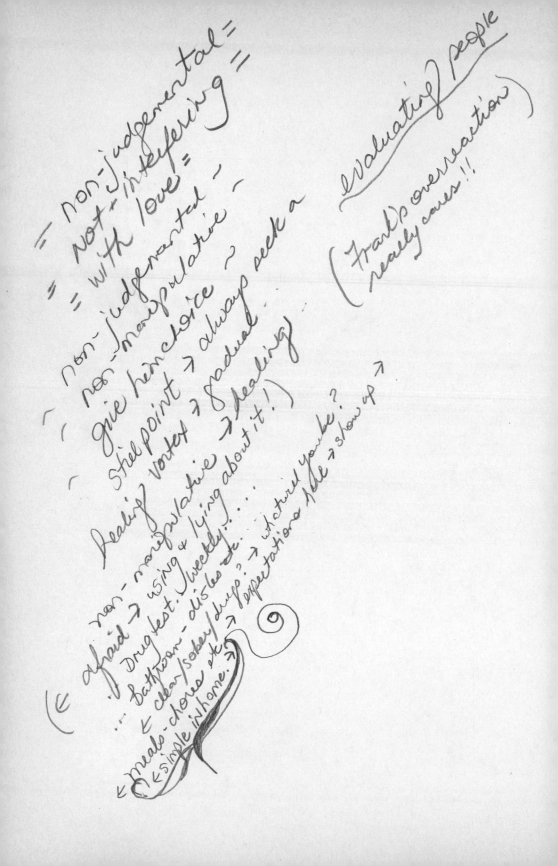

= non-judgemental =
= not interfering =
= with love =

~ non-judgemental ~
~ non-manipulative ~
~ give him choice ~

Still point → always seek a Evaluating people

(Frank's overreaction really cares!!)

Healing vortex → gradual :
non-manipulative → healing

(← afraid → using & lying about it!)
... Drug test. weekly ...
Bathroom - dishes etc ...
← clean/sober/drugs? → what will you be?
← meals - chores etc. → expectations here → show up →
← ← simple in home. →

Are your pure?? Energy ?

.. can of worms ...

.. cleanse .. yourself ..

.. disaffect me. personality .. good ...

beauty in my life ....

shall .. happy ..? .. father .. mother ..

shared truth ....

numb .. depressed ....

Frank .. supress energy coverup ...

throw shit at me —

Keep it under control .. fuel to fire.

(hurting me.) changed my life .. — illness → wakeup ..

choice pt.: toxic or life?

Suck life out of me?

SE-healthy/well-being.

(acting out) ..

numb .. high —

! pain .. destraction. !!

war → mental illness ?

Trends in your family?

what was handed down to the

through generations down ..

won't pass it on. fight it now.

won't pass it on / pass on toxicity.

sick system working ... why allow abuse ..

Bully each other ...

clear here .... Name it: walk away/

non-single life style take responsible

living single = not responsible

take care of environment / others.

(no one who gives a hoot!!)

(small steps w/ him)

: say it → little part of life ...

blame others.

(progress here.)